Cardiac Electrophysiology Without Fluoroscopy

Riccardo Proietti • Yan Wang
Yan Yao • Guo Qiang Zhong
Shu Lin Wu • Félix Ayala-Paredes
Editors

Cardiac Electrophysiology Without Fluoroscopy

Springer

Editors
Riccardo Proietti
Department of Cardiac, Thoracic
Vascular Sciences and Public Health
The University of Padua
Padua
Italy

Yan Wang
Huazhong University of Science
and Technology Tongji Hospital
Tongji Medical College
Wuhan
China

Yan Yao
Peking Union Medical College Hospital
National Center for Cardiovascular
Disease
Beijing
China

Guo Qiang Zhong
The First Affiliated Hospital of Guangxi
Medical University
Nanning
China

Shu Lin Wu
Guangdong Cardiovascular Institute
Guangzhou
Guangdong
China

Félix Ayala-Paredes
Université de Sherbrooke
Sherbrooke, QC
Canada

ISBN 978-3-030-16991-6 ISBN 978-3-030-16992-3 (eBook)
https://doi.org/10.1007/978-3-030-16992-3

This Springer imprint is published by the registered company Springer Nature Switzerland AG
The registered company address is: Gewerbestrasse 11, 6330 Cham, Switzerland

Contents

Clinical Studies of a Purely 3D Navigation in Interventional Managements of Tachyarrhythmia

1

Ahmed AlTurki and Riccardo Proietti

Introduction

Catheter ablation has become the cornerstone treatment for tachyarrhythmias over the last 20 years [1]. Firmly established as first-line therapy for the treatment of right-sided arrhythmias (atrial flutter, atrial reentrant tachycardia, and atrioventricular nodal reentrant tachycardia), catheter ablation is moving toward becoming first-line therapy for complex arrhythmias such as atrial fibrillation and ventricular tachycardia [1, 2]. These complex ablations are often prolonged and require trans-septal puncture as well as use of several catheters from multiple access sites. A major downside to such complex procedures using conventional fluoroscopy is high exposure to radiation for both the patient and the electrophysiologist [3]. Radiation exposure poses significant risks to all those exposed in the electrophysiology lab. A typical procedure results in an estimated mean total radiation dose of 16.6 mSv (ranging from 6.6 to 59.2 mSv), equivalent to 830 chest X-rays, and is associated with a lifetime risk for a fatal malignancy estimated at 0.15% for female patients and 0.21% for male patients [3, 4].

A. AlTurki (✉)
Division of Cardiology, McGill University Health Centre, Montreal, QC, Canada
e-mail: ahmed.alturki@mail.mcgill.ca

R. Proietti
Department of Cardiac, Thoracic, and Vascular Sciences, University of Padua, Padua, Italy

To counter these risks, there has been a movement toward non-fluoroscopic techniques allowing a zero or near-zero exposure [5]. These techniques have revolutionized our current practice of catheter ablation in the management of tachyarrhythmias [6]. These techniques include 3D mapping systems, remote magnetic navigation (RMN), contact force (CF) technology, and intracardiac echo (ICE). In addition to reducing radiation exposure, these techniques are thought to improve the accuracy of catheter ablation and allow the creation of an improved ablation lesion. Furthermore, these techniques reduce operator and staff fatigue due to the use of heavy-lead aprons when using fluoroscopy [7].

In this chapter, we review current technologies used for 3D navigation and their implementation and results in clinical practice as well as the state of utilization of these technologies in the targeting of different tachyarrhythmias.

Advanced 3D Electroanatomic Mapping Systems

There are variations in individual cardiac anatomy which warrant the use of a 3D electroanatomic mapping (EAM). Three-dimensional EAM systems, which were first introduced in 1997, have improved the understanding of cardiac chamber anatomy allowing precise catheter localization. EAM facilitates catheter ablation by keeping a

R. Proietti et al. (eds.), *Cardiac Electrophysiology Without Fluoroscopy*,
https://doi.org/10.1007/978-3-030-16992-3_1

catalog of activation time, voltage, and anatomic location at multiple points simultaneously and displaying them as readily understandable color-coded maps superimposed on the cardiac chamber geometry [8, 9]. Electroanatomic mapping systems can also display cardiac anatomy and sites of RF energy application with much more precision than fluoroscopic localization [9, 10]. Many arrhythmias have specific anatomic targets; electroanatomic mapping can greatly facilitate anatomic and scar-based ablation procedures [2, 11, 12]. Finally, by reducing the operator's need to use fluoroscopy to localize the mapping catheter, these systems have greatly reduced exposure to ionizing radiation [7].

Current 3D mapping systems used for electrophysiology catheter visualization include the following: CARTO (Biosense Webster Inc., Diamond Bar, CA), EnSite NavX and Mediguide technologies (Abbott, Abbott Park, IL), and Rhythmia (Boston Scientific, San Jose, CA) [9]. These EAM systems are able to integrate cardiac chamber anatomy acquired with the mapping catheter with an anatomical image that has been previously acquired with an imaging modality including fluoroscopy, MRI, or CT [13, 14]. This integrated imaging provides the electrophysiologist with an accurate rendering of cardiac anatomy to navigate catheters and perform ablation procedures [14].

One of the earliest studies using a mapping was performed by Gepstein and colleagues [15]. They used a non-fluoroscopic, catheter-based, endocardial mapping system and demonstrated highly reproducible and accurate results, both in vitro and in vivo. Gornick et al. also demonstrated the ability to place separate catheters at any site within the mapping chamber [16]. They also reported that the resolution of the 3D mapping system could be millimetric in size. The EAM systems facilitate the difficult interventional ablation procedure and can accurately navigate to a predefined site. It also shortens the fluoroscopic time and has a favorable spatial resolution [17]. In addition, after calculating and displaying the electrical activation sequence, the operator can visualize the activation sequence known as activation mapping and easily obtain the voltage information known as voltage mapping [9, 18]. Limitations of these systems include the need for patient immobility, accurate registration, and reference stability [18, 19].

Remote Magnetic Navigation

Remote magnetic navigation has been available as a tool for mapping and ablation since 2007. In that period of time, it has shown to be useful in most ablation procedures ranging from atrial flutter to ventricular tachycardia [20, 21]. Remote magnetic navigation was developed to facilitate the positioning of catheters within the heart. The system uses two computer-controlled external magnets to create and adjust an external magnetic field to guide the magnetic tip of the catheter [21]. A remote workstation, using a computer console that controls both the magnets and a motor-driven catheter, allows advancement or retraction of the catheter [20]. With a more flexible catheter tip, the catheter moves parallel to the lines of the magnetic field which are determined by the external magnet [21]. The operator can direct the catheter to the desired location within the cardiac chambers by adjusting the external magnetic field. RMN requires an electrophysiology laboratory with equipment designed specifically for magnetic guidance [22]. Potential benefits of remote magnetic navigation include more precise control of the catheter, facilitating more rapid and accurate guidance of the catheter, and significantly reduced radiation exposure [20, 22]. The softer and more flexible catheter tip theoretically reduces the risks of cardiac puncture and tamponade [21]. This lower risk comes with the possible disadvantage of smaller lesion volumes [12].

The efficacy and safety of RMN have been assessed in multiple studies especially in ablation of atrial fibrillation. In a cohort study of 356 patients, RMN did not decrease AF recurrence compared to manual navigation [23]. In addition, RMN was associated with a lower success rate of pulmonary vein isolation. However, the study showed lower procedural and fluoroscopic times as well as a trend toward a reduction in major complications [23]. In a systematic review and meta-analysis of seven studies, Proietti et al. did not demonstrate a reduction in AF recurrence or improved success of pulmonary vein isolation with RMN [24]. However, RMN was associated with a reduction in complications, procedural times, and fluoroscopic times [24]. Table 1.1 summarizes studies assessing the use of RMN in catheter ablation of AF.

More recently, RMN has been increasingly utilized for VT ablation. In a multicenter prospective observational study of 218 patients with structural heart disease, Di Biase et al. assessed the use of RMN compared to manual navigation in VT ablation in patients with ischemic cardiomyopathy [30]. In this study, RMN use was associated with a significant reduction in VT recurrence. In addition, another study showed a reduction in VT recurrence in patients with nonischemic cardio-

Table 1.1 Characteristics and results of studies assessing remote magnetic navigation in atrial fibrillation

Study first author (year)	Type of study	Population (number)	Results	Follow-up (months)
Arya (2011) [23]	Retrospective (single center)	70% Paroxysmal/30% persistent (356)	Similar freedom from AF at 6 months: 57.8% and 66.4% ($P = 0.196$). Longer procedure and ablation time with magnetic navigation 223 ± 44 min vs. 166 ± 52 min ($P < 0.0001$), and 75.4 ± 20.9 min vs. 53.2 ± 21.4 min ($P < 0.0001$).	6
Choi (2011) [25]	Retrospective (single center)	60% Persistent/40% paroxysmal (111)	Total procedure time was significantly longer (352 ± 50 min vs. 283 ± 75 min, $P < 0.0001$) and total fluoroscopy time was significantly shorter (99 ± 28 min vs. 238 ± 45 min, $P < 0.0001$) in the magnetic navigation group. Procedural success was similar in both groups (85% vs. 90%, $P = 0.08$).	3
Luthje (2011) [26]	Retrospective (single center)	67% Persistent/33% paroxysmal (161)	Procedural success and freedom from atrial fibrillation were similar in both groups (90% vs. 87%, $P = 0.6$, and 66% vs. 62%, $P = 0.8$). Magnetic navigation was associated with longer procedure duration (225.5 ± 54.6 min vs. 165.6 ± 52.4 min, $P < 0.0001$), longer ablation times (125.3 ± 46.5 min vs. 79.6 ± 28.5 min, $P < 0.0001$), and longer RF current application duration (50.4 ± 17.7 min vs. 43.9 ± 11.0 min, $P < 0.05$). However, fluoroscopy time was shorter (12, IQR = 9–17 min vs. 37, IQR = 29–44; $P < 0.0001$).	12
Miyazaki (2010) [27]	Retrospective (single center)	100% Paroxysmal (74)	Radiofrequency and procedure duration were higher in the magnetic navigation group (60 ± 27 min vs. 43 ± 16 min; $P = 0.0019$) and (246 ± 50 min vs. 153 ± 51 min; $P < 0.0001$). Freedom from atrial fibrillation was similar in both groups (69% vs. 62%, $P = 0.96$).	12
Solheim (2011) [28]	Retrospective (single center)	40% Persistent/60% paroxysmal (87)	Radiofrequency and procedure duration were higher in the magnetic navigation group (79 ± 19 min vs. 51 ± 25 min; $P < 0.001$) and (324 ± 74 min vs. 215 ± 61 min; $P < 0.001$).	4
Sorgente (2010) [29]	Retrospective (single center)	20% Persistent/80% paroxysmal (94)	Radiofrequency and procedure duration were higher in the magnetic navigation group (60 ± 27 min vs. 43 ± 16 min; $P = 0.0019$) and (246 ± 50 min vs. 153 ± 51 min; $P < 0.0001$). Freedom from atrial fibrillation was similar in both groups (66% vs. 67%, $P = 0.63$).	12

myopathy and scar-related VT [31]. Hendricks et al. also showed a significant reduction in VT recurrence with RMN in patients with idiopathic VT [32]. Turagem et al. performed a systematic review and meta-analysis of RMN versus manual navigation in VT ablation [30]. Compared to MAN, the use of RMN was associated with a 39% lower risk of VT recurrence (OR 0.61, 95% CI 0.44–0.85, $P = 0.003$). In patients with structural heart disease, there was a trend favoring lower VT recurrence with RMN versus MAN (OR 0.69, 95% CI 0.45–1.04, $P = 0.07$). In idiopathic VT, there was no significant difference between RMN and MAN (OR 0.58, 95% CI 0.31–1.1, $P = 0.1$) [30]. Studies assessing the use of RMN in VT ablation are summarized in Table 1.2. The ongoing MAGNETIC VT trial will assess if VT ablation using RMN results in superior outcomes compared to a manual approach in subjects with ischemic scar VT and low ejection fraction [37].

Ablation in patients with congenital heart disease is another avenue where RMN is important.

Table 1.2 Characteristics and results of studies assessing remote magnetic navigation in ventricular tachycardia

Study first author (year)	Type of study	Population (number)	Results	Follow-up (months)
Bauemfeind (2011) [33]	Prospective (single center)	Structural heart disease and idiopathic (83)	Magnetic navigation system was more successful for VTs (93% vs. 72%, $P < 0.05$). Less fluoroscopy was used in group MNS (30 ± 20 min vs. 35 ± 25 min, $P < 0.01$). There were no differences in procedure times and recurrence rates for the overall groups (168 ± 67 min vs. 159 ± 75 min, P = ns; 14% vs. 11%, P = ns; respectively).	15
Dinov (2012) [34]	Retrospective (single center)	Structural heart disease (102)	Acute success rate was similar in both groups (82% vs. 71%, $P = 0.246$). Remote magnetic navigation was associated with significantly shorter fluoroscopy time (13 ± 12 min vs. 32 ± 17 min, $P = 0.0001$) and ablation time (2337.59 ± 1248.22 s vs. 1589.95 ± 1047.42 s, $P = 0.049$), with similar total procedure time (157 ± 40 min vs. 148 ± 50 min, $P = 0.42$).	14
Akca (2012)	Prospective (single center)	Not available (28)	Overall recurrence rate and fluoroscopy time were significantly lower (25.0% vs. 41.4%, $P = 0.045$, and 22.8 ± 14.7 vs. 41.2 ± 10.9, $P = 0.011$) with magnetic navigation.	19
Szili-Torok (2012) [35]	Retrospective (single center)	Structural heart disease and idiopathic (113)	Higher acute success 82% vs. 66% ($P = 0.046$) and lower recurrence 24% vs. 44% ($P = 0.047$) with magnetic navigation. Overall procedural time (177 ± 79 min vs. 232 ± 99 min, $P < 0.01$) and mean patient fluoroscopy time (27 ± 19 min vs. 56 ± 32 min, $P < 0.001$) were all significantly lower using magnetic navigation.	20
Zhang (2013) [36]	Randomized (single center)	Idiopathic (30)	Procedural times were similar in both groups (131.8 ± 19.4 min and 115.1 ± 27.4; $P = 0.13$). Remote magnetic navigation was associated with 50.9% and 50.5% reduction in patients' fluoroscopic exposure and times, respectively, as well as 64% and 69% reductions in physician fluoroscopic exposure and times.	22
Hendricks (2015) [32]	Retrospective (single center)	Structural heart disease and idiopathic (198)	Procedural and ablation times were lower with magnetic navigation 150 (120–220) s vs. 190 (135–220) s and 400 (190–1065) s vs. 700 (300–1920) s. Higher acute success 88% vs. 71% ($P = 0.03$) and lower recurrence 42% vs. 57% ($P = 0.07$) with magnetic navigation.	25

Structural challenges such as the presence of baffles, conduits, patches, and shunts are better approached with RMN [38]. RMN provides several advantages in these complex congenital cases that may present with limited vascular access or difficult access to the target cardiac chambers due to previous surgical interventions [39].

Contact Force Technology

Tissue contact is critical to achieving lesion transmurality and success of radiofrequency ablation procedures. However, a delicate balance must be achieved. In power control ablation, the size and depth of ablation are directly related to the contact between the tip of the catheter and the myocardium [12]. The effectiveness of ablation may decrease if waste of resistive heating in the bloodstream occurs due to nonoptimal contact. Conversely, higher contact and excessive temperature rise may precipitate thrombus formation, steam pops, and myocardial perforation [40]. To overcome these issues, contact force-sensing catheters have been developed with the capability of monitoring in real time the degree of contact through a precision spring positioned on the tip and a sensor coil positioned on the shaft of the catheter [40].

Improving electrode-tissue contact maximizes the transfer of thermal energy to target tissue [41]. Increasing CF increases the proportion of the electrode surface in contact with the tissue. This reduces the electrode surface area that is exposed to the circulating blood pool, thus favoring greater current delivery to target tissue [40, 41]. Avitall et al. showed that increasing CF from 1 to 10 g led to greater deformation of the endocardium below the plane of the endocardial surface, which resulted in significantly greater lesion width and depth [42]. In a model, CF was demonstrated to wield as much influence on lesion size as RF power. When RF duration and power were kept constant, lesion depth, diameter, and volume increased proportionately with increasing CF. Importantly, lesion depth was greater with lower power (30 W) and moderate contact (40 g) than with higher powers (50 W) and lower contact (10 g) [42].

Contact quality is also critical. Spatiotemporal contact stability is predictive of lesion size [12]. Shah et al. showed that lesion volume was highest in constant contact, intermediate in variable contact, and lowest in intermittent contact [43]. Many factors affect spatiotemporal stability of contact: mean contact CF, cardiac and respiratory motion, catheter drift, and atrial arrhythmias [44]. The smaller lesion size that results from intermittent contact can be compensated for by increasing the duration of ablation.

Several studies have assessed the impact of contact force on procedural and clinical outcomes, mostly in catheter ablation of atrial fibrillation. Kerst et al. showed that contact force-guided and electroanatomic guided ablation is a feasible approach to achieve zero fluoroscopy. In a large retrospective study of 600 patients, contact force catheter ablation was associated with a decrease in atrial fibrillation recurrence and a decrease in total procedural time and ablation time as well as a significant reduction in fluoroscopic exposure. While there was a trend toward a lower complication rate including cardiac tamponade, this did not reach statistical significance [45]. In a meta-analysis of 11 studies including two randomized trials, Shurrab et al. showed similar findings [46]. The recurrence rate was lower with contact force (35.1% vs. 45.5%; OR 0.62, 95% CI 0.45–0.86, $P = 0.004$) as were procedural times (156 min vs. 173 min; standardized mean difference −0.85, 95% CI −1.48 to −0.21, $P = 0.009$) and fluoroscopic times (28 min vs. 36 min; standardized mean difference −0.94, 95% CI −1.66; −0.21, $P = 0.01$). There was a trend toward a decrease in major complications, but this did not reach statistical significance (1.3% vs. 1.9%; OR 0.71, 95% CI 0.29–1.73, $P = 0.45$) [46].

Intracardiac Echo

Intracardiac echocardiography (ICE) represents a major advancement in cardiac imaging and has become as indispensable part of electrophysiologic procedures [47]. ICE allows a real-time assessment of cardiac anatomy during interventional procedures and guides catheter manipulation in relation to the different anatomic structures [48]. A major advantage over transesophageal echocardiography is the ability to perform ICE by the primary operator [47].

Trans-septal puncture likely gives physicians the most pause when they consider a near-zero fluoroscopy approach. Many operators were trained using fluoroscopy to complete the critical steps of trans-septal puncture, which include placing the sheath and needle in the SVC, withdrawing the trans-septal apparatus into the level of the fossa ovalis, advancing and confirming the needle entry into the left atrium, and manipulating the dilator and sheath into the left atrium. For eliminating the need for fluoroscopy, ICE has become an indispensable tool for allowing safe trans-septal puncture. To place the guidewire and trans-septal sheath into the SVC, full visualization of the SVC right atrial junction is required. This view is obtained by positioning the ICE catheter in a neutral position in the mid-right atrium with appropriate clockwise or counterclockwise rotation to visualize the fossa ovalis and left atrium. From this position, posterior and rightward deflections are applied to fully view the SVC. Using this view, the guidewire, sheath, and trans-septal needle can be advanced into the SVC safely [49, 50].

With ICE, accurate 2D real-time and/or 3D imaging of the complex anatomy of LA and PVs is feasible [47]. Intracardiac ultrasound improves the efficacy of electrophysiological interventional procedures by exactly identifying anatomical structures and integrating this information with electrophysiological parameters and/or 3D reconstructions of CT/MRI data [51]. Early detection of periprocedural complications optimizes emergency management. Implementation of ICE in ablation procedures of AF results in reduction of fluoroscopy/procedure time, and potentially reduces complications and improves outcome [48].

Clinical Studies of Purely 3D Navigation

The abovementioned technologies have been utilized across the spectrum of ablation procedures performed in the electrophysiology lab. In a meta-analysis of ten studies in various cardiac arrhythmias that assessed the efficacy and safety of zero or near-zero fluoroscopic ablation, Yang et al. [52] found that zero or near-zero fluoroscopy ablation significantly showed reduced fluoroscopic time (standard mean difference [SMD] −1.62, 95% CI −2.20 to −1.05; $P < 0.00001$), ablation time (SMD −0.16, 95% CI −0.29 to −0.04; $P = 0.01$), and radiation dose (SMD −1.94, 95% CI −3.37 to −0.51; $P = 0.008$). This was done without any significant differences in acute or long-term success rates, complication rates, or recurrence rates [52]. Wannagat et al. showed that significant reductions in radiation exposures can be achieved in operators with varying degrees of experience (beginner, first-year fellow, second-year fellow, expert) without an increase in complications or procedure time [5]. Sadek and colleagues found that even complex ablations can be performed with zero fluoroscopy with a modest learning curve and no increase in procedural times [53]. Here, we review some of these studies in the context of the various arrhythmias. These studies are summarized in Table 1.3.

Atrial Flutter

Typical atrial flutter is an atrial arrhythmia in which catheter ablation is first-line therapy. The arrhythmia is maintained by a reentry mechanism in which the area between the tricuspid valve annulus and inferior vena cava forms a critical isthmus, known as the cavotricuspid isthmus, that is targeted for ablation [74]. Deutsch et al. demonstrated that complete elimination of fluoroscopy is feasible, safe, and effective during radiofrequency catheter ablation of atrial flutter [54]. The authors, in a study of 460 patients, compared techniques involving as low as reasonably achievable (ALARA) fluoroscopy and non-fluoroscopic techniques including electroanatomic mapping [54]. In another study, Schoene et al. used 3D mapping in 20 patients undergoing catheter ablation of the cavotricuspid isthmus and found no difference in freedom from recurrences, safety, and procedure duration while achieving a significant reduction

Table 1.3 Characteristics and results of studies reporting on purely 3D navigation

Study first author (year)	Type of study	Cardiac arrhythmia targeted (number)	Results	Follow-up (months)
Deutsch (2017) [54]	Prospective cohort study	Atrial flutter (460)	In the zero-fluoroscopy groups, the procedure time decreased (45.4 ± 17.6 and 47.2 ± 15.7 min vs. 52.6 ± 23.7 and 59.8 ± 24.0 min, $P < 0.01$) as compared to the as low as reasonably possible (ALARA) groups. In the zero-fluoroscopy groups, 91% and 98% of the procedures were performed with complete elimination of fluoroscopy and were associated with a significant reduction in fluoroscopy exposure (from 0.2 ± 1.1 and 0.3 ± 1.6 to 7.7 ± 6.0 min and 9.1 ± 7.2 min, $P < 0.001$) in the ALARA groups. No major complications were observed in either groups.	None
Schoene (2015) [55]	Randomized controlled trial	Atrial flutter (40)	Bidirectional isthmus block was achieved in all patients. Fluoroscopy time was significantly reduced in the zero-fluoroscopy group (0.3, IQR 0.2–0.5 min) when compared with the conventional group (5, IQR 4.2–11.5; $P < 0.001$). This resulted in a significant reduction in radiation dose in patients randomized to zero-fluoroscopy (17.4, IQR 11; 206.6 cGy cm) vs. the conventional group (418.4, IQR 277; 812.2 cGy cm; ($P < 0.001$). There were no significant differences in procedure duration between the zero-fluoroscopy group (49.5, IQR 37; 65 min) when compared with the conventional group (33.5, IQR 26.3; 55.5 min; $P = 0.053$). No adverse events were recorded. Freedom from atrial flutter at 6 months of follow-up was 19/20 (95%) in the zero-fluoroscopy and 18/20 (90%) in the conventional group, which was not statistically significant.	6
Alvarez (2011) [56]	Retrospective cohort study	Atrial flutter (80)	Success was obtained in 98.8% of the procedures; in 1 patient it was necessary to implant a pacemaker for sinus node dysfunction and 4 patients experienced minor complications. In 75 procedures (90.4%), fluoroscopy was not required.	None
Kopelman (2003) [57]	Randomized controlled trial	AVNRT (20)	Acute procedural success was 100% in both groups, with no complications. Although there were no differences in time taken for pre- and post-ablation electrophysiological evaluations, in the zero-fluoroscopy group, the ablation portion of the procedure showed a substantial reduction in duration (12.6 ± 6.8 min vs. 35.9 ± 18.3 min; $P < 0.001$) and fluoroscopic exposure (0.7 ± 0.5 min vs. 9.6 ± 5.0 min; $P < 0.001$) compared with the fluoroscopic group. This was reflected in reduced total procedure time (83.6 ± 23.6 min vs. 114 ± 19.3 min; $P = 0.008$) and total fluoroscopic exposure (4.2 ± 1.4 min vs. 15.9 ± 6.4 min; $P < 0.001$). Zero fluoroscopy was associated with a lower number (2.7 ± 1.6 vs. 5 ± 2.8; $P = 0.018$), duration (165.3 ± 181.6 s vs. 341 ± 177.7 s; $P = 0.013$), and total energy delivery (24.3 ± 3.1 W vs. 28.7 ± 4.5 W; $P = 0.042$) of radiofrequency applications. There were no acute or long-term complications or arrhythmia recurrence in either group	9
Luani (2018) [58]	Prospective cohort study	AVNRT/AVRT (25)	All EPS in the AVNRT subgroup could be accomplished without the need for fluoroscopy. Three patients (12%) required fluoroscopy during ablation. Mean EPS duration in the AVNRT subgroup was 99.8 ± 39.6 min, ICE-guided catheter placement 11.9 ± 5.8 min, time needed for diagnostic evaluation 27.1 ± 10.8 min, and cryo-application duration 26.3 ± 30.8 min.	None

(continued)

Table 1.3 (continued)

Study first author (year)	Type of study	Cardiac arrhythmia targeted (number)	Results	Follow-up (months)
Casella (2011) [59]	Retrospective cohort study	AVNRT/AVRT/ Atrial flutter (50)	In 38/50 cases (76%), a zero fluoroscopy approach was successfully attained. In the remaining 12/50 cases (24%), fluoroscopy use was limited to 122 ± 80 s, with a correspondingly low radiation exposure (dose area product 1.3 ± 1.1 mGy m). All procedures were acutely successful, with a procedural time of 113 ± 37 min, and without incurring in any major complication. Over a mean follow-up of 12 ± 3 months, there was one recurrence of AVRT and one of atrial flutter.	12
Clark (2008) [60]	Case series	AVRT (10)	All patients had acutely successful ablations, and none required the use of fluoroscopy. Mean procedure time was 4.4 h, with a range of 3.2–7.2 h. There were no complications. One patient (10%) had recurrence.	6
Scaglione (2015) [61]	Retrospective cohort study	AVRT (44)	Ablation without the use of fluoroscopy was successfully performed in every patient (33 with radiofrequency and 11 with cryoenergy). No complication occurred. There were seven recurrences (16%), of which three (43%) of them were successfully re-ablated without fluoroscopy.	16
Balli (2018) [62]	Retrospective cohort study	AVNRT/AVRT (109)	The mean procedure time was 109.8 ± 46 min, and the acute procedural success rate was 100%. Recurrence was noted in one patient (1%).	13
Bigelow (2014) [62]	Retrospective cohort study	AVNRT/AVRT (524)	Mean procedure time was 142 min (range 42–402 min). There were no complications. Twenty-five patients (5%) required the use of fluoroscopy, mostly as part of simultaneous diagnostic or interventional catheterization procedures. There was only one instance (0.2%) in which fluoroscopy was used when not anticipated at the start of the procedure.	None
Casella (2016) [63]	Randomized controlled trial	AVNRT/AVRT (262)	Zero fluoroscopy approach was associated with a significant reduction in patients' radiation dose (0 mSv, IQR 0–0.08 mSv vs. 8.87 mSv, IQR 3.67–22.01; $P < 0.00001$), total fluoroscopy time (0 s, IQR 0–12 s vs. 859 s, IQR 545–1346; $P < 0.00001$), and operator radiation dose (1.55 μS vs. 25.33 μS per procedure; $P < 0.001$).	12
Reddy (2010) [64]	Case series	Atrial fibrillation (20)	In all patients, single ($n = 18$) or dual ($n = 2$) transseptal access was successfully achieved. The left atrial-pulmonary vein anatomy was rendered using either a circular (14 patients) or a penta-array (6 patients) catheter in 22 ± 10 min; CT image integration was used in 11 patients. Using 49 ± 18 ablation lesions/patient, electrical isolation was achieved in 38/39 ipsilateral PV-isolating lesion sets (97%). The procedure time was 244 ± 75 min.	None
Razminia (2014) [65]	Case series	Atrial fibrillation (5)	A total of 20 pulmonary veins were identified and successfully isolated (100%) with the guidance of intracardiac echocardiography and three-dimensional electroanatomic mapping. No fluoroscopy was used for the procedures. There were no major procedural adverse events	None
Bulava (2015) [66]	Randomized controlled trial	Atrial fibrillation (80)	The total procedure duration and application time in both the zero-fluoroscopy and fluoroscopy groups were comparable (92.5 ± 22.9 min vs. 99.9 ± 15.9 min, $P = 0.11$, and 1785 ± 548 s vs. 1755 ± 450 s, $P = 0.79$, respectively). Zero fluoroscopic time was achieved in all patients in the zero-fluoroscopy group with the exception of one patient, where 8 s of fluoroscopy was needed to assess proper position of the guidewire in the femoral vein. No serious procedure-related complications were recorded and no differences in arrhythmia-free survival at 12 months were found between the groups.	12

Huo (2015) [67]	Randomized controlled trial	Atrial fibrillation (80)	Fluoroscopy time (10.42, IQR 8.45–12.46 min) vs. (1.45, IQR 1.05–2.22 min; $P < 0.001$) and radiation doses (2440, IQR 1593–3091 cGy cm) vs. 652 (IQR 326–1489 cGy cm; $P < 0.001$) in the zero-fluoroscopy group were significantly greater than those in the fluoroscopy group. The majority of reduction of radiation exposure was achieved after transseptal puncture, and near-zero fluoroscopic exposure procedure time did not differ significantly (1.39, IQR 1.18–2.10 h) vs. (1.37, IQR 1.17–1.50 h; $P = 0.362$). During follow-up, 61 patients (76.3%) had no recurrence of atrial arrhythmias. The recurrence rate between the 2 groups did not differ.	6
McCauley (2016) [68]	Case series	Atrial fibrillation (7)	Zero fluoroscopy procedure time was 183.9 ± 33.7 min versus 293.13 ± 129.9 min for conventional group controls ($P = 0.05$). Fluoroscopy time was 17.5 ± 14.1 min in zero-fluoroscopy patients versus 73.4 ± 50.3 min in controls ($P = 0.01$). AF recurrence in zero-fluoroscopy patients was 14% versus 25% in controls	12
Zhang (2017) [69]	Randomized controlled trial	Atrial fibrillation (342)	In group 1 (zero fluoroscopy), the average fluoroscopy time before LA reconstruction was similar to that in group 2 (conventional) (2.8 ± 0.4 min vs. 2.4 ± 0.6 min, $P = 0.75$). The average fluoroscopy time during ablation was significantly lower than that in group 2 (0 min vs. 7.6 ± 1.3 min, $P < 0.001$). The total X-ray exposure dose of the procedure in group 1 was significantly lower than that in group 2 (19.6 ± 9.4 mGy vs. 128.7 ± 62.5 mGy, respectively, $P < 0.001$). Kaplan-Meier analysis indicated that there were no statistical differences in the probability of freedom from atrial fibrillation recurrence at 12 months between group 1 and group 2 ($P = 0.152$). The success rate after a single ablation procedure and without drugs (Class I/III AAD) at 12 months was not significantly different between the 2 groups (67.6%, 95% confidence interval [CI]: 62–79.5% in group 1 and 68.9%, 95% CI: 63–80.7% in group 2, $P = 0.207$). Procedural related adverse events showed no significant different incidence between group 1 and group 2. A multivariate logistic regression analysis of risk factors was performed to evaluate the effectiveness outcome, which demonstrated that the percentage of contact force (within the investigator-selected work ranges) during therapy was significantly associated with positive outcomes (odds ratio: 3.68; 95% CI: 1.65–10.6, $P = 0.008$), whereas the LA dimension was negatively associated with effectiveness outcomes (odds ratio: 0.72; 95% CI: 0.52–0.84, $P = 0.016$).	12
Sommer (2018) [70]	Prospective cohort study	Atrial fibrillation (1000)	The median procedure time was 120 min, median fluoroscopy time was 0.90 min, and the median fluoroscopy dose was 345.1 cGy cm^2. Stratification of the first 750 patients (group 1) and the last 250 (group 2) cases showed significant improvement in the median procedure time (140–110 min) and reduction in the median fluoroscopy time (6–0.5 min) and the median dose (2263–151.9 cGy cm^2). The overall complication rate was 2.0%.	3
Cano (2016) [71]	Prospective cohort study	Ventricular tachycardia (41)	Median total fluoroscopy time and effective dose of 6.08 (1.51–12.36) min and 2.15 (0.58–8.22) mSv, respectively. Patients with ischemic VT had lower radiation exposure than patients with nonischemic VT (total fluoroscopy time, 2.53 [1.22–11.22] min versus 8.51 [5.55–17.34] min; $P = 0.016$). Epicardial access was associated with significantly higher levels of radiation exposure. Complications occurred in 4.9% patients, none of them being related to the use of the image integration tool. A near-zero fluoroscopy ablation could be performed in 14 of 44 procedures (32%), 43% of ischemic VT procedures, and 50% of procedures with endocardial access only.	None

(continued)

Table 1.3 (continued)

Study first author (year)	Type of study	Cardiac arrhythmia targeted (number)	Results	Follow-up (months)
Wang (2017) [72]	Prospective cohort study	Ventricular tachycardia (489)	The completely zero fluoroscopy approach was successful in 163 (100%) patients for electrophysiological study, and in 151 patients (94.4%) for arrhythmia ablation with 9 cases having to switch to the conventional approach due to the need for coronary angiography. There was no significant difference between the zero fluoroscopy approach and conventional approach in procedural success rate (84.1% vs. 85.4%, respectively), arrhythmia recurrence (1.9% vs. 2.2%), or severe complications (0.6% vs. 0.9%). The medical staffs using the zero fluoroscopy approach did not wear heavy protective apparels, and thus experienced significantly less fatigue compared with those using the conventional approach (2.1 ± 0.7 vs. 3.9 ± 1.6, $P < 0.05$).	
Akca (2012) [73]	Retrospective cohort study	Ventricular tachycardia (36)	In 31 patients, ablation was successful, with an endpoint of non-inducibility (86%). The success rate for congenital heart disease complexity of types I, II, and III was 50%, 88%, and 89%, respectively. The mean procedure and fluoroscopy time was 216 ± 101 and 40 ± 34 min, respectively. The number of radiofrequency applications was 42 ± 47. No major complications related to the procedures occurred. Of the patients, 67% remained free of recurrence during a mean follow-up of 26 ± 4 months. Recurrence developed in 0%, 16%, and 45% of patients with congenital heart disease types I, II, and III, respectively	26

in radiation exposure [55]. Alvarez and colleagues reported the results of an observational study patients referred for atrial flutter ablation that utilized EnSite-NavX™ system to provide an almost zero fluoroscopy approach [56]. One or two diagnostic catheters and a cooled-tip ablation catheter were used in each procedure with the endpoint for success being bidirectional cavo-tricuspid isthmus block. Eighty-three ablation procedures were performed in 80 patients (82.5% men, 61 ± 10 years of age). Success was obtained in 98.8% of the procedures with the only major complication being the requirement of a pacemaker in one patient for sinus node dysfunction. In 90.4% of cases, fluoroscopy was not required, with visualization of the diagnostic catheters being the commonest reason for fluoroscopy use. Procedural time was similar to that seen using a conventional approach [56]. Macias et al. [75] showed that a zero fluoroscopy approach using the CARTO system yielded similar results to when using the EnSite-NavX with both systems leading to a high rate of procedural success and low rates of complications and recurrences. Both mapping systems allowed operators to avoid fluoroscopy in a very high percentage of cases, 90% [75].

AVNRT/AVRT

Atrioventricular-nodal reentry tachycardia (AVNRT) is a common supraventricular tachycardia and is also treated with catheter ablation as first-line therapy. Kopelman et al. were able to achieve a fourfold decrease in fluoroscopy duration using electroanatomic mapping and other non-fluoroscopic techniques [57]. Importantly, this did not compromise procedural efficacy and safety. Luani et al. demonstrated the safety and feasibility of using a zero fluoroscopy, ICE-guided approach to AVNRT ablation in 25 patients [58]. Similarly, Álvarez et al. [76] prospectively enrolled 100 patients with AVNRT who underwent catheter ablation by fluoroscopic versus non-fluoroscopic approaches. Procedural success was similar using the non-fluoroscopic approach (100%) and the fluoroscopic approach (96%) with no difference in complications, procedure, and ablation duration [76]. After an initial learning curve, catheter ablation of AVNRT can be performed in a similar timeframe using non-fluoroscopic technique [77]. Casella et al. [59] reported a case series of 50 patients who underwent electrophysiological testing and ablation for AVNRT and AVRT guided by electroanatomic mapping. In 78% of cases, acute procedural success was achieved with zero fluoroscopy while the remainder required only minimal fluoroscopy. In addition, there were no major complications and, over a 12-month period, only two cases of recurrence [59]. Clark et al. [60] reported a case series of ten patients with AVRT and accessory pathways mapped to the left side using the NavX system. All ten patients underwent successful ablation, and none required the use of fluoroscopy. Only one patient had a recurrence and there were no complications [60]. Scaglione et al. [61] also reported the results of a case series with 44 patients with accessory pathways, of which almost half were left sided and AVRT. In this case series, electroanatomic mapping was provided using the CARTO system, and ablation without the use of fluoroscopy was successfully performed in every patient without any complication [61]. Similar to the traditional approach with radiofrequency, Balli et al. [78] showed that AVRT can be successfully ablated using cryoablation and electroanatomic mapping without recurrence or complications. Bigelow et al. [62] reported their extensive 8-year experience, with 524 consecutive patients, in performing ablation of right-sided and left-sided supraventricular arrhythmias using a near-zero fluoroscopy approach with the EnSite system. There were no complications with procedure times as expected and no unanticipated use of fluoroscopy (except in one case) [62].

In a prospective, multicenter, randomized controlled trial that enrolled 262 patients with supraventricular arrhythmias who were randomized to a minimal fluoroscopy approach utilizing electroanatomic mapping compared to a conventional fluoroscopic approach, Casella and colleagues [63] found that a minimal fluoroscopy approach was associated with a significant reduction in patients' radiation dose (0 mSv, interquartile range 0–0.08 mSv vs. 8.87 mSv, interquartile range 3.67–22.01; $P < 0.00001$), total fluoroscopy time (0 s, interquartile range 0–12 s vs. 859 s, interquartile range 545–1346; $P < 0.00001$), and operator radiation dose (1.55 μS vs. 25.33 μS per procedure; $P < 0.001$). Stec et al. went one step further in implementing a zero-X-ray approach in which staff no longer used lead aprons. There were 188 patients (mean age, 45 ± 21 years; 55% women) included in the zero-X-ray approach who were then compared to 714 consecutive patients referred for a simplified approach using X-rays (age, 52 ± 18 years; 55% women). The procedure times (63 ± 26 min vs. 63 ± 29 min, $P > 0.05$), major complications (0% vs. 0%, $P > 0.05$), and acute (98% vs. 98%, $P > 0.05$) and long-term (93% vs. 94%, $P > 0.05$) success rates were similar between the two groups [63].

Atrial Fibrillation

Atrial fibrillation is the most common arrhythmia in older adults. Catheter ablation of atrial fibrillation is a relatively complex procedure. The full range of techniques are required to shift this procedure to a zero fluoroscopy approach. Reddy et al. [64] evaluated the feasibility and safety of pulmonary vein isolation with zero fluoroscopy use, using a combination of three-dimensional EAM and ICE. In this case series of 20 consecutive patients with paroxysmal atrial fibrillation, right-sided mapping required 5.5 ± 2.6 min. Trans-septal access was successfully achieved in all patients. Left-sided anatomy was visualized using either a circular (14 patients) or a penta-array (6 patients) catheter in 22 ± 10 min; CT image integration was used in 11 patients. Using 49 ± 18 ablation lesions, electrical isolation was achieved in 38 out of 39 ipsilateral PV-isolating lesion sets (97%). The procedure time was 244 ± 75 min. There were no complications [64]. Non-fluoroscopic atrial fibrillation ablation is also feasible using cryoballoon ablation [65].

Bulava and colleagues [66] performed a randomized trial of eight patients who randomized to fluoroscopic or non-fluoroscopic (using CARTO mapping and ICE) pulmonary vein isolation. The total procedure duration and radiofrequency application time in both groups were comparable (92.5 ± 22.9 min vs. 99.9 ± 15.9 min, $P = 0.11$, and 1785 ± 548 s vs. 1755 ± 450 s, $P = 0.79$, respectively). Zero fluoroscopic time was achieved in all patients in the non-fluoroscopic group apart from one patient, where 8 s of fluoroscopy was needed to assess proper position of the guidewire in the femoral vein. No serious procedure-related complications were recorded and no differences in arrhythmia-free survival at 12 months were found between the groups [66]. In a randomized trial of 80 patients, the use of 3D mapping in AF catheter ablation led to a significant reduction in fluoroscopy duration [67]. The use of CF catheters improves the quality of the ablation lesion [12] and imaging performed prior to the imaging such as magnetic resonance imaging may significantly improve ablation accuracy [79]. The main step limiting a zero fluoroscopy approach in AF ablation is the trans-septal puncture [51]. As mentioned, the mastering of ICE is essential for performing this step with little to no fluoroscopy. McCauley et al. showed that a zero fluoroscopy approach using EAM and ICE is safe and effective [68].

Zhang and colleagues [69] assessed the feasibility of zero fluoroscopy during reconstruction left atrium and atrial fibrillation ablation in 342 consecutive patients with paroxysmal atrial fibrillation. Patients were randomly divided into two groups after LA angiography: in the first group, reconstruction of the left atrium and isolation of the pulmonary veins were performed using EAM while the second group used both fluoroscopy and EAM. Total X-ray exposure dose of the procedure in first was significantly lower than that in latter group (19.6 ± 9.4 mGy vs. 128.7 ± 62.5 mGy, respectively, $P < 0.001$). There were no statistical differences in procedural success, the probability of freedom from atrial arrhythmia recurrence at 12 months, or complications between the two groups [69]. One of the largest experiences of zero-fluoroscopy atrial fibrillation ablation reported was performed by Sommer and colleagues [70]. In this prospective 1000 patient registry, the authors assessed the feasibility of zero-fluoroscopy ablation in terms of reduction in procedural and radiation time as well as safety aspects. The study showed that, in a cohort of 1000 patients (62.9 ± 11 years; 72% men; left ventricular ejection fraction 57%; and left atrial diameter 43.2 mm), the median procedure time was 120 min, median fluoroscopy time was 0.90 min, the median fluoroscopy dose was 345.1 cGy cm^2, and the overall complication rate was 2.0%. Stratification by operator experience (initial 75% of patients compared to last 25%) showed significant improvement in the median procedure time (from 140 to 110 min) and reduction in the median fluoroscopy time (from 6 to 0.5 min) and the median dose (from 2263 to 151.9 cGy cm^2) [70].

Ventricular Tachycardia

Catheter ablation of ventricular tachycardia is increasingly utilized. The VANISH trial has demonstrated the superiority of catheter ablation compared to escalation of anti-arrhythmic drug therapy in patients already receiving therapy [80]. In a subsequent trial, catheter ablation is currently being tested as first-line therapy for ventricular tachycardia (NCT02830360). Electroanatomic mapping has become a critical component of ventricular tachycardia ablation [51]. Cano et al. [71] compared radiation exposure in a case series of 41 patients with ventricular tachycardia (22 ischemic and 19 nonischemic) who underwent a catheter ablation using a minimal fluoroscopy approach; the authors compared the type of cardiomyopathy and the use of epicardial access. The use of the electroanatomical mapping system (CARTO) resulted in low levels of radiation exposure: median total fluoroscopy time and effective dose of 6.08 (1.51–12.36) min and 2.15 (0.58–8.22) mSv, respectively. Patients with ischemic cardiomyopathy had lower radiation exposure than patients with nonischemic ventricular tachycardia (total fluoroscopy time, 2.53 [1.22–11.22] min vs. 8.51 [5.55–17.34] min; $P = 0.016$). Epicardial access was associated with significantly higher levels of radiation exposure. A near-zero fluoroscopy ablation could be performed in 32% of cases [71]. Wang and colleagues [72] aimed to assess the safety and efficacy of a zero fluoroscopy approach, without the use of lead aprons, compared to a conventional approach for catheter ablation of idiopathic ventricular tachycardia in a prospective cohort study of seven centers. The zero fluoroscopy approach was successful in 163 (100%) patients for the electrophysiological study, and in 151 patients (94.4%) for ventricular tachycardia ablation with 9 patients having to switch to the conventional approach due to the need for coronary angiography. There was no significant difference between the two approaches in procedural success rate (84.1% vs. 85.4%), arrhythmia recurrence (1.9% vs. 2.2%), or major complications (0.6% vs. 0.9%) [72]. Several small studies have shown the feasibility and safety of a near-zero fluoroscopy approach to catheter ablation of ventricular tachycardia, including a study in complex congenital patients [73].

Conclusion

There has been considerable development and improvement in non-fluoroscopic techniques. 3D mapping, RMN, CF sensing, and ICE have all contributed to the safety and efficacy of purely 3D navigational procedures with zero or near-zero fluoroscopic exposure. Further studies are needed to assess the long-term outcomes of catheter ablation with purely 3D navigation.

References

1. Calkins H, Hindricks G, Cappato R, Kim YH, Saad EB, Aguinaga L, et al. 2017 HRS/EHRA/ECAS/APHRS/SOLAECE expert consensus statement on catheter and surgical ablation of atrial fibrillation. Heart Rhythm. 2017;14(10):e275–444.
2. AlTurki A, Marshall HJ, Proietti R. Targeting non-pulmonary vein triggers during atrial fibrillation ablation: is the game worth the candle? Curr Opin Cardiol. 2018;33(1):50–7.
3. Nair GM, Nery PB, Redpath CJ, Sadek MM, Birnie DH. Radiation safety and ergonomics in the electrophysiology laboratory: update on recent advances. Curr Opin Cardiol. 2016;31(1):11–22.
4. Sarkozy A, De Potter T, Heidbuchel H, Ernst S, Kosiuk J, Vano E, et al. Occupational radiation exposure in the electrophysiology laboratory with a focus on personnel with reproductive potential and during pregnancy: a European Heart Rhythm Association (EHRA)

consensus document endorsed by the Heart Rhythm Society (HRS). Europace. 2017;19(12):1909–22.
5. Wannagat S, Loehr L, Lask S, Volk K, Karakose T, Ozcelik C, et al. Implementation of a near-zero fluoroscopy approach in interventional electrophysiology: impact of operator experience. J Interv Card Electrophysiol. 2018;51(3):215–20.
6. Hill KD, Einstein AJ. New approaches to reduce radiation exposure. Trends Cardiovasc Med. 2016;26(1):55–65.
7. Heidbuchel H, Wittkampf FH, Vano E, Ernst S, Schilling R, Picano E, et al. Practical ways to reduce radiation dose for patients and staff during device implantations and electrophysiological procedures. Europace. 2014;16(7):946–64.
8. Lo LW, Chen SA. Three-dimensional electroanatomic mapping systems in catheter ablation of atrial fibrillation. Circ J. 2010;74(1):18–23.
9. Nedios S, Sommer P, Bollmann A, Hindricks G. Advanced mapping systems to guide atrial fibrillation ablation: electrical information that matters. J Atr Fibrillation. 2016;8(6):1337.
10. Christoph M, Wunderlich C, Moebius S, Forkmann M, Sitzy J, Salmas J, et al. Fluoroscopy integrated 3D mapping significantly reduces radiation exposure during ablation for a wide spectrum of cardiac arrhythmias. Europace. 2015;17(6):928–37.
11. AlTurki A, Huynh T, Dawas A, AlTurki H, Joza J, Healey JS, et al. Left atrial appendage isolation in atrial fibrillation catheter ablation: a meta-analysis. J Arrhythm. 2018;34(5):478–84.
12. AlTurki A, Proietti R. Remote magnetic navigation versus contact force technology: the two faces of the ablation lesion. Pacing Clin Electrophysiol. 2018;41(5):447–9.
13. Kistler PM, Earley MJ, Harris S, Abrams D, Ellis S, Sporton SC, et al. Validation of three-dimensional cardiac image integration: use of integrated CT image into electroanatomic mapping system to perform catheter ablation of atrial fibrillation. J Cardiovasc Electrophysiol. 2006;17(4):341–8.
14. Kistler PM, Rajappan K, Jahngir M, Earley MJ, Harris S, Abrams D, et al. The impact of CT image integration into an electroanatomic mapping system on clinical outcomes of catheter ablation of atrial fibrillation. J Cardiovasc Electrophysiol. 2006;17(10):1093–101.
15. Gepstein L, Hayam G, Ben-Haim SA. A novel method for nonfluoroscopic catheter-based electroanatomical mapping of the heart. In vitro and in vivo accuracy results. Circulation. 1997;95(6):1611–22.
16. Gornick CC, Adler SW, Pederson B, Hauck J, Budd J, Schweitzer J. Validation of a new noncontact catheter system for electroanatomic mapping of left ventricular endocardium. Circulation. 1999;99(6):829–35.
17. Khaykin Y, Oosthuizen R, Zarnett L, Wulffhart ZA, Whaley B, Hill C, et al. CARTO-guided vs. NavX-guided pulmonary vein antrum isolation and pulmonary vein antrum isolation performed without 3-D mapping: effect of the 3-D mapping system on procedure duration and fluoroscopy time. J Interv Card Electrophysiol. 2011;30(3):233–40.
18. de Groot NM, Schalij MJ, Zeppenfeld K, Blom NA, Van der Velde ET, Van der Wall EE. Voltage and activation mapping: how the recording technique affects the outcome of catheter ablation procedures in patients with congenital heart disease. Circulation. 2003;108(17):2099–106.
19. Graham AJ, Orini M, Lambiase PD. Limitations and challenges in mapping ventricular tachycardia: new technologies and future directions. Arrhythmia Electrophysiol Rev. 2017;6(3):118–24.
20. Da Costa A, Lafond P, Romeyer-Bouchard C, Gate-Martinet A, Bisch L, Nadrouss A, et al. Remote magnetic navigation and arrhythmia ablation. Arch Cardiovasc Dis. 2012;105(8):446–53.
21. Aagaard P, Natale A, Briceno D, Nakagawa H, Mohanty S, Gianni C, et al. Remote magnetic navigation: a focus on catheter ablation of ventricular arrhythmias. J Cardiovasc Electrophysiol. 2016;27(Suppl 1):S38–44.
22. Burkhardt JD. Remote magnetic navigation for ventricular ablation: did the machine win this round? J Interv Card Electrophysiol. 2017;48(1):5–7.
23. Arya A, Zaker-Shahrak R, Sommer P, Bollmann A, Wetzel U, Gaspar T, et al. Catheter ablation of atrial fibrillation using remote magnetic catheter navigation: a case-control study. Europace. 2011;13(1):45–50.
24. Proietti R, Pecoraro V, Di Biase L, Natale A, Santangeli P, Viecca M, et al. Remote magnetic with open-irrigated catheter vs. manual navigation for ablation of atrial fibrillation: a systematic review and meta-analysis. Europace. 2013;15(9):1241–8.
25. Choi MS, Oh Y-S, Jang SW, Kim JH, Shin WS, Youn H-J, et al. Comparison of magnetic navigation system and conventional method in catheter ablation of atrial fibrillation: is magnetic navigation system is more effective and safer than conventional method? Korean Circ J. 2011;41(5):248–52.
26. Lüthje L, Vollmann D, Seegers J, Dorenkamp M, Sohns C, Hasenfuss G, et al. Remote magnetic versus manual catheter navigation for circumferential pulmonary vein ablation in patients with atrial fibrillation. Clin Res Cardiol. 2011;100(11):1003–11.
27. Miyazaki S, Shah AJ, Xhaet O, Derval N, Matsuo S, Wright M, et al. Remote magnetic navigation with irrigated tip catheter for ablation of paroxysmal atrial fibrillation. Circ Arrhythm Electrophysiol. 2010;3(6):585–9.
28. Solheim E, Off MK, Hoff PI, De Bortoli A, Schuster P, Ohm O-J, et al. Remote magnetic versus manual catheters: evaluation of ablation effect in atrial fibrillation by myocardial marker levels. J Interv Card Electrophysiol. 2011;32(1):37–43.
29. Sorgente A, Chierchia GB, Capulzini L, Yazaki Y, Muller-Burri A, Bayrak F, et al. Atrial fibrillation ablation: a single center comparison between remote magnetic navigation, cryoballoon and conventional manual pulmonary vein isolation. Indian Pacing Electrophysiol J. 2010;10(11):486–95.
30. Turagam MK, Atkins D, Tung R, Mansour M, Ruskin J, Cheng J, et al. A meta-analysis of manual versus remote magnetic navigation for ventricular

tachycardia ablation. J Interv Card Electrophysiol. 2017;49(3):227–35.
31. Gökoğlan Y, Mohanty S, Gianni C, Santangeli P, Trivedi C, Güneş MF, et al. Scar homogenization versus limited-substrate ablation in patients with nonischemic cardiomyopathy and ventricular tachycardia. J Am Coll Cardiol. 2016;68(18):1990–8.
32. Hendriks AA, Akca F, Dabiri Abkenari L, Khan M, Bhagwandien R, Yap SC, et al. Safety and clinical outcome of catheter ablation of ventricular arrhythmias using contact force sensing: consecutive case series. J Cardiovasc Electrophysiol. 2015;26(11):1224–9.
33. Bauernfeind T, Akca F, Schwagten B, de Groot N, Van Belle Y, Valk S, et al. The magnetic navigation system allows safety and high efficacy for ablation of arrhythmias. Europace. 2011;13(7):1015–21.
34. Dinov B, Schonbauer R, Wojdyla-Hordynska A, Braunschweig F, Richter S, Altmann D, et al. Long-term efficacy of single procedure remote magnetic catheter navigation for ablation of ischemic ventricular tachycardia: a retrospective study. J Cardiovasc Electrophysiol. 2012;23(5):499–505.
35. Szili-Torok T, Schwagten B, Akca F, Bauernfeind T, Abkenari LD, Haitsma D, et al. Catheter ablation of ventricular tachycardias using remote magnetic navigation: a consecutive case-control study. J Cardiovasc Electrophysiol. 2012;23(9):948–54.
36. Zhang F, Yang B, Chen H, Ju W, Kojodjojo P, Cao K, et al. Magnetic versus manual catheter navigation for mapping and ablation of right ventricular outflow tract ventricular arrhythmias: a randomized controlled study. Heart Rhythm. 2013;10(8):1178–83.
37. Di Biase L, Tung R, Szili-Torok T, Burkhardt JD, Weiss P, Tavernier R, et al. MAGNETIC VT study: a prospective, multicenter, post-market randomized controlled trial comparing VT ablation outcomes using remote magnetic navigation-guided substrate mapping and ablation versus manual approach in a low LVEF population. J Interv Card Electrophysiol. 2017;48(3):237–45.
38. Roy K, Gomez-Pulido F, Ernst S. Remote magnetic navigation for catheter ablation in patients with congenital heart disease: a review. J Cardiovasc Electrophysiol. 2016;27(Suppl 1):S45–56.
39. Suman-Horduna I, Babu-Narayan SV, Ernst S. Remote navigation for complex arrhythmia. Arrhythm Electrophysiol Rev. 2013;2(1):53–8.
40. Rordorf R, Sanzo A, Gionti V. Contact force technology integrated with 3D navigation system for atrial fibrillation ablation: improving results? Expert Rev Med Devices. 2017;14(6):461–7.
41. Gerstenfeld EP. Contact force-sensing catheters: evolution or revolution in catheter ablation technology? Circ Arrhythm Electrophysiol. 2014;7(1):5–6.
42. Avitall B, Mughal K, Hare J, Helms R, Krum D. The effects of electrode-tissue contact on radiofrequency lesion generation. Pacing Clin Electrophysiol. 1997;20(12 Pt 1):2899–910.
43. Shah DC, Namdar M. Real-time contact force measurement: a key parameter for controlling lesion creation with radiofrequency energy. Circ Arrhythm Electrophysiol. 2015;8(3):713–21.
44. Shah DC, Lambert H, Nakagawa H, Langenkamp A, Aeby N, Leo G. Area under the real-time contact force curve (force-time integral) predicts radiofrequency lesion size in an in vitro contractile model. J Cardiovasc Electrophysiol. 2010;21(9):1038–43.
45. Jarman JWE, Panikker S, Das M, Wynn GJ, Ullah W, Kontogeorgis A, et al. Relationship between contact force sensing technology and medium-term outcome of atrial fibrillation ablation: a multicenter study of 600 patients. J Cardiovasc Electrophysiol. 2015;26(4):378–84.
46. Shurrab M, Di Biase L, Briceno DF, Kaoutskaia A, Haj-Yahia S, Newman D, et al. Impact of contact force technology on atrial fibrillation ablation: a meta-analysis. J Am Heart Assoc. 2015;4(9):e002476.
47. Saliba W, Thomas J. Intracardiac echocardiography during catheter ablation of atrial fibrillation. Europace. 2008;10(Suppl 3):iii42–7.
48. Biermann J, Bode C, Asbach S. Intracardiac echocardiography during catheter-based ablation of atrial fibrillation. Cardiol Res Pract. 2012;2012:921746.
49. Mitchell-Heggs L, Lellouche N, Deal L, Elbaz N, Hamdaoui B, Castanie JB, et al. Transseptal puncture using minimally invasive echocardiography during atrial fibrillation ablation. Europace. 2010;12(10):1435–8.
50. Shalganov TN, Paprika D, Borbás S, Temesvári A, Szili-Török T. Preventing complicated transseptal puncture with intracardiac echocardiography: case report. Cardiovasc Ultrasound. 2005;3:5.
51. Gaita F, Guerra PG, Battaglia A, Anselmino M. The dream of near-zero X-rays ablation comes true. Eur Heart J. 2016;37(36):2749–55.
52. Yang L, Sun G, Chen X, Chen G, Yang S, Guo P, et al. Meta-analysis of zero or near-zero fluoroscopy use during ablation of cardiac arrhythmias. Am J Cardiol. 2016;118(10):1511–8.
53. Sadek MM, Ramirez FD, Nery PB, Golian M, Redpath CJ, Nair GM, et al. Completely nonfluoroscopic catheter ablation of left atrial arrhythmias and ventricular tachycardia. J Cardiovasc Electrophysiol. 2019;30:78–88.
54. Deutsch K, Sledz J, Mazij M, Ludwik B, Labus M, Karbarz D, et al. Maximum voltage gradient technique for optimization of ablation for typical atrial flutter with zero-fluoroscopy approach. Medicine (Baltimore). 2017;96(25):e6939.
55. Schoene K, Rolf S, Schloma D, John S, Arya A, Dinov B, et al. Ablation of typical atrial flutter using a non-fluoroscopic catheter tracking system vs. conventional fluoroscopy—results from a prospective randomized study. Europace. 2015;17(7):1117–21.
56. Alvarez M, Tercedor L, Herrera N, Munoz L, Galdeano RS, Valverde F, et al. Cavotricuspid isthmus catheter ablation without the use of fluoroscopy as a first-line treatment. J Cardiovasc Electrophysiol. 2011;22(6):656–62.
57. Kopelman HA, Prater SP, Tondato F, Chronos NA, Peters NS. Slow pathway catheter ablation of atrioventricular nodal re-entrant tachycardia guided by electroanatomical mapping: a randomized

comparison to the conventional approach. Europace. 2003;5(2):171–4.
58. Luani B, Zrenner B, Basho M, Genz C, Rauwolf T, Tanev I, et al. Zero-fluoroscopy cryothermal ablation of atrioventricular nodal re-entry tachycardia guided by endovascular and endocardial catheter visualization using intracardiac echocardiography (Ice&ICE Trial). J Cardiovasc Electrophysiol. 2018;29(1):160–6.
59. Casella M, Pelargonio G, Dello Russo A, Riva S, Bartoletti S, Santangeli P, et al. "Near-zero" fluoroscopic exposure in supraventricular arrhythmia ablation using the EnSite NavX mapping system: personal experience and review of the literature. J Interv Card Electrophysiol. 2011;31(2):109–18.
60. Clark J, Bockoven JR, Lane J, Patel CR, Smith G. Use of three-dimensional catheter guidance and transesophageal echocardiography to eliminate fluoroscopy in catheter ablation of left-sided accessory pathways. Pacing Clin Electrophysiol. 2008;31(3):283–9.
61. Scaglione M, Ebrille E, Caponi D, Siboldi A, Bertero G, Di Donna P, et al. Zero-fluoroscopy ablation of accessory pathways in children and adolescents: CARTO3 electroanatomic mapping combined with RF and cryoenergy. Pacing Clin Electrophysiol. 2015;38(6):675–81.
62. Bigelow AM, Smith G, Clark JM. Catheter ablation without fluoroscopy: current techniques and future direction. J Atrial Fibrillation. 2014;6(6):1066.
63. Casella M, Dello Russo A, Pelargonio G, Del Greco M, Zingarini G, Piacenti M, et al. Near zerO fluoroscopic exPosure during catheter ablAtion of supRavenTricular arrhYthmias: the NO-PARTY multicentre randomized trial. Europace. 2016;18(10):1565–72.
64. Reddy VY, Morales G, Ahmed H, Neuzil P, Dukkipati S, Kim S, et al. Catheter ablation of atrial fibrillation without the use of fluoroscopy. Heart Rhythm. 2010;7(11):1644–53.
65. Razminia M, Demo H, Arrieta-Garcia C, D'Silva OJ, Wang T, Kehoe RF. Nonfluoroscopic ablation of atrial fibrillation using cryoballoon. J Atrial Fibrillation. 2014;7(1):1093.
66. Bulava A, Hanis J, Eisenberger M. Catheter ablation of atrial fibrillation using zero-fluoroscopy technique: a randomized trial. Pacing Clin Electrophysiol. 2015;38(7):797–806.
67. Huo Y, Christoph M, Forkmann M, Pohl M, Mayer J, Salmas J, et al. Reduction of radiation exposure during atrial fibrillation ablation using a novel fluoroscopy image integrated 3-dimensional electroanatomic mapping system: a prospective, randomized, single-blind, and controlled study. Heart Rhythm. 2015;12(9):1945–55.
68. McCauley MD, Patel N, Greenberg SJ, Molina-Razavi JE, Safavi-Naeini P, Razavi M. Fluoroscopy-free atrial transseptal puncture. Eur J Arrhythm Electrophysiol. 2016;2(2):57–61.
69. Zhang JQ, Yu RH, Liang JB, Long Y, Sang CH, Ma CS, et al. Reconstruction left atrium and isolation pulmonary veins of paroxysmal atrial fibrillation using single contact force catheter with zero X-ray exposure: a CONSORT study. Medicine (Baltimore). 2017;96(41):e7726.
70. Sommer P, Bertagnolli L, Kircher S, Arya A, Bollmann A, Richter S, et al. Safety profile of near-zero fluoroscopy atrial fibrillation ablation with non-fluoroscopic catheter visualization: experience from 1000 consecutive procedures. Europace. 2018;20:1952–8.
71. Cano O, Andres A, Osca J, Alonso P, Sancho-Tello MJ, Olague J, et al. Safety and feasibility of a minimally fluoroscopic approach for ventricular tachycardia ablation in patients with structural heart disease: influence of the ventricular tachycardia substrate. Circ Arrhythm Electrophysiol. 2016;9(2):e003706.
72. Wang Y, Chen GZ, Yao Y, Bai Y, Chu HM, Ma KZ, et al. Ablation of idiopathic ventricular arrhythmia using zero-fluoroscopy approach with equivalent efficacy and less fatigue: a multicenter comparative study. Medicine (Baltimore). 2017;96(6):e6080.
73. Akca F, Bauernfeind T, Witsenburg M, Dabiri Abkenari L, Cuypers JA, Roos-Hesselink JW, et al. Acute and long-term outcomes of catheter ablation using remote magnetic navigation in patients with congenital heart disease. Am J Cardiol. 2012;110(3):409–14.
74. Cosío FG. Atrial flutter, typical and atypical: a review. Arrhythmia Electrophysiol Rev. 2017;6(2):55–62.
75. Macias R, Uribe I, Tercedor L, Jimenez-Jaimez J, Barrio T, Alvarez M. A zero-fluoroscopy approach to cavotricuspid isthmus catheter ablation: comparative analysis of two electroanatomical mapping systems. Pacing Clin Electrophysiol. 2014;37(8):1029–37.
76. Álvarez M, Tercedor L, Almansa I, Ros N, Galdeano RS, Burillo F, et al. Safety and feasibility of catheter ablation for atrioventricular nodal re-entrant tachycardia without fluoroscopic guidance. Heart Rhythm. 2009;6(12):1714–20.
77. Gist K, Tigges C, Smith G, Clark J. Learning curve for zero-fluoroscopy catheter ablation of AVNRT: early versus late experience. Pacing Clin Electrophysiol. 2011;34(3):264–8.
78. Balli S, Kucuk M, Orhan Bulut M, Kemal Yucel I, Celebi A. Transcatheter cryoablation procedures without fluoroscopy in pediatric patients with atrioventricular nodal reentrant tachycardia: a single-center experience. Acta Cardiol Sin. 2018;34(4):337–43.
79. Faletti R, Rapellino A, Barisone F, Anselmino M, Ferraris F, Fonio P, et al. Use of oral gadobenate dimeglumine to visualise the oesophagus during magnetic resonance angiography in patients with atrial fibrillation prior to catheter ablation. J Cardiovasc Magn Reson. 2014;16:41.
80. Sapp JL, Wells GA, Parkash R, Stevenson WG, Blier L, Sarrazin JF, et al. Ventricular tachycardia ablation versus escalation of antiarrhythmic drugs. N Engl J Med. 2016;375(2):111–21.

Radiation Exposure and Safety for the Electrophysiologist

2

Darbhamulla V. Nagarajan, Ahmed AlTurki, and Sabine Ernst

Introduction

Ever since the first ablation procedure was performed by Dr. Scheinman in 1981 the field of interventional electrophysiology has made significant progress [1]. Electrophysiology (EP) studies and radiofrequency catheter ablation (RFCA) procedures are widely performed worldwide. Radiofrequency ablation has been established as a first-line treatment for supraventricular arrhythmias and one of the accepted treatment modalities for more complex atrial and ventricular arrhythmias [2–4]. Traditionally, EP procedures are performed in cardiac catheter laboratories and fluoroscopy is used as the key imaging modality to guide positioning cardiac catheters. As a consequence, electrophysiologists are exposed to considerable ionising radiation as scatter emitted by their patients (Fig. 2.1) [5]. In fact electrophysiologists seem to have even higher amount of radiation exposure compared to other medical personnel including interventional radiologists [5–7]. Several reports about possible radiation-related serious complications amongst cardiologists who were previously exposed to ionising radiation have heightened the awareness about the need for better understanding and optimal utilisation of available technologies in cardiac catheter labs [8–10]. Females comprise 11% of electrophysiology trainees as well as a significant proportion of electrophysiology lab personnel [11]. Misconceptions regarding the risk of occupational radiation exposure on pregnancy may lead to changes in family and career planning. Proper monitoring is essential to prevent harm to both the foetus and the mother.

D. V. Nagarajan
Department of Cardiology, Royal Brompton and Harefield Hospital, National Heart and Lung Institute, Imperial College London, London, UK

Department of Cardiology, Doncaster and Bassetlaw Hospitals NHS Foundation Trust, Doncaster, UK
e-mail: v.nagarajan@nhs.net

A. AlTurki
Division of Cardiology, McGill University Health Centre, Montreal, QC, Canada
e-mail: ahmed.alturki@mail.mcgill.ca

S. Ernst (✉)
Department of Cardiology, Royal Brompton and Harefield Hospital, National Heart and Lung Institute, Imperial College London, London, UK
e-mail: s.ernst@rbht.nhs.uk

Quantification of Ionising Radiation

Radiation exposure can be quantified using different measures. Commonly used terminology includes absorbed dose, cumulative air kerma, dose area product (DAP) also referred to as kerma area product (KAP), equivalent dose, personal dose equivalent and effective dose. These terms are defined by the International Commission on Radiological Protection (ICRP) [12].

R. Proietti et al. (eds.), *Cardiac Electrophysiology Without Fluoroscopy*, https://doi.org/10.1007/978-3-030-16992-3_2

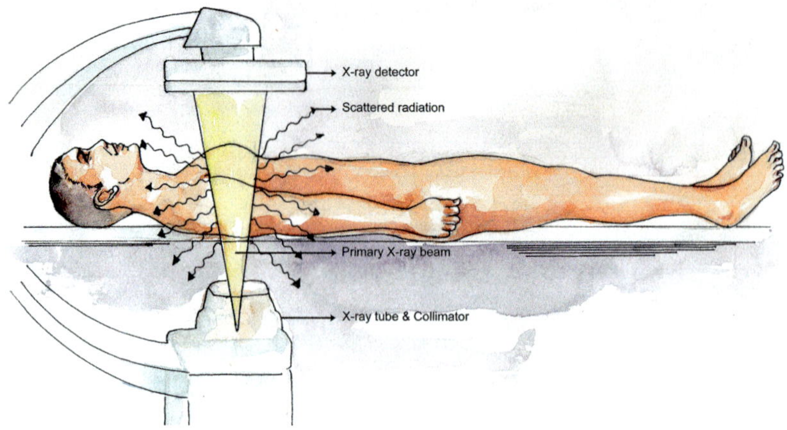

Fig. 2.1 Diagrammatic representation of X-ray equipment and scatter radiation in an EP lab. Please note that the X-ray beam is emitted from under the table, making the under-table protection apron very important

Absorbed dose is the energy absorbed per unit mass of the absorbing tissue. It is expressed in grey units. One grey (Gy) equates to one joule of energy per kilogram of absorbing tissue.

Cumulative air kerma is a quantitative measure of X-ray energy delivered to air at the interventional reference point (15 cm from the isocentre in the direction of the focal spot).

DAP is a product of the radiation dose to air and cross-sectional X-ray beam area at any given distance from the X-ray source. It is independent of the distance from the X-ray source. DAP is expressed as Gy cm^2.

Equivalent dose is a measure of biological effect of ionising radiation. To allow comparisons of the risk of harm due to different ionising radiations, each type of radiation is assigned a radiation weighting factor (W_R) as a measure of its biological effect. Equivalent dose is the product of absorbed dose and radiation weighting factor. Equivalent dose is measured in sieverts (Sv) and denotes potency of radiation (for example one grey of gamma rays is equivalent to 1 Sv whilst one grey of alpha rays is equivalent to 20 Sv).

Effective dose (ED) takes into consideration the potency as well as the probability of a tissue being affected per unit dose of radiation (e.g. the same amount of equivalent dose would equate to 20 times more equivalent dose to ovaries compared to skin). Effective dose is a tissue-weighted sum of all equivalent dose in different tissues of human body. Radio sensitivity in human tissues is highest in highly mitotic or undifferentiated tissues such as bone marrow, lens, basal epidermis and gonads. It reduces with age and as a consequence young children exposed to radiation are much more likely to be affected than the older ones [13, 14]. Effective doses are related to the whole-body risk associated with any given deposition of ionising radiation in an individual.

Personal dose equivalent is measured by the personal occupational dosimeters and is expressed in millisieverts. It gives an estimate of the organ doses.

Hazards from Exposure to Ionising Radiation

The harmful effects of ionising radiation are well known and can be classified as stochastic and deterministic effects.

Stochastic effects are not related to a particular threshold level of radiation exposure; however the risk of their occurrence increases with a lifetime cumulative increase in radiation exposure and severity independent of the dose. Typical example of a stochastic effect of ionising radiation is the risk of developing malignancy and genetic effect being the other. Stochastic risk from exposure to ionising radiation can be expressed using the concept of "effective dose", a term first used by Wolfgang Jacobi in 1975 [15].

The excessive relative risk of cancer mortality according to International Commission of Radiological Protection (ICRP) is 5% per Sv and 0.2% per Sv for heritable effects.

Dose area product has been shown to correlate well with the total ionising energy imparted to a patient and total scatter radiation and therefore to the risk of stochastic effects such as malignancy both to patient and medical workers [16–22].

Deterministic effects only occur once a threshold of exposure has been exceeded. The severity of deterministic effects increases as the dose of exposure increases. Deterministic effects are caused by significant cell damage or death. The physical effects will occur when the cell death burden is large enough to cause obvious functional impairment of a tissue or an organ. Radiological measurement that has been used to estimate deterministic effects is cumulative air kerma (Gy). Some of the recognised deterministic effects of radiation include erythema, necrosis and epilation of skin, cataract, reduced fertility and acute radiation syndrome. The skin and eyes are most vulnerable to X-rays with a suggested threshold radiation dose (for deterministic effects) of 2 Gy and 500 μGy, respectively [23–26].

Monitoring Radiation Exposure in Electrophysiology Lab

The ICRP recommends the use of two personal dosimeters for staff exposed to radiation: one to be worn on the trunk of the body inside lead apron at about waist level and the other worn outside lead apron at collar or left shoulder. Inside dosimeter estimates radiation to internal organs including reproductive organs. However it may be an overestimate as it does not account for further attenuation of radiation through superficial tissues [11]. The outer dosimeter estimates radiation exposure to thyroid, lens, head and neck.

Female medical personnel working in cardiac labs should be encouraged to declare pregnancy as early as possible as it would help monitor ED to foetus. Additional dosimeter at the level of abdomen could be used to assess foetal exposure [27].

Compliance with dosimeter use is essential and should be made mandatory. Passive dosimeters are usually read monthly. Records of exposure are kept for as long as required by national legislation/guidelines, and may depend on the type of radiation worker. Please note that it is not generally possible to establish whether an individual's cancer has been caused by radiation exposure. The causal relationship between radiation exposure and cancer incidence is only detectable through statistical analysis of large population samples. In some very rare circumstances it may be possible to conclude (on balance of probabilities) that an individual's cancer is linked to their occupational exposure. This might be possible when the cancer is rare in the general population but observed in disproportionate numbers in an occupational group having very specific exposures to radiation, and the individual in question has had the specific exposure.

Historical Data About Radiation Exposure in Electrophysiology Procedures

Most of the studies looking at radiation exposure in electrophysiology labs are patient centric with main focus on the radiation exposure to the patient [28–30]. Very few studies were aimed at physician radiation exposure [7, 31, 32]. Higher radiation exposure both to the patient and physician was noted with complex ablation procedures [33, 34]. It was also observed that there was operator variability; however average operator dose was quantitatively related to average patient dose. It was also noted that there was reduction in radiation exposure over time with development of newer non-fluoroscopic three-dimensional navigation and electroanatomical mapping systems [35].

Electrophysiologists have been shown to have high radiation exposure with a median of 4.3 mSv per year (3.5–6.1) whilst interventional cardiologists averaged 3.3 mSv (2.0–19.6 mSv) and average background radiation received by a European resident is around 2.1 mSv per year [7, 36]. Casella and colleagues examined the

Table 2.1 Radiation exposure of various electrophysiological procedures [37]

Procedure	Mean effective dose (mSv) 2010	Mean effective dose (mSv) 2016	Trend	Significance (*P*-value) of trend from 2010 to 2016
Electrophysiological study	1.0	0.5	−50%	Significant
Pacemaker/implantable cardioverter defibrillator implantation	1.8	1.0	−44%	Significant
Cardiac resynchronisation therapy	16.0	7.5	−53%	Not significant
SVT ablation	5.4	2.2	−59%	Significant
Atrial flutter ablation	11.0	3.2	−71%	Significant
Atrial fibrillation ablation	34.0	7.3	−79%	Significant
Ventricular tachycardia ablation	38.9	10.0	−74%	Significant

trend in radiation exposure amongst the various electrophysiological procedures in a retrospective study of 8150 patients over a 7-year period. There was a significant decrease in radiation exposure in all procedures except cardiac resynchronisation therapy. This demonstrates the remarkable improvement in procedural influences, protective equipment, as well as operator experience and compliance with protection protocols. Radiation exposures of the various electrophysiological procedures in the year 2010 and 2016 are summarised in Table 2.1. The fact that vast improvement was seen in ablation procedures and specially complex ablations, namely atrial fibrillation and ventricular tachycardia ablations, is testament to the increasing use of non-fluoroscopic techniques and their ability to reduce radiation exposure [37].

Measures to Reduce Radiation Exposure in Electrophysiology Laboratory

There are three principles that govern the use of radiation in the electrophysiology lab: responsibility, justification and optimisation. It is the physician's responsibility to limit the exposure to radiation by utilising the knowledge of procedural, operator and patient influences on radiation exposure. The use and dose of radiation must be justified in view of the patient's clinical context. The benefits of the procedure and the need for fluoroscopy must be carefully weighed against the risk of exposure to radiation. In addition, all factors must be optimised to ensure the minimum exposure to radiation without compromising the safety and efficacy of the procedure [38].

Various measures to reduce radiation exposure during electrophysiology procedures can be grouped under the following categories which include

1. Awareness and education resulting in a change in culture
2. Use of protective gear in cath labs (including thyroid shields, lead glasses, etc.)
3. Effective use of radiological views
4. Effective use of available fluoroscopic technology (such as collimation and lower pulse rates)
5. Effective adaptation and implementation of local and national policies
6. Effective use of mapping systems and newer technologies in electrophysiology labs
7. Continued research to facilitate eventual zero-radiation procedures

Awareness and Education Resulting in a Change in Culture

Unlike other professionals such as professional pilots involved with radiation exposure electrophysiologists seem to be less educated about radiation hazards and ways to minimise them [35]. Electrophysiology trainees need to be educated about awareness and need to use radiation as low as reasonably achievable (ALARA principle) [39, 40], a concept that has been proposed by the International Commission for Radiation Protection to guide responsible radiation use.

Education about radiation exposure hazards and ways to reduce it should start very early in electrophysiology training and should be made mandatory. Electrophysiologists should be well equipped to utilise alternative non-fluoroscopic imaging modalities at every possible stage during the procedure. Proper documentation of radiation doses and compliance with dosimeters should be ensured by the local authorities. It has been shown that use of fluoroscopy is not strictly a function of experience and that the awareness of the harm correlated with X-rays and the presence of a background in radiation safety are the cornerstones for reducing radiation exposure in interventional cardiology [41, 42].

Use of Protective Gear in Cath Labs (Fig. 2.2)

Lead aprons (minimum of 0.5 mm lead equivalence in front and 0.25 mm at the rear) have been shown to reduce radiation dose by over 95% for the operator [43, 44]. In addition, wearing a thyroid shield and lead glasses or the use of a radiation protection cabin and avoiding direct hand exposure help reduce radiation doses significantly. Professional cataract is a well-known problem in invasive cardiology workers and is distinguished from naturally occurring cataract forms as it occurs in the posterior pole of the lens [45, 46]. Use of protective eyewear (leaded glasses with side panels) is highly recommended [47, 48]. Under-table lead shielding and over-table glass shielding help reduce scatter radiation to the operator and hence should be used routinely during EP procedures.

Effective Use of Radiological Views

For a given amount of beam energy the resultant image quality is inversely proportional to the

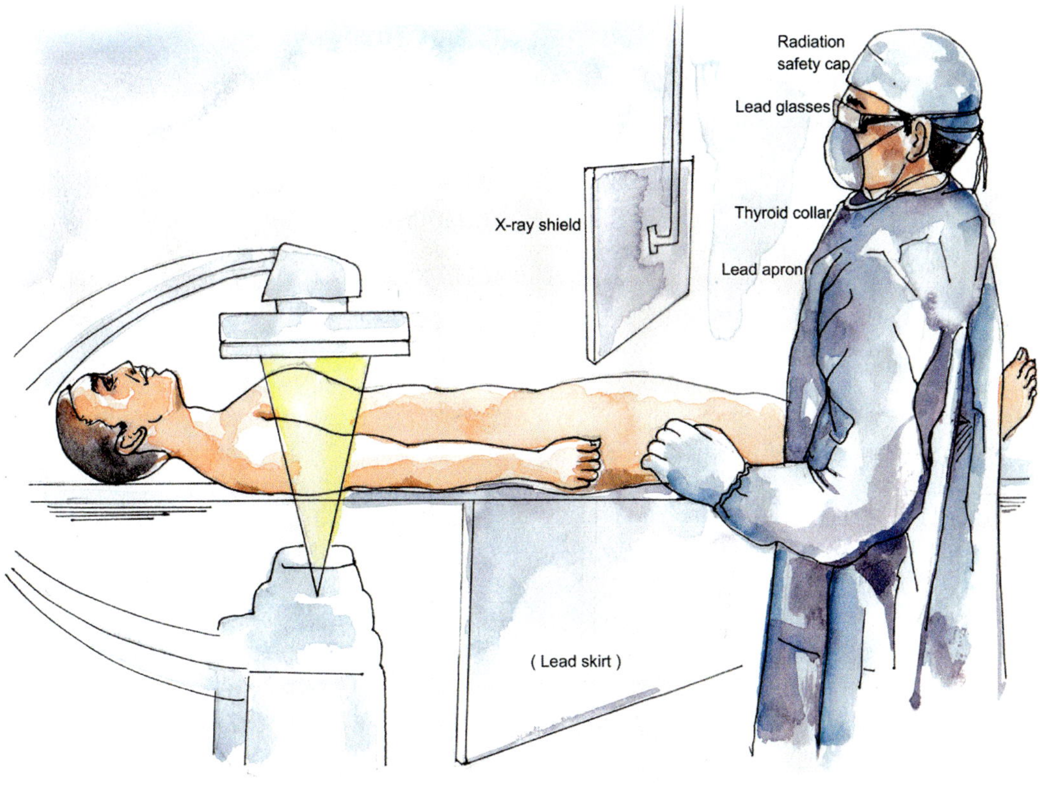

Fig. 2.2 Diagrammatic representation of protective equipment used in an EP lab

amount of tissue and distance it has to traverse. In lateral (or craniocaudal) angulations, X-rays cross more tissues, which increases attenuation and decreases image quality [49]. To compensate, the system increases the beam energy to maintain image quality. As a result there is more radiation to the patient as well as operator. The operator receives most of the radiation as a result of scatter from the patient. The operator is likely to receive higher radiation dose when standing on the same side of the patient as the tube (as a result of scatter from the patient) [50] and therefore when operating from right side of the patient the operator receives more radiation in a left lateral view compared to the right lateral view. Traditionally when ablation is carried out most operators view catheter position in a left anterior oblique view. Care should be taken that lead shied is protecting the operator during these lateral angulated views. Overall one should be mindful of the fact that higher radiation is being used during the use of angulated views [51]. Also operators have to be cautious using angulated views in patients with high body mass index as it would result in much higher doses of radiation [52].

Effective Use of Available Fluoroscopic Technology

Electrophysiologists can reduce radiation to the patient and scatter radiation for themselves in turn by effective use of available fluoroscopic technology. Effective use of various strategies available with modern X-ray units can considerably reduce radiation dose without significant change in fluoroscopy time. Use of lower pulse frequency and shorter pulse durations has been shown to reduce radiation dose [36, 53, 54]. This can be achieved by using lower frame rates such as 3–4 fps. Removal of the secondary radiation grid and programming an ultra-low pulsed fluoroscopy rate during ablation procedures were associated with significant reductions in radiation exposure [36]. Confining the X-ray beam to small area of interest can be achieved by using collimation. Collimation reduces DAP as it reduces cross-sectional area at any given distance from the source. During interventional electrophysiology procedure collimation has been shown to significantly reduce radiation exposure without compromising on the image quality. These benefits have been more marked in simple ablation procedures where smaller areas are of interest during ablation [55]. Asymmetric collimation can achieve another 60–80% reduction compared with normal collimation [56]. Whilst fluoroscopy is used for catheter placement, cine is used to acquire and store images. Cine acquisitions account for majority of radiation exposure despite representing a smaller fraction of X-ray tube operation time [57, 58]. Cine acquisitions can be minimised or even avoided by using the stored fluoroscopy feature (saving the last fluoroscopic loop) [59].

The X-ray tube output is proportional to the distance between the tube and the detector. The detector should therefore be lowered onto the patient throughout the procedure (Fig. 2.3). A 15% reduction in radiation dose was noted with a combination of elevation of table and lowering detector by 10 cm [60]. Frame rate settings are programmable between 25–30 and 6 fps. Still lower frame rates may be achieved by using triggered fluoroscopy. Lower frame rates are linearly related to lower radiation doses.

Effective Adaptation and Implementation of Local and National Policies

European Commission has recognised the need to educate and train medical personnel involved in procedures using ionising radiation. The current Medical Exposure Directive (MED) outlines the justification and optimisation of radiological procedures, distribution of responsibilities, training of medical staff, procedural aspects and equipment use. Under the EURATOM Treaty the European Commission is responsible for the protection of patients and other individuals in medical facilities [61]. It does this by consistently updating the Basic Safety Standards Directive which regulates, amongst other items, the safe use of ionising radiation in medical applications.

Directive 2013/59/Euratom—protection against ionising radiation—states that the member states

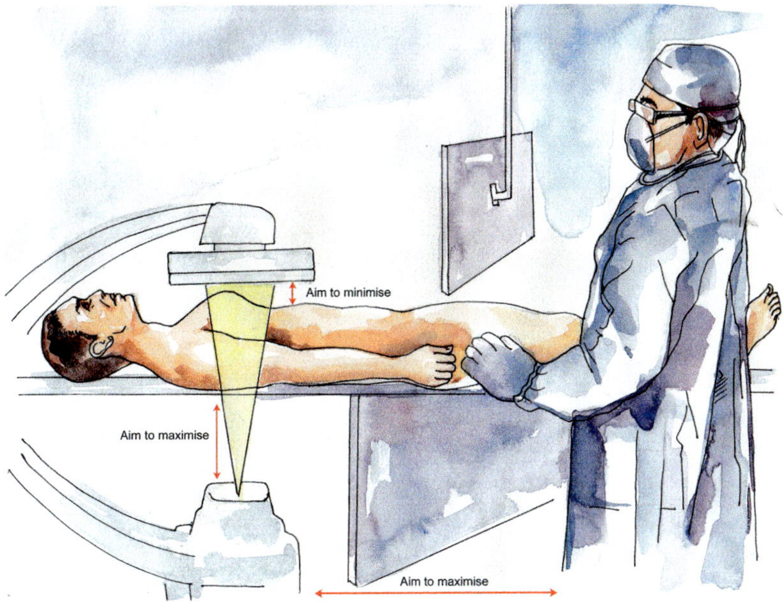

Fig. 2.3 Diagrammatic representation of possible ways to reduce scatter radiation in an EP lab. Scattered radiation can be reduced by reducing the X-ray field size, the path length of the X-ray beam through the patient (i.e. projection) and the exposure parameters (e.g. pulse rate). The patient-detector distance is minimised and the focus-patient distance is maximised (within the constraints of available focus-to-detector distances) in the first instance to reduce magnification (image quality) and patient dose. The lower patient dose arises from lower exposure parameters, which in turn reduces scatter. In the case of interventional X-ray units with an isocentre, the focus-patient distance is essentially determined by the unit's geometry; the operator however is able to control the position of the detector

system of radiation protection shall be based on the principles of justification (benefits outweigh risks) and optimisation (exposure to as few, and as low as possible: dose constraints) and

Dose limitations (on the individual's level) are as follows:

- For effective dose limit: 20 mSv in any single year
- In special circumstances: up to 50 mSv in a single year (the average annual dose over any 5 consecutive years must not exceed 20 mSv)
- Eyes: 20 mSv in a year or 100 mSv in any 5 consecutive years
- Skin and extremities: 500 mSv per year

The onus of medical staff's awareness and protection from radiation exposure lies with the employer. Accordingly, the major cardiovascular associations have published detailed recommendations about X-ray use and suggested practical ways to reduce it [62].

Effective Use of Mapping Systems and Newer Technologies in Electrophysiology Labs

Electroanatomic mapping systems (EMS) have been developed for facilitating catheter localisation, three-dimensional cardiac chamber description, obtaining three-dimensional electrical activation sequences and voltage map within a cardiac chamber (Fig. 2.4). The two EMS that are mostly used include the NavX system (St. Jude/Abbott) which uses low-amplitude high-frequency current fields [63] and CARTO (Biosense Webster) which uses magnetic fields and impedance measurements for catheter localisation [64]. These are also called "non-fluoroscopic" mapping systems as they do not utilise fluoroscopy. Whilst EMS greatly facilitates identification of appropriate ablation sites during complex ablation procedures, operators need greater understanding of underlying principles and appropriate experience in

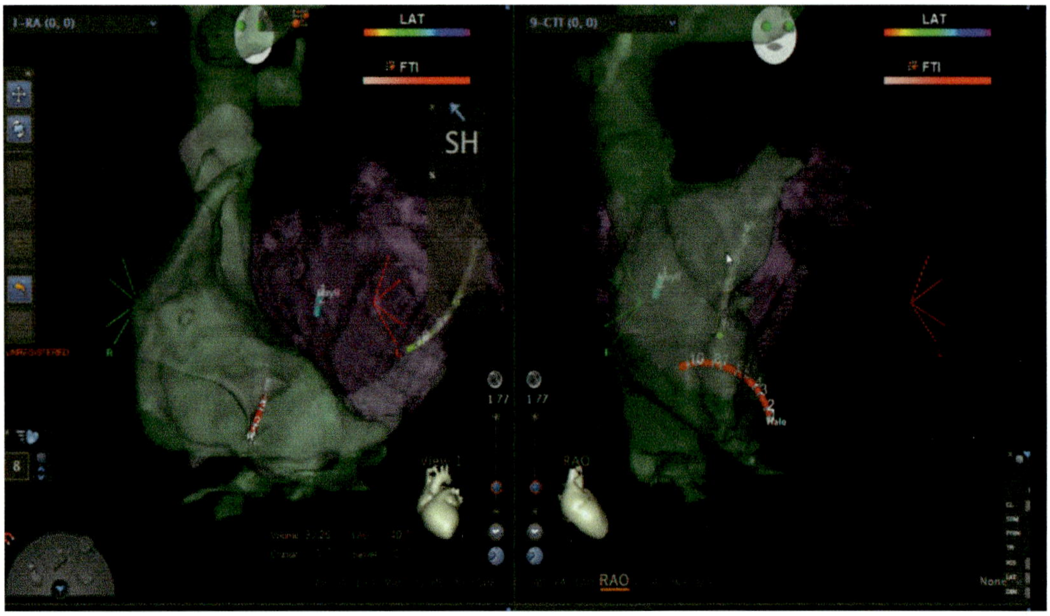

Fig. 2.4 Electroanatomical mapping (CARTO) image showing transseptal puncture being carried out without using fluoroscopy. The transseptal needle tip is visualised as a catheter which can be located in real time on corresponding 3D projections

their use. Use of EMS has been shown to reduce radiation dose during ablation procedures [53, 65, 66]. EMS can be further enhanced by integration of 3D imaging obtained using cardiac MRI or CT prior to procedure [67].

Remote navigation systems have been developed on the premise that it would provide better precision movement of ablation catheter and improve outcomes by enabling more effective lesions. The only system currently in use allows remote navigation by moving special catheter by a static magnetic field [68] (Niobe system from Stereotaxis). Whilst remote navigation does not reduce the radiation dose for the patient, it can facilitate near-zero radiation for the operator. However, as the image integration of the system allowed for better orientation of the operator, significant reduction of the patient's radiation exposure has been demonstrated for a number of different arrhythmias [68–70].

Continued Innovation to Facilitate Eventual Zero-Radiation Procedures

Whilst near-zero-radiation ablation procedures have been shown to be feasible amongst paediatric population they are still a work in progress amongst adult cohorts. In our experience it has been feasible to perform complex ablation procedures (including transseptal punctures) using no fluoroscopy with the aid of EMS and alternate imaging modalities such as transoesophageal echocardiography. The key step in transseptal punctures is to visualise the transseptal needle, which can be "faked" on the EMS system [71]. By using a radiofrequency needle (NRG, Baylis Medical) with an isolated tip that serves as small electrode, the exact location of the needle tip on the 3D reconstruction of the right atrium can be achieved.

Radiation Effects on Fertility and Pregnancy

Radiation is toxic to tissues including reproductive organs. However, data is unfortunately scarce in humans. The testes are very sensitive to ionising radiation and therefore sperm count data provide a useful source of information on the effect of ionising radiation on the testes. In a study of healthy volunteer prisoners, aged 22–50 years, who were scheduled to undergo vasectomy, radiation exposure as low as 150 mGy resulted in significant suppression in sperm production [72]. In addition, there was transient abolition of sperm production in most men after exposure to a dose of 500 mGy, with higher doses leading to more prolonged suppression of spermatogenesis. Higher doses also lead to histological changes in the testes [72]. With regard to sperm quality, exposure to ionising radiation in male healthcare workers leads to a significant decrease in sperm quality as evidenced by decreased motility, decreased viability and altered morphological features [73]. Based on the available data, Rowley and colleagues adjudged that short-term exposure to ionising radiation of the magnitude of 110–150 mGy results in transient loss of spermatogenesis, whilst exposure to larger doses of 2000 mGy or higher over a prolonged period may lead to male infertility [74].

The exposure of a pregnant operator to ionising radiation continues to be a difficult issue to handle. As a conservative measure, the radiation dose recorded on the dosimeter inside the apron, which should be worn on the abdomen, is used to estimate the radiation exposure of the foetus. Whilst the mother's abdomen will provide some shielding, this should not be taken into account [62]. Low doses of radiation as would be expected from operators who are properly protected and follow all of the abovementioned recommendations to reduce exposure do not pose an increased risk of prenatal complications or malformations beyond the incidence seen in the general population [75]. Therefore, proper and precise monitoring is essential to ensure that such doses are not exceeded. Current guidelines emphasise that the highest risk occurs in the first trimester, which is the time of organogenesis. Malformations are known to occur with exposures of around 100 mGy [75]. Current guidelines state that at the recommended exposure levels, malformations should not occur. Furthermore, current data suggests no alterations in mental development of children who are exposed to radiation at recommended doses in utero [62]. The greatest uncertainty resides in the risk of childhood malignancy in children, who are exposed to radiation at recommended doses in utero. However, based on the currently available data, there appears to be a small increase in risk which is of uncertain significance [75]. Further research in this area would certainly be welcome.

Current guidelines recommend that the dose of radiation after declaration of pregnancy not exceed 1 mSv. However, the authors state that this does not preclude the electrophysiologist from continuing to work in the electrophysiology lab. In order to do so, the guidelines recommend that the following occur: (1) the electrophysiologist should understand the risks of further radiation exposure and willingly elect to continue working in the electrophysiology lab; (2) to monitor the dose to the foetus, an extra dosimeter should be worn at the level of the abdomen monthly; the exposure dose values should be relayed to the electrophysiologist on a regular basis; (3) the electrophysiologist must be aware of all the aforementioned methods to reduce radiation exposure and should attempt to regulate her workload in fluoroscopy-guided procedures; and (4) a dedicated radiation monitoring and protection programme should exist in the hospital, led by a competent expert [27].

The pregnant electrophysiologist should employ constant radiation awareness, appropriate use of monitoring and radioprotection measures to minimise exposure to the lowest possible level during pregnancy [62]. A significantly greater amount of scattered radiation occurs during device implantation compared to ablation procedures. Therefore, great care should be taken to optimise positioning and shielding in order to reduce radiation exposure. A two-piece wrap around lead skirt and vest should be used with a minimum of 0.5 mm lead equivalence in the front [62]. As mentioned, 3D mapping systems, remote navigation systems as well as protection cabins should be utilised when available [76].

Summary and Outlook for the Future

Using all the options of modern fluoroscopy systems and wearing all personal protection gear available, daily work in the EP lab can be performed without significant increase of the professional risk. However, it is in the greatest personal interest of every operator to protect himself or herself as much as possible and apply ALARA principle whenever possible. Using all available 3D imaging information and applying ZERO-radiation techniques if possible is only a matter of dedicated training. Low personal exposure for the operator always equates to low exposure for the patient and vice versa, such that any attempt of radiation reduction will always benefit both parties. Future 3D EMS should aim to eliminate the need to use X-rays completely, which would open the opportunity to perform invasive procedures outside cath labs.

References

1. Scheinman MM, Morady F, Hess DS, Gonzalez R. Catheter-induced ablation of the atrioventricular junction to control refractory supraventricular arrhythmias. JAMA. 1982;248:851.
2. Al-Khatib SM, Stevenson WG, Ackerman MJ, et al. 2017 AHA/ACC/HRS guideline for management of patients with ventricular arrhythmias and the prevention of sudden cardiac death: a report of the American College of Cardiology/American Heart Association Task Force on Clinical Practice Guidelines and the Heart Rhythm Society. Heart Rhythm. 2018;15:e190–e252 [published online ahead of print 30 Oct 2017]. https://doi.org/10.1016/j.hrthm.2017.10.035.
3. Calkins H, Hindricks G, Cappato R, et al. 2017 HRS/EHRA/ECAS/APHRS/SOLAECE expert consensus statement on catheter and surgical ablation of atrial fibrillation: executive summary. Europace. 2018;20(1):157–208.
4. Page RL, Joglar JA, Caldwell MA, et al. 2015 ACC/AHA/HRS guideline for the management of adult patients with supraventricular tachycardia: a report of the American College of Cardiology/American Heart Association Task Force on Clinical Practice Guidelines and the Heart Rhythm Society. J Am Coll Cardiol. 2016;67:e27–e115.
5. Kim KP, Donald LM, Balter S, Kleinerman RA, Linet MS, Kwon D, et al. Occupational radiation doses to operators performing cardiac catheterization procedures. Health Phys. 2008;94:211–27.
6. Picano E, Vañó E, Rehani MM, Cuocolo A, Mont L, Bodi V, Bar O, Maccia C, Pierard L, Sicari R, Plein S, Mahrholdt H, Lancellotti P, Knuuti J, Heidbuchel H, Di Mario C, Badano LP. The appropriate and justified use of medical radiation in cardiovascular imaging: a position document of the ESC Associations of Cardiovascular Imaging, Percutaneous Cardiovascular Interventions and Electrophysiology. Eur Heart J. 2014;35:665–72.
7. Venneri L, Rossi F, Botto N, Andreassi MG, Salcone N, Emad A, Lazzeri M, Gori C, Vano E, Picano E. Cancer risk from professional exposure in staff working in cardiac catheterization laboratory: insights from the national research council's biological effects of ionizing radiation VII report. Am Heart J. 2009;157:118–24.
8. Buchanan GL, Chieffo A, Mehilli J, Mikhail GW, Mauri F, Presbitero P, et al. The occupational effects of interventional cardiology: results from the WIN for safety survey. EuroIntervention. 2012;8:658–63.
9. Marinskis G, Bongiorni MG, Dagres N, Lewalter T, Pison L, Blomstrom-Lundqvist C. Scientific Initiative Committee, European Heart Rhythm Association. X-ray exposure hazards for physicians performing ablation procedures and device implantation: results of the European Heart Rhythm Association survey. Europace. 2013;15:444–6.
10. Roguin A, Goldstein J, Bar O. Brain tumours among interventional cardiologists: a cause for alarm? Report of four new cases from two cities and a review of the literature. EuroIntervention. 2012;7(9):1081–6.
11. Sarkozy A, De Potter T, Heidbuchel H, Ernst S, Kosiuk J, et al. Occupational radiation exposure in the electrophysiology laboratory with a focus on personnel with reproductive potential and during pregnancy: a European Heart Rhythm Association (EHRA) consensus document endorsed by the Heart Rhythm Society (HRS). Europace. 2017;19(12):1909–22.
12. ICRP. Compendium of dose coefficients based on ICRP publication 60. ICRP publication 119. Ann ICRP. 2012;41(Suppl).
13. Modan B, Keinan L, Blumstein T, et al. Cancer following cardiac catheterization in childhood. Int J Epidemiol. 2000;29:424–8.
14. Pearce MS, Salotti JA, Little MP, et al. Radiation exposure from CT scans in childhood and subsequent risk of leukaemia and brain tumours: a retrospective cohort study. Lancet. 2012;380:499–505.
15. Jacobi W. The concept of effective dose—a proposal for the combination of organ doses. Radiat Environ Biophys. 1975;12:101–9.
16. Shrimpton PC, Wall BF, Jones DG, Fisher ES. The measurement of energy imparted to patients during diagnostic X-ray examinations using the Diamentor exposure-area product meter. Phys Med Biol. 1984;29:1199–208.
17. Heron J. Estimation of effective dose to the patient during medical X-ray examinations from measurements of the dose-area product. Phys Med Biol. 1992;37:2117–26.
18. Theocharopoulos N, Perisinakis K, Damilakis J, Varveris H, Gourtsoyiannis N. Comparison of four methods for assessing patient effective dose from radiological examinations. Med Phys. 2002;29:2070–9.
19. Jaco JW, Miller DL. Measuring and monitoring radiation dose during fluoroscopically guided procedures. Tech Vasc Interv Radiol. 2010;13:188–93.
20. Schueler BA, Vrieze TJ, Bjarnason H, Stanson AW. An investigation of operator exposure in interventional radiology. Radiographics. 2006;26:1533–41.
21. Servomaa A, Karppinen J. The dose-area product and assessment of the occupational dose in interventional radiology. Radiat Prot Dosim. 2001;96:235–6.
22. Williams JR. Scatter dose estimation based on dose-area product and the specification of radiation barriers. Br J Radiol. 1996;69:1032–7.

23. Koenig TR, Mettler FA, Wagner LK. Skin injuries from fluoroscopically guided procedures: part 2, review of 73 cases and recommendations for minimizing dose delivered to patient. AJR Am J Roentgenol. 2001;177:13–20.
24. Wagner LK, McNeese MD, Marx MV, et al. Severe skin reactions from interventional fluoroscopy: case report and review of the literature. Radiology. 1999;213:773–6.
25. Koenig TR, Wolff D, Mettler FA, et al. Skin injuries from fluoroscopically guided procedures: part 1, characteristics of radiation injury. AJR Am J Roentgenol. 2001;177:3–11.
26. Ciraj-Bjelac O, Rehani MM, Sim KH, et al. Risk for radiation induced cataract for staff in interventional cardiology: is there reason for concern? Catheter Cardiovasc Interv. 2010;76:826–34.
27. Rehani MM, Ciraj-Bjelac O, Vano E, Miller DL, Walsh S, Giordano BD, et al. International Commission on Radiological Protection. ICRP publication 117. Radiological protection in fluoroscopically guided procedures performed outside the imaging department. Ann ICRP. 2010;40:1–102.
28. Kovoor P, Ricciardello M, Collins L, Uther JB, Ross DL. Risk to patients from radiation associated with radiofrequency ablation for supraventricular tachycardia. Circulation. 1998;98:1534–40.
29. Lickfett L, Mahesh M, Vasamreddy C, et al. Radiation exposure during catheter ablation of atrial fibrillation. Circulation. 2004;110:3003–10.
30. Rosenthal LS, Mahesh M, Beck TJ, et al. Predictors of fluoroscopy time and estimated radiation exposure during radiofrequency catheter ablation procedures. Am J Cardiol. 1998;82:451–8.
31. Balter S. Stray radiation in the cardiac catheterisation laboratory. Radiat Prot Dosim. 2001;94:183.
32. Vano E. Radiation exposure to cardiologists: how it could be reduced. Heart. 2003;89:1123.
33. Macle L, Weerasooriya R, Jais P, et al. Radiation exposure during radiofrequency catheter ablation for atrial fibrillation. Pacing Clin Electrophysiol. 2003;26:288–91.
34. Voskoboinik A, Kalman ES, Savicky Y, Sparks PB, Morton JB, Lee G, Kistler PM, Kalman JM. Reduction in radiation dose for atrial fibrillation ablation over time: a 12-year single-center experience of 2344 patients. Heart Rhythm. 2017;14:810–6.
35. Sporton SC, Earley MJ, Nathan AW, Schilling RJ. Electroanatomic versus fluoroscopic mapping for catheter ablation procedures: a prospective randomized study. J Cardiovasc Electrophysiol. 2004;15:310–5.
36. Rogers DP, England F, Lozhkin K, Lowe MD, Lambiase PD, Chow AW. Improving safety in the electrophysiology laboratory using a simple radiation dose reduction strategy: a study of 1007 radiofrequency ablation procedures. Heart. 2011;97(5):366–70.
37. Casella M, Dello Russo A, Russo E, Catto V, Pizzamiglio F, Zucchetti M, et al. X-ray exposure in cardiac electrophysiology: a retrospective analysis in 8150 patients over 7 years of activity in a modern, large-volume laboratory. J Am Heart Assoc. 2018;7(11):e008233.
38. Vom J, Williams I. Justification of radiographic examinations: what are the key issues? J Med Radiat Sci. 2017;64(3):212–9.
39. Chambers CE, Fetterly KA, Holzer R, Lin PJ, Blankenship JC, Balter S, et al. Radiation safety program for the cardiac catheterization laboratory. Catheter Cardiovasc Interv. 2011;77(4):546–56.
40. Ernst S, Castellano I. Radiation exposure and safety for the electrophysiologist. Curr Cardiol Rep. 2013;15(10):402.
41. Fetterly KA, Mathew V, Lennon R, Bell MR, Holmes DR Jr, Rihal CS. Radiation dose reduction in the invasive cardiovascular laboratory: implementing a culture and philosophy of radiation safety. JACC Cardiovasc Interv. 2012;5:866–73.
42. Estner HL, Grazia Bongiorni M, Chen J, Dagres N, Hernandez-Madrid A, Blomstrom-Lundqvist C. Use of fluoroscopy in clinical electrophysiology in Europe: results of the European Heart Rhythm Association Survey. Europace. 2015;17:1149–52.
43. Miller DL, Vano E, Bartal G, Balter S, Dixon R, Padovani R, Schueler B, Cardella JF, de Baere T. Occupational radiation protection in interventional radiology: a joint guideline of the Cardiovascular and Interventional Radiology Society of Europe and the Society of Interventional Radiology. Cardiovasc Intervent Radiol. 2010;33:230–9.
44. de Souza E, de Macedo Soares JP. Occupational and technical correlations of interventional radiology. J Vasc Bras. 2008;7:341–50.
45. Vano E, Kleiman NJ, Duran A, Rehani MM, Echeverri D, Cabrera M. Radiation cataract risk in interventional cardiology personnel. Radiat Res. 2010;174:490–5.
46. Ciraj-Bjelac O, Rehani M, Minamoto A, Sim KH, Liew HB, Vano E. Radiation-induced eye lens changes and risk for cataract in interventional cardiology. Cardiology. 2012;123:168–71.
47. Jacob S, Donadille L, Maccia C, Bar O, Boveda S, Laurier D, Bernier MO. Eye lens radiation exposure to interventional cardiologists: a retrospective assessment of cumulative doses. Radiat Prot Dosim. 2013;153:282–93.
48. Principi S, Delgado Soler C, Ginjaume M, Beltran Vilagrasa M, Rovira Escutia JJ, Duch MA. Eye lens dose in interventional cardiology. Radiat Prot Dosim. 2015;165:289–93.
49. Hirshfeld JW Jr, Balter S, Brinker JA, et al. ACCF/AHA/HRS/SCAI clinical competence statement on physician knowledge to optimize patient safety and image quality in fluoroscopically guided invasive cardiovascular procedures. J Am Coll Cardiol. 2004;44:2259–82.
50. Theocharopoulos N, Damilakis J, Perisinakis K, Manios E, Vardas P, Gourtsoyiannis N. Occupational exposure in the electrophysiology laboratory: quantifying and minimizing radiation burden. Br J Radiol. 2006;79:644–51.

51. Beston S, Efstathopolous EP, Katritsis D, Faulkner K, Panayiotakis G. Patient radiation doses during cardiac catheterization procedures. Br J Radiol. 1998;71(846):634–9.
52. Agarwal S, Parashar A, Bajaj NS, et al. Relationship of beam angulation and radiation exposure in the cardiac catheterization laboratory. JACC Cardiovasc Interv. 2014;7:558–66.
53. Wittkampf FH, Wever EF, Vos K, Geleijns J, Schalij MJ, van der Tol J, et al. Reduction of radiation exposure in the cardiac electrophysiology laboratory. Pacing Clin Electrophysiol. 2000;23:1638–44.
54. Davies AG, Cowen AR, Kengyelics SM, Moore J, Pepper C, Cowan C, et al. X-ray dose reduction in fluoroscopically guided electrophysiology procedures. Pacing Clin Electrophysiol. 2006;29:262–71.
55. Walters TE, Kistler PM, Morton JB, Sparks PB, Halloran K, Kalman JM. Impact of collimation on radiation exposure during interventional electrophysiology. Europace. 2012;14(11):1670.
56. De Buck S, La Gerche A, Ector J, et al. Asymmetric collimation can significantly reduce patient radiation dose during pulmonary vein isolation. Europace. 2012;14:437–44.
57. Betsou S, Efstathopoulos EP, Katritsis D, Faulkner K, Panayiotakis G. Patient radiation doses during cardiac catheterization procedures. Br J Radiol. 1998;71:634–9.
58. Efstathopoulos E, Karvouni E, Kottou S, et al. Patient dosimetry during coronary interventions: a comprehensive analysis. Am Heart J. 2004;147:468–75.
59. Olcay A, Guler E, Karaca IO, Omaygenc MO, Kizilirmak F, Olgun E, Yenipinar E, Cakmak HA, Duman D. Comparison of fluoro and cine coronary angiography: balancing acceptable outcomes with a reduction in radiation dose. J Invasive Cardiol. 2015;27:199–202.
60. JCS Joint Working Group. Guidelines for radiation safety in interventional cardiology (JCS 2006). Digest version. Circ J. 2010;74:2760–85.
61. Smith PH. EC directive: 97/43/Euratom. Br J Radiol. 1998;71:108.
62. Heidbuchel H, Wittkampf FH, Vano E, Ernst S, Schilling R, Picano E, Mont L, Jais P, de Bono J, Piorkowski C, Saad E, Femenia F. Practical ways to reduce radiation dose for patients and staff during device implantations and electrophysiological procedures. Europace. 2014;16:946.
63. Wittkampf F, Wever E, Derksen R, Wilde A, Ramanna H, Hauer R, et al. LocaLisa: new technique for real-time 3-dimensional localization of regular intracardiac electrodes. Circulation. 1999;99:1312–7.
64. Gepstein L, Hayam G, Ben-Haim SA. A novel method for nonfluoroscopic catheter-based electroanatomical mapping of the heart. In vitro and in vivo accuracy results. Circulation. 1997;95:1611–22.
65. Kottkamp H, Hugl B, Krauss B, Wetzel U, Fleck A, Schuler G, et al. Electromagnetic versus fluoroscopic mapping of the inferior isthmus for ablation of typical atrial flutter: a prospective randomized study. Circulation. 2000;102:2082–6.
66. Earley MJ, Showkathali R, Alzetani M, Kistler PM, Gupta D, Abrams DJ, et al. Radiofrequency ablation of arrhythmias guided by non-fluoroscopic catheter location: a prospective randomized trial. Eur Heart J. 2006;27:1223–9.
67. Reddy VY, Malchano ZJ, Neuzil P. Early clinical experience with CARTO-merge for integration of 3D-CT imaging with real-time mapping to guide catheter ablation of atrial fibrillation. Heart Rhythm. 2005;2:S160.
68. Ernst S, Ouyang F, Linder C, et al. Initial experience with remote catheter ablation using a novel magnetic navigation system: magnetic remote catheter ablation. Circulation. 2004;109(12):1472–5.
69. Ueda A, Suman-Horduna I, Mantziari L, Gujic M, Marchese P, Ho SY, Babu-Narayan SV, Ernst S. Contemporary outcomes of supraventricular tachycardia ablation in congenital heart disease: a single-center experience in 116 patients. Circ Arrhythm Electrophysiol. 2013;6:606–13.
70. Schwagten BK, Szili-Torok T, Rivero-Ayerza M. Usefulness of remote magnetic navigation for ablation of ventricular arrhythmias originating from outflow regions. Neth Heart J. 2009;17:245–9.
71. Guarguali S, Cazzoli I, Kempny A, Gatzoulis M, Ernst S. A new technique for zero fluoroscopy atrial fibrillation ablation without the use of intracardiac echocardiography. J Am Coll Cardiol Clin Electrophysiol. 2018;4:1647–8.
72. Clifton DK, Bremner WJ. The effect of testicular x-irradiation on spermatogenesis in man. A comparison with the mouse. J Androl. 1983;4(6):387–92.
73. Kumar D, Salian SR, Kalthur G, Uppangala S, Kumari S, Challapalli S, et al. Semen abnormalities, sperm DNA damage and global hypermethylation in health workers occupationally exposed to ionizing radiation. PLoS One. 2013;8(7):e69927.
74. Rowley MJ, Leach DR, Warner GA, Heller CG. Effect of graded doses of ionizing radiation on the human testis. Radiat Res. 1974;59(3):665–78.
75. The 2007 Recommendations of the International Commission on Radiological Protection. ICRP publication 103. Ann ICRP. 2007;37(2–4):1–332.
76. AlTurki A, Proietti R. Remote magnetic navigation versus contact force technology: the two faces of the ablation lesion. Pacing Clin Electrophysiol. 2018;41(5):447–9.

Ablation Energy Sources: Principles and Utility in Ablation Without Fluoroscopy

3

Clarence Khoo

Introduction

While the advent of the electrophysiology study in the 1960s–1970s provided the clinician with the ability to probe the behavior of intracardiac conduction and thereby elucidate the mechanisms of cardiac arrhythmias, therapeutic interventions were limited to open surgical techniques [1]. It was not until the development of catheter-based ablation modalities that percutaneous therapeutic options for arrhythmia management became widely available. Initial catheter ablation techniques utilized the delivery of direct-current (DC) shocks to the area of interest, which were both limited in efficacy and capable of significant harm, including cardiac perforation and unintended collateral injury [1, 2]. Presently, the primary energy sources used in catheter ablation are radiofrequency energy and cryothermal energy. In this chapter, we review how these energy sources have been harnessed in the ablation of cardiac arrhythmias, along with their use in the setting of fluoroscopic reduction.

C. Khoo (✉)
Section of Cardiology, University of Manitoba, Winnipeg, MB, Canada
e-mail: ckhoo@sbgh.mb.ca

Radiofrequency Energy

Radiofrequency (RF) energy has become the most widely used modality for the ablation of cardiac arrhythmias. When alternating current is delivered to an antenna, electromagnetic energy at wavelengths similar to radio waves can be generated. By allowing this energy to conduct through tissue, *radiofrequency energy* can be harnessed for lesion generation. By utilizing high-frequency stimulation, tissue heating and damage can occur in the absence of cardiac myocyte depolarization; as a result, proarrhythmia due to radiofrequency is avoided [3].

RF energy delivery during catheter ablation is transmitted from the metal electrode of the catheter to the grounding pad, traversing intervening tissue in the process. Every component of this electrical circuit contributes to the impedance of the system, and as the current passes through the tissue, energy is lost proportional to the impedance of the component. The energy expended traversing the impedance is dissipated as heat. While RF energy is expended along the entire course of its journey from the electrode-tissue interface to the grounding pad, due to the small surface area of the electrode compared to the grounding pad, the current density is highest at the electrode, with tissue heating thus occurring predominantly at the ablation site. A large proportion of delivered energy, however, is delivered to the surrounding blood pool, as a result of

R. Proietti et al. (eds.), *Cardiac Electrophysiology Without Fluoroscopy*,
https://doi.org/10.1007/978-3-030-16992-3_3

both the lower impedance of blood and a larger surface area of contact between the electrode and blood compared to the electrode and tissue [3].

Resistive heating occurring by impedance-mediated voltage drop results in a fairly shallow area of effect, limited largely to the first 1–1.5 mm of tissue depth [4]. Deeper tissue heating occurs via conduction of heat, which requires time to allow for sufficient penetration of energy to occur. Delayed results of ablation can thereby be seen even after RF application is halted, in a phenomenon referred to as thermal latency. While lesion depth can be increased by raising RF power, formation of coagulum once tissue temperatures approach 100 °C limits further energy delivery. Excessive heating of the tissue can also produce high-pressure steam vapor beneath the surface, which can then produce a "steam pop"—rupturing either into the endocardium, thus forming a crater, or into the pericardial space [2, 5]. Tissue temperatures between 50 and 90 °C delivered over at least 60 s provide ideal conditions for lesion formation [3, 4]. Convective cooling of the electrode tip by blood moving past the electrode tip reduces local tissue temperature and allows for greater energy delivery to the tissue of interest.

Irrigated tip RF catheters (Fig. 3.1) are designed to overcome limitations in lesion size formation by providing even more cooling of the tissue-electrode interface, allowing for greater energy delivery and even greater lesion depth. When compared to nonirrigated ablation catheters, irrigated catheters produce lesions that are larger in volume and greater in depth, and are less likely to cause rises in impedance, coagulum formation, steam pops, or crater formation [6]. Aside from these advantages, irrigated RF catheters also allow for effective ablation in areas with poor blood flow and convective cooling, such as in myocardial trabeculation or within the coronary sinus.

At the cellular level, the effects of RF energy are dependent on the achieved tissue temperatures, with reversible loss of excitability seen in the 45–50 °C range, followed by permanent loss once tissue temperatures exceed ~54 °C [3]. Acutely, the local tissue undergoes protein denaturation with formation of a layer of fibrin. If tissue temperatures approach boiling point, char, thrombus, and coagulum may also be found. Surrounding a core of coagulation necrosis is a penumbra of hemorrhagic tissue and inflammation. With maturation, this forms a well-demarcated lesion comprised of fibrosis and chronic inflammatory infiltrates. However, some variability in maturation can occur at the transition zone of the acute lesion, with either

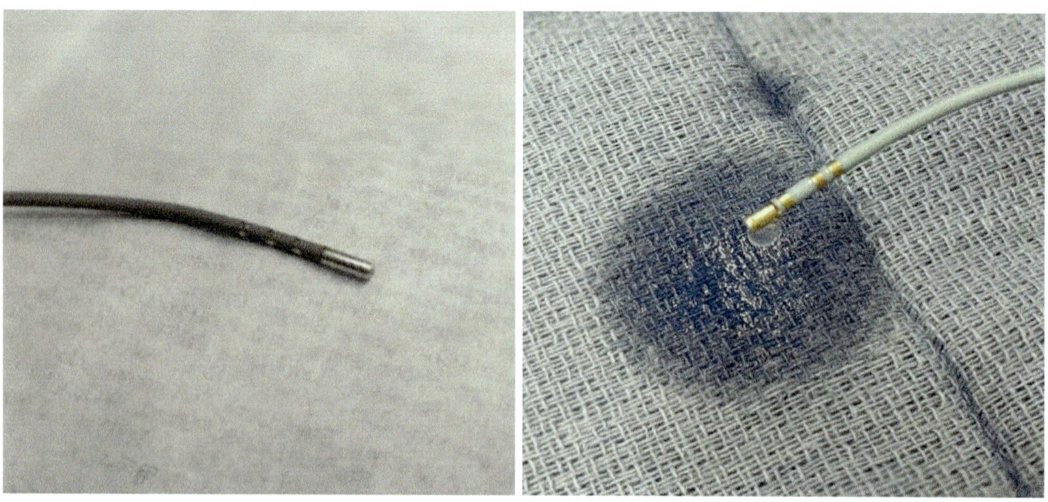

Fig. 3.1 Radiofrequency (RF) ablation catheter tips. Left—nonirrigated 8 mm RF ablation catheter. Right—Irrigated 3.5 mm RF ablation catheter. Note ejection of saline via ports at distal end of catheter tip

progressive inflammatory changes and necrosis resulting in what may be referred to as lesion expansion, or healing of the tissue resulting in recovery of function [3].

Multielectrode RF ablation catheters designed specifically for pulmonary vein isolation (PVI) allow for rapid ablation from multiple electrodes situated on the catheter. These systems utilize phased RF energy, whereby ablation can occur simultaneously in either a unipolar (vs. grounding pad) or a bipolar fashion (vs. another electrode on the catheter). Lesion depth is provided by unipolar ablation, while confluent lesions between electrodes are provided by bipolar ablation [7]. Deflectable, circular multielectrode catheters are designed for ablation at the antrum of pulmonary veins, while multielectrode catheters preformed in specific geometric shapes facilitate mapping and modification of left atrial substrate [8]. A higher rate of silent cerebral ischemic events has been observed with PVI with multielectrode RF catheters [9, 10]. Saline-irrigated systems have been introduced to curtail this increased incidence of silent cerebral microemboli [2].

Cryoablation

Cryoablation utilizes cryothermal energy to produce tissue freezing and subsequent lesion formation. Generation of cryothermal energy is reliant on the Joule-Thomson effect, where precooled liquid refrigerant is delivered to the catheter tip and allowed to rapidly decompress and expand, resulting in a fall in temperature. This allows for catheter tip temperatures to approach −75 °C or lower. With relatively mild tissue cooling (0 to −20 °C), ice crystals form in the extracellular space, resulting in osmotic shift of water out of cells. This produces reversible cellular damage initially, but can become irreversible following prolonged cooling. With deeper cooling (<−40 °C), intracellular crystals form, resulting in direct damage to cardiac myocytes and cell death. Vasoconstriction also occurs with the temperature drop, and may persist for hours after thawing. This leads to ischemia-mediated necrosis [3, 11]. While the freeze is the most obvious means of lesion formation, the thaw and rewarming phase also contributes to tissue injury. Thawing of intracellular ice crystals further damages cellular organelles, while hyperemia leads to edema formation and an inflammatory response [3]. As a result, freezing followed by thawing followed by another freeze (a freeze-thaw-freeze cycle) is usually performed to maximize the results of cryoablation.

Similar to RF ablation, the tissue adjacent to the catheter tip experiences the most effective ablation effect, as intense local cooling results in tissue damage occurring typically within the first 30 s of ablation. More peripheral areas not only receive comparatively less cooling, but the effect is also delayed; thus, these regions are more likely to recover following rewarming. Unlike RF lesions that benefit from high surrounding blood flow and convective cooling to improve power delivery and thus generate larger lesions, cryoablation lesions suffer from convective warming as it may limit tissue freezing. As a result, cryoablation fares better in areas of low blood flow [3]. Compared to lesions produced by RF ablation, cryoablation lesions generally demonstrate less endothelial damage and thrombus formation [3, 11].

Cryoablation provides certain advantages over RF ablation. Formation of ice at the catheter tip during cryothermal energy application results in the catheter becoming firmly attached to the ablation area. This is known as *cryoadherence*, and allows for catheter stability despite cardiorespiratory motion. As noted above, mild cooling allows for reversible disruption of myocyte function, and this can be harnessed via *cryomapping*. By cooling the tissue to −30 °C for no more than 60 s, electrophysiologic testing can be performed to assess the effects of tissue disruption, and full cryoablation subsequently applied if the desired effect is observed. If either an undesired effect or a lack of response is seen, cryomapping can be stopped, with full recovery of tissue function. Coupled with more dense and better demarcated lesions, cryoablation allows for an increased margin of safety when ablating areas in close proximity to vital cardiac structures due to its potentially reversible, more compact lesions [3, 11].

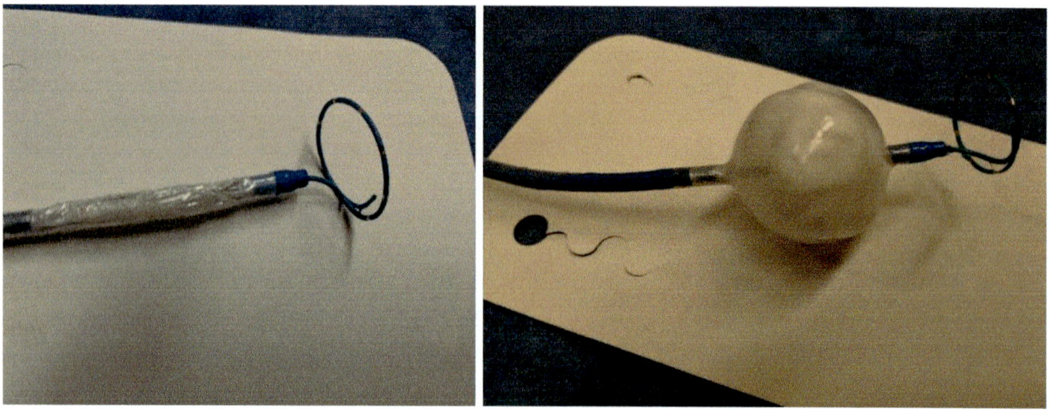

Fig. 3.2 Cryoballoon ablation catheter. Left—cryoballoon deflated with circular multipolar mapping catheter extruding from distal end. Right—cryoballoon inflated with active cryoablation application. Note the formation of ice cap on the side of the balloon closest to the circular mapping catheter

Disadvantages with this energy source, however, are at times an extension of their potential benefits. Procedural duration may be increased due to the time required to provide sufficient cooling of the tissue, as up to 240 s is provided per ablation lesion. Completion of a full freeze-thaw-freeze cycle may then be required, further lengthening procedural time [12]. Recurrences may also be more likely, as permanent lesions require accurate catheter placement such that the region of interest receives sufficient cooling from the catheter tip as opposed to reversible stunning.

The cryoballoon (Fig. 3.2) is a specialized tool that harnesses cryothermal energy for PVI procedures. Once the balloon is inflated within the left atrium, it can be maneuvered into the antrum of the pulmonary vein. An appropriate seal between the balloon and the pulmonary vein is confirmed, followed by introduction of cryorefrigerant into the balloon, resulting in circumferential ablation of the antrum of the vein.

Other Energy Sources

In clinical practice, RF and cryothermal energy sources serve as the primary modalities harnessed for the ablation of cardiac arrhythmias. However, a handful of other energy sources have been investigated for their potential use in this arena. While these alternative energy sources either have failed to establish clinical utility or serve a very specific niche, they nonetheless deserve mention.

Laser Energy

Laser energy delivers photons to the target tissue which are absorbed by molecules in the tissue known as chromophores, exciting them and thereby creating thermal injury [5]. Balloon-based systems using laser energy are available for PVI. Once deployed within the antrum of the pulmonary vein, direct visualization of the endocardial surface is achieved via endoscopic views from within the balloon. Laser energy can then be delivered from the catheter shaft within the balloon to create a circumferential lesion around the vein [2, 13]. The efficacy of this strategy appears comparable to the use of other energy modalities, with a potentially favorable risk of complications [13, 14].

Microwave Energy

Microwave energy, when applied to cardiac tissue, causes kinetic excitement of water molecules, thereby causing intermolecular friction and generation of heat. Unlike RF ablation, there is no reliance on resistive heating, and thus energy can be delivered at a distance from the delivery source without direct contact [3, 5]. Despite initial attempts to bring microwave ablation into routine clinical practice, difficulties in the incorporation of this technology in catheter designs have limited its utility [3].

Ultrasound Energy

High-frequency sound waves can be focused on the tissue of interest to produce tissue injury at a distance from the delivery source. Ultrasound energy produces thermal heating upon attenuation within cardiac tissue. On top of this, microcavitation results from the generation of microbubbles within the tissue that expand and collapse violently, further causing cellular injury. High-intensity focused ultrasound (HIFU) can produce intramural lesions in the absence of tissue contact or injury to intervening structures [15]. Attempts to introduce HIFU into atrial fibrillation ablation have been limited due to the persistence of gaps within linear lesions produced by the technique, as well as a number of complications including unintended collateral injury to the phrenic nerve and esophagus [5, 16]. In addition, complications may result from cavitation in much the same way as steam pops during RF ablation, including cardiac perforation and tamponade [15]. The narrow therapeutic window with HIFU has thus to-date limited its routine clinical use [14, 16].

Considerations with Fluoroscopic Reduction in Selection of Ablation Energy Sources

Fluoroscopy has been the mainstay for visualization of catheter position during ablation procedures. Attempts at fluoroscopic reduction have employed a number of different strategies, some of which apply more readily to some ablation energy sources than others. We review below some of these strategies and their utility with different energy sources.

Electroanatomical Mapping

The advent of electroanatomical mapping (EAM) has allowed for fluoroscopic reduction by allowing for the accurate determination and portrayal of catheter position in three-dimensional space. By superimposing functional electrical data onto a 3D representation of the heart, both anatomy and electrophysiology can be displayed simultaneously [2]. In order to register on current EAM systems, catheters require either an active electrode (in impedance-based systems) or proprietary location sensors (in electromagnetic sensor-based systems); however, some combination of these two localization systems are currently employed by leading EAM systems. As a result, in the absence of any limitations posed by technical considerations, zero-fluoroscopy ablation can be achieved with comparable efficacy using either RF or cryothermal energy using available EAM systems [17].

Limitations of EAM systems may still exist with certain ablation energy types, however, and may influence the choice of ablation energy if zero-fluoroscopy ablation is desired. Unlike RF ablation, EAM support for cryothermal ablation is somewhat less universal. Certain EAM setups that require proprietary location sensors on its ablation catheter may need to be "tricked" into recognizing cryoablation catheters [17, 18]. On the other hand, the absence of electrodes or proprietary sensors on the inflatable balloon on certain PVI ablation systems may limit the exclusive use of EAM systems in visualizing adequate balloon positioning, unless intracardiac echocardiography is simultaneously used (see below).

Intracardiac Echocardiography

Intracardiac echocardiography (ICE), when integrated with EAM systems, can facilitate generation of anatomical geometries by translating echocardiographic images into anatomical shells. Moreover, it can be used to confirm catheter tip position when anatomically complex structures that are poorly defined by routine EAM are encountered (e.g., papillary muscles).

As noted earlier, ICE can also be used to visualize catheter components not usually visible with EAM, most notably deployment of the cryoballoon in the pulmonary vein antrum during PVI. Once positioned, the adequacy of balloon seal can also be determined without fluoroscopy by using color flow Doppler imaging to look for leaks. In addition, as phrenic nerve palsy is a known complication of cryoballoon PVI, ICE can also be employed to directly visualize diaphragmatic excursion in place of fluoroscopy [19]. By combining ICE with EAM, zero-fluoroscopy cryoballoon PVI procedures may thus be safely performed [18].

Contact Force

Contact force (CF) determination is yet another technologic innovation that can aid in fluoroscopic reduction. Adequate tissue-electrode contact is highly sought after in order to ensure sufficient ablation energy delivery to the tissue of interest to produce desired lesion depth and durability. While tactile feedback and surrogate markers including local electrogram attenuation and impedance drops provide some indication of this, fluoroscopy is conventionally relied upon to confirm motion of the catheter tip as it is held in contact with the endocardium [20].

By detecting either force transduced by spring-based sensors or changes in interference patterns of reflected light by deformation of the catheter tip, CF can be measured. Studies have confirmed that increased CF correlates with improved tissue contact and results in higher tissue temperatures during ablation, improved catheter stability, and larger lesion size [20]. When used for PVI procedures, this has been shown to translate to lower recurrence rates and shorter procedural times, with a trend towards reduced complications [21].

Fluoroscopy can thereby be avoided when CF is used in conjunction with EAM, as this can be employed to not only determine tissue-electrode contact, but also confirm accuracy of created geometry and warn against potential cardiac perforation [2]. A meta-analysis comparing the use of CF ablation catheters with conventional ablation catheters in PVI showed a significant reduction in fluoroscopic time by ~20% [21]. Currently, contact force technology is available only for radiofrequency ablation catheters.

Conclusions

The advent of numerous safe and efficacious ablation energy sources that may be delivered via a steerable catheter has provided the clinician the tools to effect electrophysiologic change and thereby treat arrhythmias. Cardiac electrophysiologists who wield these tools need to be aware of their unique therapeutic attributes, including both their comparative strengths and limitations. With the promulgation of low- and zero-fluoroscopic ablation procedures, an appreciation must also be developed of how facilely each energy source may be incorporated into these procedures. By recognizing the limitations in the use of a given energy source in fluoroscopic reduction, strategies may be employed to circumvent any barriers or an alternative energy source may be selected. Furthermore, as more novel energy sources are harnessed, fluoroscopic reduction will need to be presciently incorporated.

References

1. Joseph JP, Rajappan K. Radiofrequency ablation of cardiac arrhythmias: past, present and future. QJM. 2012;105:303–14.
2. Andrade JG, Rivard L, Macle L. The past, the present, and the future of cardiac arrhythmia ablation. Can J Cardiol. 2014;30:S431–41.
3. Issa Z. Ablation energy sources. In: Issa ZF, Miller JM, Zipes DP, editors. Clinical arrhythmology and electrophysiology: a companion to Braunwald's heart disease. 1st ed. Philadelphia, PA: Saunders Elsevier; 2009.
4. Wittkampf FH, Nakagawa H. RF catheter ablation: lessons on lesions. Pacing Clin Electrophysiol. 2006;29:1285–97.
5. Cummings JE, Pacifico A, Drago JL, Kilicaslan F, Natale A. Alternative energy sources for the ablation of arrhythmias. Pacing Clin Electrophysiol. 2005;28:434–43.
6. Dorwarth U, Fiek M, Remp T, et al. Radiofrequency catheter ablation: different cooled and noncooled electrode systems induce specific lesion geometries and adverse effects profiles. Pacing Clin Electrophysiol. 2003;26:1438–45.

7. Kiss A, Sandorfi G, Nagy-Balo E, Martirosyan M, Csanadi Z. Phased RF ablation: results and concerns. J Atr Fibrillation. 2015;8:1240.
8. Andrade JG, Dubuc M, Rivard L, et al. Efficacy and safety of atrial fibrillation ablation with phased radiofrequency energy and multielectrode catheters. Heart Rhythm. 2012;9:289–96.
9. Herrera Siklody C, Deneke T, Hocini M, et al. Incidence of asymptomatic intracranial embolic events after pulmonary vein isolation: comparison of different atrial fibrillation ablation technologies in a multicenter study. J Am Coll Cardiol. 2011;58:681–8.
10. Gaita F, Leclercq JF, Schumacher B, et al. Incidence of silent cerebral thromboembolic lesions after atrial fibrillation ablation may change according to technology used: comparison of irrigated radiofrequency, multipolar nonirrigated catheter and cryoballoon. J Cardiovasc Electrophysiol. 2011;22:961–8.
11. Skanes AC, Klein G, Krahn A, Yee R. Cryoablation: potentials and pitfalls. J Cardiovasc Electrophysiol. 2004;15:S28–34.
12. Manusama R, Timmermans C, Limon F, Philippens S, Crijns HJ, Rodriguez LM. Catheter-based cryoablation permanently cures patients with common atrial flutter. Circulation. 2004;109:1636–9.
13. Schade A, Krug J, Szollosi AG, El Tarahony M, Deneke T. Pulmonary vein isolation with a novel endoscopic ablation system using laser energy. Expert Rev Cardiovasc Ther. 2012;10:995–1000.
14. Filgueiras-Rama D, Merino JL. The future of pulmonary vein isolation—single-shot devices, remote navigation or improving conventional radiofrequency delivery by contact monitoring and lesion characterisation? Arrhythm Electrophysiol Rev. 2013;2:59–64.
15. Laughner JI, Sulkin MS, Wu Z, Deng CX, Efimov IR. Three potential mechanisms for failure of high intensity focused ultrasound ablation in cardiac tissue. Circ Arrhythm Electrophysiol. 2012;5:409–16.
16. Neven K, Schmidt B, Metzner A, et al. Fatal end of a safety algorithm for pulmonary vein isolation with use of high-intensity focused ultrasound. Circ Arrhythm Electrophysiol. 2010;3:260–5.
17. Scaglione M, Ebrille E, Caponi D, et al. Zero-fluoroscopy ablation of accessory pathways in children and adolescents: CARTO3 electroanatomic mapping combined with RF and cryoenergy. Pacing Clin Electrophysiol. 2015;38:675–81.
18. Patel N. Experience with arctic front advance cryoablation system for paroxysmal atrial fibrillation in an established fluoroless EP lab. EP Lab Digest. 2016;16(3).
19. Su W, Kowal R, Kowalski M, et al. Best practice guide for cryoballoon ablation in atrial fibrillation: the compilation experience of more than 3000 procedures. Heart Rhythm. 2015;12:1658–66.
20. Shah DC, Namdar M. Real-time contact force measurement: a key parameter for controlling lesion creation with radiofrequency energy. Circ Arrhythm Electrophysiol. 2015;8:713–21.
21. Shurrab M, Di Biase L, Briceno DF, et al. Impact of contact force technology on atrial fibrillation ablation: a meta-analysis. J Am Heart Assoc. 2015;4:e002476.

3D Mapping and Reduction in Radiation Exposure

4

Isabelle Nault

Principles of 3D Mapping Systems

Mapping systems rely on two technologies to achieve localization of catheters: electromagnetic mapping and current or impedance-based mapping.

Electromagnetic location technology uses a magnetic field emitter positioned external to the patient and sensor patches on the patient. A metal coil, embedded within the catheter tip, generates a current when exposed to the magnetic field, which size is dependant upon the strength of the magnetic field and the orientation of the coil within the field. The information is then integrated by the system and graphically displayed on the screen. The catheter is located and visualized by the system with a precision of ≤ 1 mm. An electromagnetic system is independent from physiologic changes that may occur during the procedure. The use of navigation-enabled specific catheters is necessary.

Advantages of the electromagnetic mapping technology are enhanced precision in localization, spatial resolution, and accuracy with the anatomic model. Disadvantages are the need to use dedicated sensor-enabled catheters only, loss of precision if the patient moves, and extra time needed to construct the virtual anatomic shell.

I. Nault (✉)
IUCPQ, Québec, QC, Canada
e-mail: isabelle.nault@criucpq.ulaval.ca

Current or impedance-based technology uses a signal of low current and high frequency through the catheters or the patches on the patient's body to locate each catheter within the body of the patient. The accuracy of this system is dependant upon impedance changes that may occur physiologically during the procedure (i.e., development of tissue edema or significant fluid shifts). This is an open architecture that allows any catheter to be visualized.

Advantages of the impedance-based technology are its rapidity in constructing a geometry, the flexibility to use any catheter, and stability even with movement of the patient. Disadvantages include less accuracy in spatial localization and loss of precision if the reference catheter moves.

Initially, mapping systems used either electromagnetic location or impedance-based location. Carto™ was based on magnetic technology and EnSite™ was based on impedance. There were therefore significant differences between the two mainly used systems [1].

Nowadays, all major 3D mapping systems integrate both technologies, Rhythmia™ (Boston Scientific) (Fig. 4.1), Carto3™ (Biosense Webster) (Fig. 4.2), and EnSite Precision™ (Abbott) (Fig. 4.3), and all use a combination of impedance and electromagnetic mapping. All systems therefore require a system-dedicated sensor-enabled catheter, but other catheters can also be used in combination that do not necessarily have sensors. The map is built either with a multipolar

R. Proietti et al. (eds.), *Cardiac Electrophysiology Without Fluoroscopy*,
https://doi.org/10.1007/978-3-030-16992-3_4

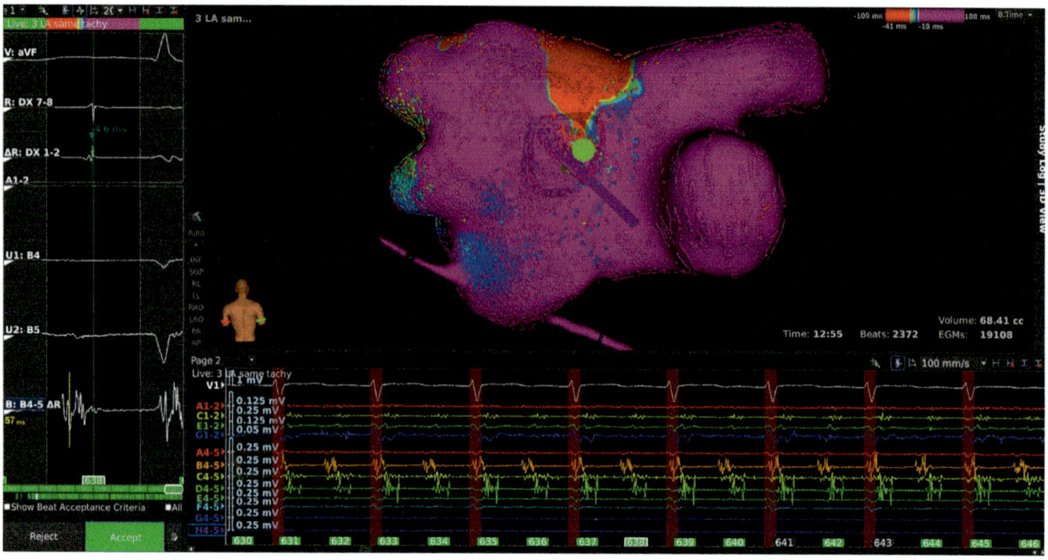

Fig. 4.1 Activation map using Rhythmia™ system (Boston Scientific) along with Orion™ multipolar high-density mapping catheter

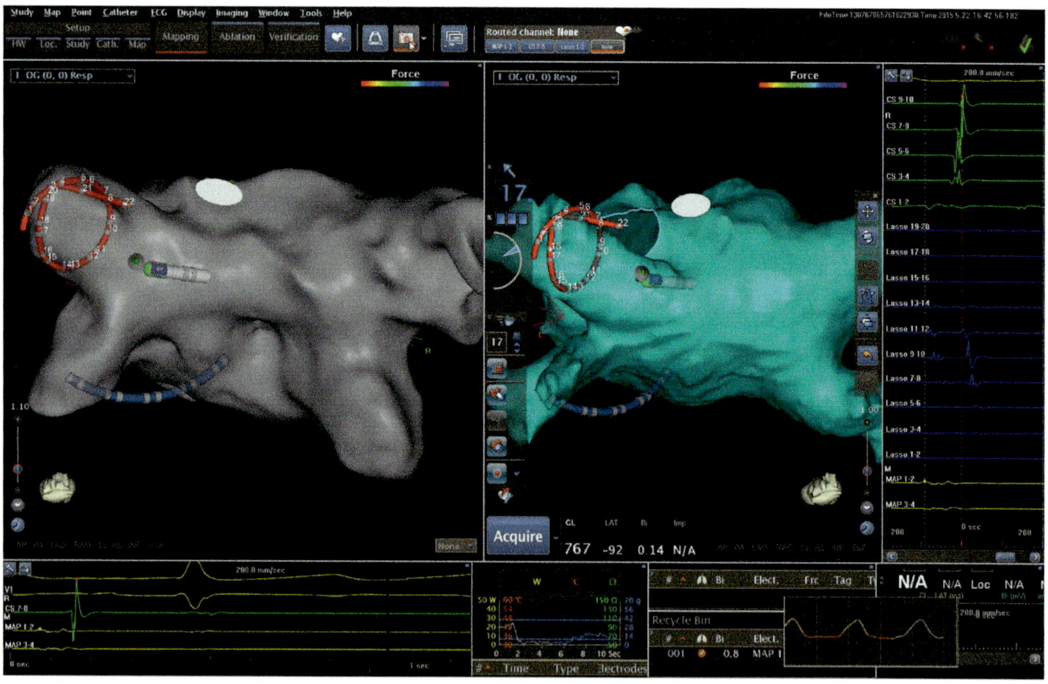

Fig. 4.2 Integration of magnetic resonance imaging (MRI) scan of the left atrium to the anatomic map acquired with Carto3™ (Biosense Webster)

mapping catheter or with the ablation catheter. Anatomic landmarks such as the inferior vena cava, the superior vena cava, and the His bundle are identified and tagged. Depending on the comfort of the operator with the 3D mapping system and his knowledge of the anatomy, the use of fluoroscopy while establishing the landmarks is optional. Once access to the chamber of interest in which arrhythmia will be mapped and/or ablated is secured, a more detailed map of this chamber is

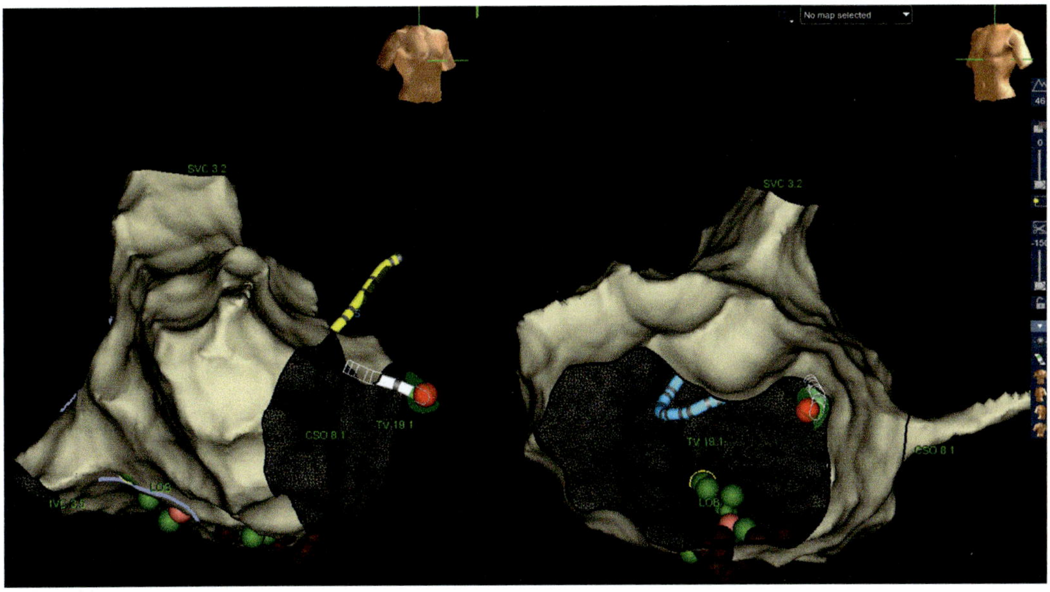

Fig. 4.3 Mapping of the right atrium and ablation of cavo-tricuspid isthmus in a patient with typical atrial flutter using a zero fluoroscopy approach with EnSite Precision™ (Abott)

constructed. Points are taken and integrated by the system inside the heart chamber being mapped and are graphically shown on the screen to form a virtual shell of the cavity. Clues such as electrogram timing and amplitude, electrogram morphology, and impedance are used to define the borders of the chamber and the different anatomical structures. When available, contact force information helps to define tissue contact. The anatomy constructed is then used to guide navigation within the virtual shell. The use of 3D mapping has proven to reduce the use of fluoroscopy [2, 3] and even eliminate the need for fluoroscopy in some cases by some operators especially dedicated to reduce radiation exposure [4–8]. Such procedures have been performed safely with good outcomes [9–11]. For standard noncomplex procedures (supraventricular tachycardia, atrial tachycardia), the complication rates using a nonfluoroscopy approach were 0.85% [11] and 0.8% [9]. The complication rate during atrial fibrillation ablation using a near-zero fluoroscopy approach was 2% in a cohort of 1000 patients, which is comparable to or even lower than the complication rate observed using a conventional approach [10, 12].

Long-term success of ablation of different tachyarrhythmias was 90.8% in a cohort with zero-fluoroscopy procedures [9].

Anatomic Reconstruction

Anatomic reconstruction is most useful for procedures in which the ablation is guided by anatomy such as pulmonary vein isolation for atrial fibrillation, slow pathway ablation for AVNRT (atrioventricular nodal reciprocating tachycardia), or cavotricuspid isthmus ablation for typical atrial flutter (Fig. 4.4).

Activation Mapping

In patients with active ongoing arrhythmia, activation mapping helps to identify the mechanism of arrhythmia (reentry versus focal) and the site of origin of a focus or the critical isthmus in case of a reentrant mechanism. The activation map can be constructed during or after the acquisition of the anatomy by integrating the timing of electrogram at each point compared to a fix reference point. Color is attributed to each point according to its timing compared to the fix reference, colors blue and purple meaning far, late or “cold” related to the reference, getting closer or “heating up” to shades of yellow, and orange and then red to the earliest activation points (white in some systems). Activation mapping is performed

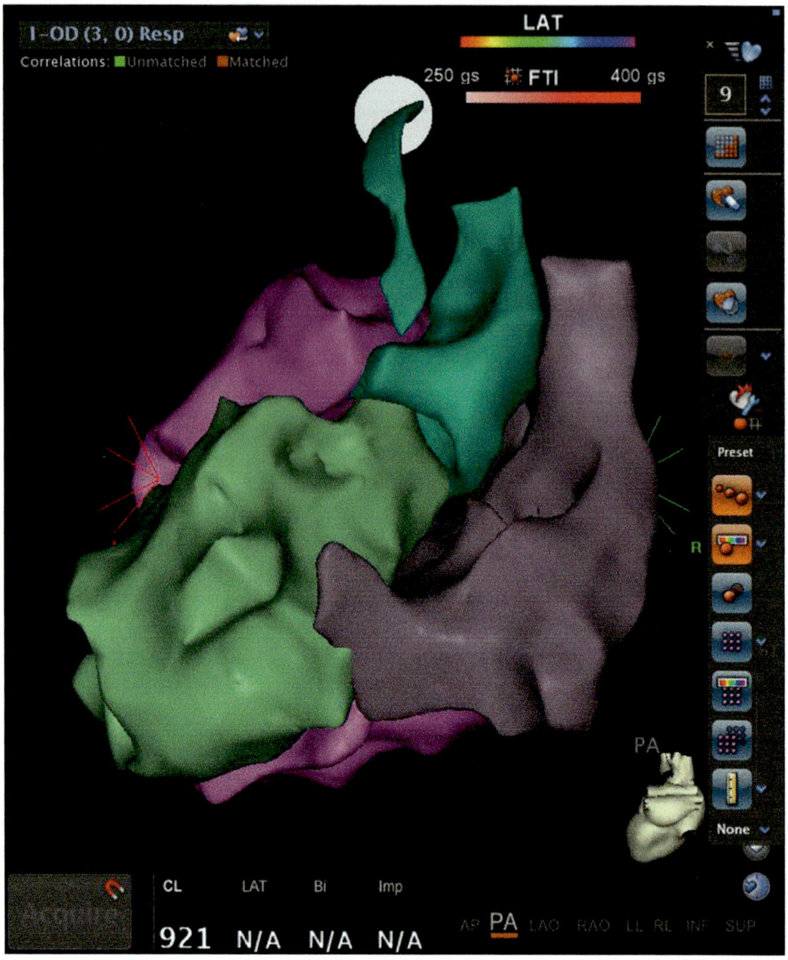

Fig. 4.4 Anatomic reconstruction of the right atrium, right ventricle, aorta, and left ventricle using Carto 3™ without using fluoroscopy

for atrial tachycardia, atrial flutter, premature atrial contractions, stable ventricular tachycardia, and premature ventricular contraction ablation (Fig. 4.5). It can also be used for accessory pathway-mediated reentrant arrhythmias.

Voltage Mapping

To construct a voltage map, signal amplitude is collected at each point. In the ventricle, scar border zone is defined by endocardial amplitude signal 0.5–1.5 mV [13]. Color coding according to the voltage of the signal visually defines endomyocardial scar. This type of map is used in patients with scar-related ventricular tachycardia and atrial arrhythmias and in some isolated cases to guide endomyocardial biopsy [14] or to help with diagnostic such as arrhythmogenic right ventricular tachycardia [15]. In both voltage and activation maps, the density of points collected is important to have adequate resolution and to locate with precision focus or isthmus of the tachycardia.

Ripple Mapping

Ripple mapping is voltage and activation mapping integrated and displayed as moving bars instead of colors [16–18]. The bars are perpendicular to the surface and dynamically protrude out according to the activation time of the local potential. Their length is proportional to the voltage amplitude. The final graphical display is a propagation map.

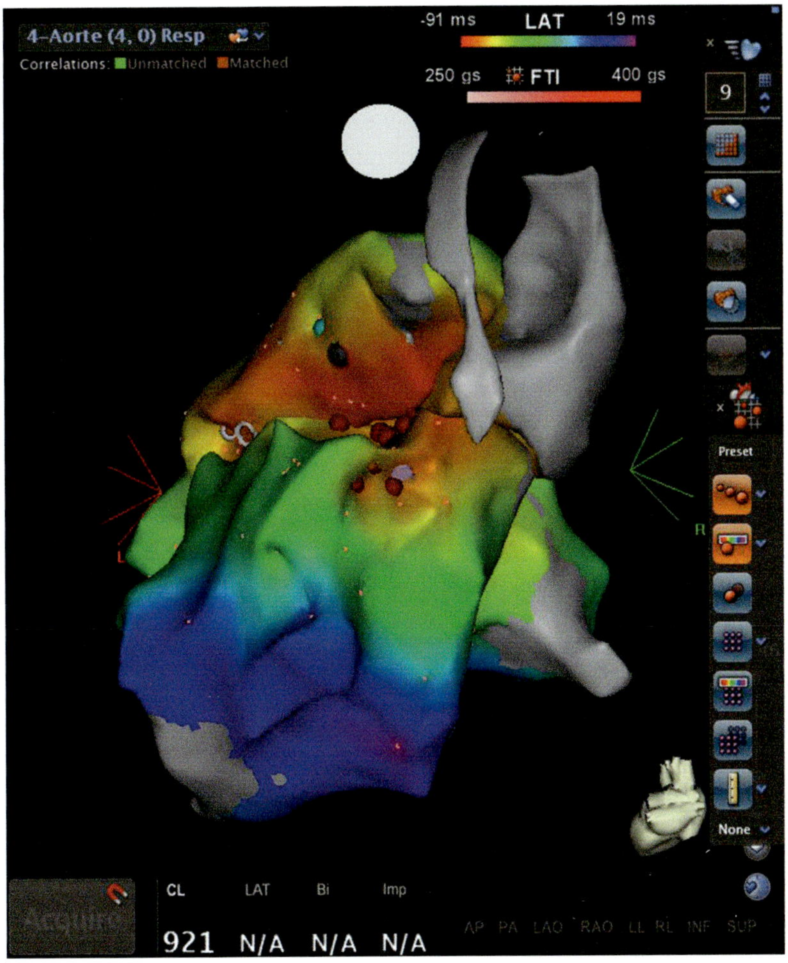

Fig. 4.5 Activation mapping of a PVC arising from the interventricular septum, with activation earliest in the left ventricle and successful elimination after ablation in the right and left ventricle on each side of the septum. The map was created with Carto3™ using no fluoroscopy

All these maps can be performed with minimal or no fluoroscopy since navigation and point collection are performed within the virtual anatomy with excellent reliability. It is even more valuable to reduce radiation in cases of multiple arrhythmias where several maps need to be constructed.

Image Integration

Carto3™ (Biosense Webster) and EnSite Precision™ (Abbott) systems can integrate computed tomography (CT), magnetic resonance imaging (MRI), or rotational angiography images and merge them with the anatomy constructed by the 3D mapping system. It has the advantage to identify unusual anatomies, such as additional pulmonary veins, or anatomical variants such as a common venous pulmonary trunk. It also helps in defining borders such as pulmonary vein antrum. However, care needs to be taken to acquire imaging close to the time of the procedure and during similar rhythm as volume may vary with time and with underlying rhythm. Image integration contributes to reduce or eliminate fluoroscopy during the ablation procedure; however to reduce radiation exposure to the patient and not only to the staff, imaging modalities not using ionizing radiation, such as MRI, should be preferred.

Intracardiac Ultrasound

Intracardiac ultrasound can be used in order to reduce fluoroscopy [19]. Please refer to other chapters for details. However intracardiac ultrasound can also be integrated with the Carto™ system using the CartoSound™ module [20]. Images obtained by the intracardiac ultrasound are used to draw the borders or the walls of the mapped cavity. It is especially useful to draw inner structures such as papillary muscles in the left ventricle or the ridge between the left pulmonary veins and the left atrial appendage in the left atrium and to assess catheter location and catheter stability on such structures. Moreover, points obtained by the mapping catheter are integrated in the ultrasound anatomic images and the location of the catheter is visualized on the ultrasound environment.

Additional Features

Different additional features are available to help ablation procedures. Pacemapping is facilitated by matching a template of the spontaneous or induced arrhythmia and the paced morphology at different points. The Paso™ (Carto, Biosense Webster) or Automap™ (Abbott) modules compare the pacemapped QRS morphology to that of the ventricular tachycardia or premature ventricular beat and calculates a matching score. Both QRS are superimposed so visual assessment of each lead concordance is facilitated. The use of such automated matching improves pacemapping precision compared to visual assessment only [21].

Automated fractionation mapping and complex and fractionated atrial electrogram (CFAE) mapping are also provided by 3D mapping system [22]. The usefulness of such mapping and ablation in patients with atrial fibrillation is still a controversial area [23].

During ablation, all mapping systems tag ablation points. Tags can be manually appointed or can be automatically appointed according to preset criteria such as contact force, energy, and time. Ablation tags are useful to assess lesion contiguity and to recall exact point location.

Differences Between Available Systems

Although the different available 3D mapping and navigation systems share similar basic technology, the different platforms all have distinctive characteristics. The Rhythmia™ system with its dedicated Orion™ multipolar (64 poles) catheter can create ultrahigh-density maps with superior resolution (Fig. 4.1). Carto3™ and EnSite Precision™ each has proprietary modules and functions; for example the CartoSound™ module integrating intracardiac ultrasound with 3D mapping as discussed above is distinctive to Carto™. Both Carto3™ and EnSite Precision™ have contact force-sensing catheter display, available for the ablation catheter.

Advantages of 3D Mapping-Only Ablation (Zero Fluoroscopy Approach)

The use of 3D mapping systems allow to work in a minimal or even no radiation environment. Other advantages include: the need for less localisation catheters since anatomical landmarks can be marked within the anatomic reconstruction, easier and more precise recall of areas of interest whether it is during activation mapping or voltage mapping, visual integration of all collected information. It also saves time if more than one arrythmia needs to be targeted and reduce the risk of having to reschedule a procedure because of unexpected complexity.

Limitations of Current Technology

With most 3D systems only the tip of the catheter is depicted within the map. For almost all instances, it is sufficient, but if the catheter loops inside the vascular system, there is little clue (unexpected extra length of the catheter already inside the vessel, abnormal transmission of force or torque to the catheter) to detect it with the 3D mapping system; future design will help to allow better visualization of a longer distal part of the catheters.

The left atrium is accessed via transseptal using a long sheath and transseptal needle. Future design allowing to visualize the introducer on the mapping system would simplify left atrial access and minimize the need for radiation.

Remote Navigation

Remote magnetic navigation Stereotaxis™ is integrated with 3D mapping (Carto™). Remote robotic navigation Hansen™ is also used in conjunction with 3D mapping. The mapping principles are the same; only catheter steering is done remotely. Radiation to the operator can be significantly reduced since he/she can work remotely outside the field of radiation, and the use of 3D mapping reduces radiation exposure to the patient.

Conclusion

3D mapping is now part of many EP procedures. All systems share fundamental technology, magnetic and impedance; however each system has unique characteristics that differentiate one from another. The optimized use of 3D mapping significantly reduced radiation exposure during EP procedures [24]. As the EP community is getting more and more conscious of deleterious effect of radiation exposure, 3D mapping for navigation, anatomic reconstruction, voltage, and anatomic mapping is increasingly performed by several operators and centers across the world.

References

1. Khaykin Y, Oosthuizen R, Zarnett L, Wulffhart ZA, Whaley B, Hill C, et al. CARTO-guided vs. NavX-guided pulmonary vein antrum isolation and pulmonary vein antrum isolation performed without 3-D mapping: effect of the 3-D mapping system on procedure duration and fluoroscopy time. J Interv Card Electrophysiol. 2011;30(3):233–40.
2. Christoph M, Wunderlich C, Moebius S, Forkmann M, Sitzy J, Salmas J, et al. Fluoroscopy integrated 3D mapping significantly reduces radiation exposure during ablation for a wide spectrum of cardiac arrhythmias. Europace. 2015;17(6):928–37.
3. Estner HL, Deisenhofer I, Luik A, Ndrepepa G, von Bary C, Zrenner B, et al. Electrical isolation of pulmonary veins in patients with atrial fibrillation: reduction of fluoroscopy exposure and procedure duration by the use of a non-fluoroscopic navigation system (NavX). Europace. 2006;8(8):583–7.
4. Yang L, Sun G, Chen X, Chen G, Yang S, Guo P, et al. Meta-analysis of zero or near-zero fluoroscopy use during ablation of cardiac arrhythmias. Am J Cardiol. 2016;118(10):1511–8.
5. Calkins H, Hindricks G, Cappato R, Kim YH, Saad EB, Aguinaga L, et al. 2017 HRS/EHRA/ECAS/APHRS/SOLAECE expert consensus statement on catheter and surgical ablation of atrial fibrillation. Heart Rhythm. 2017;14(10):e275–444.
6. Prolic Kalinsek T, Jan M, Rupar K, Razen L, Antolic B, Zizek D. Zero-fluoroscopy catheter ablation of concealed left accessory pathway in a pregnant woman. Europace. 2017;19(8):1384.
7. Karbarz D, Stec PJ, Deutsch K, Sledz J, Stec S. Zero-fluoroscopy catheter ablation of symptomatic preexcitation from non-coronary cusp during pregnancy. Kardiol Pol. 2017;75(12):1351.
8. Huang X, Chen Y, Huang Z, He L, Liu S, Deng X, et al. Catheter radiofrequency ablation for arrhythmias under the guidance of the Carto 3 three-dimensional mapping system in an operating room without digital subtraction angiography. Medicine (Baltimore). 2018;97(25):e11044.
9. Giaccardi M, Mascia G, Paoletti Perini A, Giomi A, Cartei S, Milli M. Long-term outcomes after "Zero X-ray" arrhythmia ablation. J Interv Card Electrophysiol. 2019;54:43–8.
10. Sommer P, Bertagnolli L, Kircher S, Arya A, Bollmann A, Richter S, et al. Safety profile of near-zero fluoroscopy atrial fibrillation ablation with non-fluoroscopic catheter visualization: experience from 1000 consecutive procedures. Europace. 2018;20:1952–8.
11. Alvarez M, Bertomeu-Gonzalez V, Arcocha MF, Morina P, Tercedor L, Ferrero de Loma A, et al. Nonfluoroscopic catheter ablation. Results from a prospective multicenter registry. Rev Esp Cardiol (Engl Ed). 2017;70(9):699–705.
12. Cappato R, Calkins H, Chen SA, Davies W, Iesaka Y, Kalman J, et al. Updated worldwide survey on the methods, efficacy, and safety of catheter ablation for human atrial fibrillation. Circ Arrhythm Electrophysiol. 2010;3(1):32–8.
13. Hsia HH, Lin D, Sauer WH, Callans DJ, Marchlinski FE. Anatomic characterization of endocardial substrate for hemodynamically stable reentrant ventricular tachycardia: identification of endocardial conducting channels. Heart Rhythm. 2006;3(5):503–12.
14. D'Amario D, Leone AM, Narducci ML, Smaldone C, Lecis D, Inzani F, et al. Human cardiac progenitor cells with regenerative potential can be isolated and characterized from 3D-electro anatomic guided endomyocardial biopsies. Int J Cardiol. 2017;241:330–43.
15. Corrado D, Basso C, Leoni L, Tokajuk B, Bauce B, Frigo G, et al. Three-dimensional electroanatomic voltage mapping increases accuracy of diagnosing arrhythmogenic right ventricular cardiomyopathy/dysplasia. Circulation. 2005;111(23):3042–50.
16. Linton NW, Koa-Wing M, Francis DP, Kojodjojo P, Lim PB, Salukhe TV, et al. Cardiac ripple mapping: a novel three-dimensional visualization method for use with electroanatomic mapping of cardiac arrhythmias. Heart Rhythm. 2009;6(12):1754–62.
17. Luther V, Cortez-Dias N, Carpinteiro L, de Sousa J, Balasubramaniam R, Agarwal S, et al. Ripple mapping: Initial multicenter experience of an intui-

tive approach to overcoming the limitations of 3D activation mapping. J Cardiovasc Electrophysiol. 2017;28(11):1285–94.
18. Luther V, Linton NW, Koa-Wing M, Lim PB, Jamil-Copley S, Qureshi N, et al. A prospective study of ripple mapping in atrial tachycardias: a novel approach to interpreting activation in low-voltage areas. Circ Arrhythm Electrophysiol. 2016;9(1):e003582.
19. Enriquez A, Saenz LC, Rosso R, Silvestry FE, Callans D, Marchlinski FE, et al. Use of intracardiac echocardiography in interventional cardiology: working with the anatomy rather than fighting it. Circulation. 2018;137(21):2278–94.
20. Khaykin Y, Skanes A, Wulffhart ZA, Gula L, Whaley B, Oosthuizen R, et al. Intracardiac ECHO integration with three dimensional mapping: role in AF ablation. J Atr Fibrillation. 2008;1(2):32.
21. Moak JP, Sumihara K, Swink J, Hanumanthaiah S, Berul CI. Ablation of the vanishing PVC, facilitated by quantitative morphology-matching software. Pacing Clin Electrophysiol. 2017;40(11):1227–33.
22. Wu J, Estner H, Luik A, Ucer E, Reents T, Pflaumer A, et al. Automatic 3D mapping of complex fractionated atrial electrograms (CFAE) in patients with paroxysmal and persistent atrial fibrillation. J Cardiovasc Electrophysiol. 2008;19(9):897–903.
23. Jadidi AS, Arentz T. A decade of CFAE mapping: still seeking more specific tools to identify sources and substrate of persistent atrial fibrillation. Arrhythm Electrophysiol Rev. 2015;4(2):108.
24. Lehrmann H, Jadidi AS, Minners J, Keyl C, Hochholzer W, Carrapatoso F, et al. Important reduction of the radiation dose for pulmonary vein isolation using a multimodal approach. Europace. 2018;20(2):279–87.

Catheter Placement and Model Reconstruction

5

Yan Wang

Abbreviations

AP Anterior posterior
LAO Left anterior oblique
PA Posterior anterior
PVA Pulmonary vein antrum
RAO Right anterior oblique
RVOT Right ventricular outflow tract
SVT Supraventricular tachycardia

Introduction

Electrophysiological study and catheter ablation procedures are traditionally performed using fluoroscopic guidance, which can be associated with considerable radiation exposure that is potentially harmful to the patients and the medical staffs. Protective lead apparel can only partially reduce harmful radiation to medical staffs and the patients are still left at risk of radiation exposure. It has been estimated that 1 h of radiation exposure is associated with a rise of 0.1% in the lifetime risk of developing a fatal malignancy [1].

Y. Wang (✉)
Cardiovascular Division, Tongji Hospital, Tongji Medical College, Huazhong University of Science and Technology, Wuhan, China
e-mail: newswangyan@tjh.tjmu.edu.cn

R. Proietti et al. (eds.), *Cardiac Electrophysiology Without Fluoroscopy*,
https://doi.org/10.1007/978-3-030-16992-3_5

In the past decade, more and more reports suggest that electrophysiological study and catheter ablation procedures can be performed without fluoroscopic guidance just using three-dimensional navigation system [2–11]. Here we introduce the tips and points about catheter placement and model reconstruction without fluoroscopic guidance.

Catheter Placement

Navigation Systems

Both three-dimensional navigation systems including electric-field mapping system (e.g., EnSite NavX™) and electric-magnetic mapping system (e.g., Carto™) can be used for zero-fluoroscopic electrophysiological study and ablation.

Relevant Preparation

1. Apparatus for pressure measurement
   (a) Extension tube with stopcock: A tube is routinely used for pump injection; the tube comprises a male Luer slip connector at one end and a female Luer slip connector at another end; the male connector is used for collecting a needle and the female collector is for collecting a stopcock or a syringe (Figs. 5.1 and 5.2).

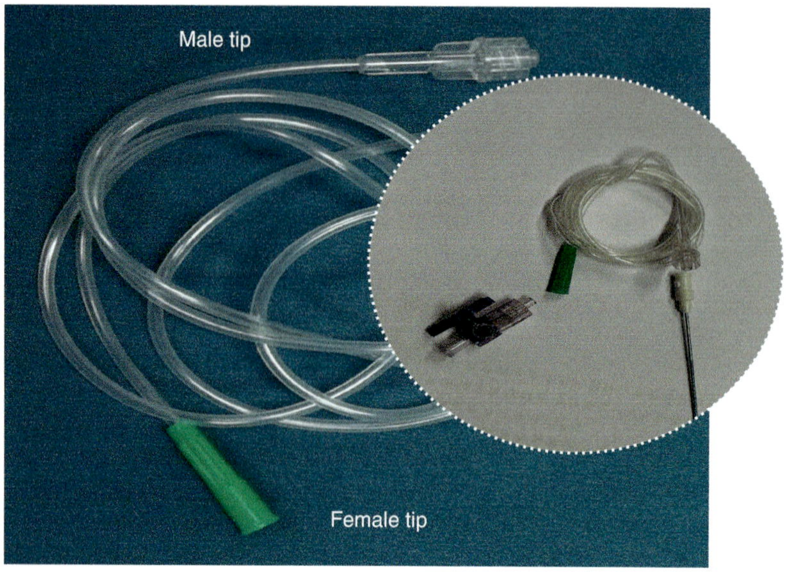

Fig. 5.1 An extension tube is utilized for pressure measurement or simplified blood return test. The male connector is used for collecting a needle; the female collector is used for collecting a stopcock or a syringe

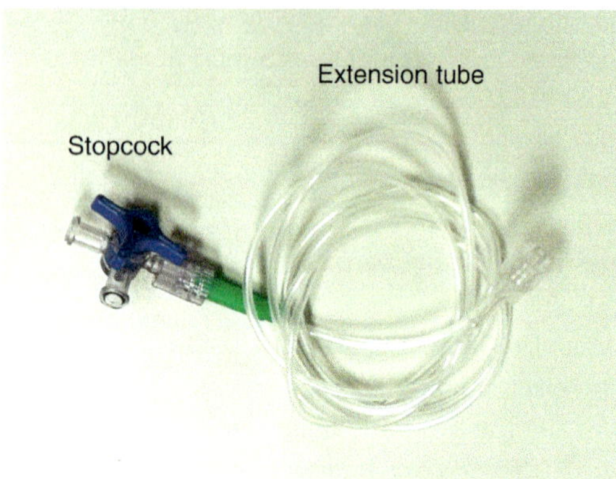

Fig. 5.2 The extension tube is collected with a stopcock and is filled with natural solution before puncture

(b) Portable manometer (optional): A manometer is used for pressure measurement by collecting the needle with an extension tube.
(c) Invasive blood pressure monitoring system and transducers (optional): A system is routinely used for manometer during coronary angiography.

2. Monopolar guide wire (optional): The tip of monopolar guide wire is conductive and it extends to a conductive metal tail through which a three-dimensional navigation system can be collected.
3. Clip-pin or clip-clip adaptor with cable (optional): The alligator style clip can be attached to the conductive tail of a monopolar guide wire and the pin can be inserted in the pin box of a three-dimensional navigation system. A clip-clip cable can be used for navigation if a clip-pin cable is not available. Thus, the operator needs to manually make a pin. Peel the plastic shroud of the pins of a cable designed for linking diagnostic electrophysiological catheter and collect the clip to the peeled pin and finally insert the "clip-peeled pin" assembly into the pin box (Fig. 5.3).

Confirmation of Venous Access

A real venous access is particularly important, especially when a subclavian vein or an internal jugular vein is punctured; mechanic compression is difficult to achieve hemostasis in those veins; a surgery might be required in case of bleeding.

Under fluoroscopic guidance, a real venous access can be confirmed by the following manifestations: (1) the characteristic color of venous blood and (2) the consistent venous rout of a J-shaped wire revealed by fluoroscopy.

Without fluoroscopic guidance, a venous access can be verified by the following tips:

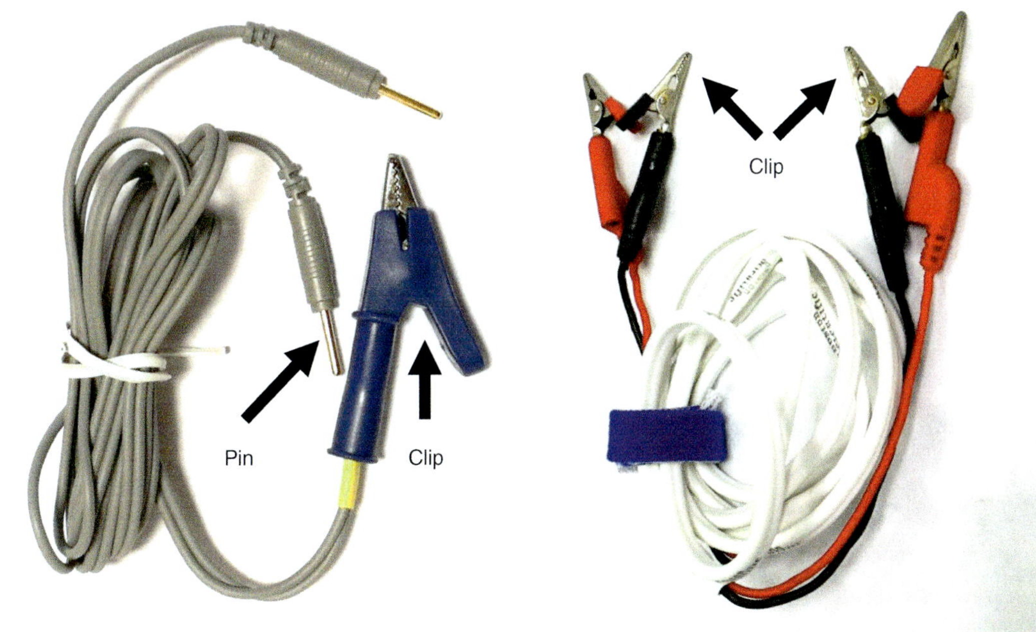

Fig. 5.3 A clip-pin adaptor with cable is utilized for three-dimensional navigation; the conductive tail of a monopolar guide wire is collected with the alligator-style clip and the pin is inserted into the pin box of the navigation system. A clip-clip cable can be used for navigation, and the operator needs to manually make a pin in this situation. Peel the plastic shroud of the pins of a cable designed for linking diagnostic electrophysiological catheter, collect the clip to the peeled pin, and finally insert the "clip-peeled pin" assembly into the pin box

Pressure Measurement

The pressure in the punctured vessel can be evaluated by the following methods:

1. Blood return test: A venous access can be confirmed if the blood flows back to the needle when you just lift the extension tube filled with natural solution (Figs. 5.4 and 5.5).
2. Portable manometer: A portable manometer can measure the pressure within the punctured lumen via an "extension tube" collected to the needle and help you to verify a venous access.
3. Transducer and invasive blood pressure monitoring system: The pressure can be measured using transducer and invasive blood pressure monitoring system via an "extension tube" collected to the needle.

Interference Test

The test is often used to confirm a correct venous access when a subclavian vein or an internal jugular vein is punctured for introducing a catheter with fixed curve into coronary sinus [2].

Using electroanatomic navigation system, this technique can be applied according to the following steps:

1. A catheter with fixed curve is advanced to the right atrium via femoral vein and then a rough model is constructed.
2. The tip of catheter is placed at the middle of right atrium via three-dimensional navigation system (e.g., EnSite NavX™).
3. A subclavian vein or an internal jugular vein is punctured, and then a J-shaped guide wire is inserted into the needle and collected to a three-dimensional navigation system via a clip-pin cable. The push-and-pull manipulation of guide wire may lead to passive movement of the catheter placed at right atrium; additionally, rotation of the catheter may touch the J-shaped wire and lead to interference signal seen in the screen (Fig. 5.6).

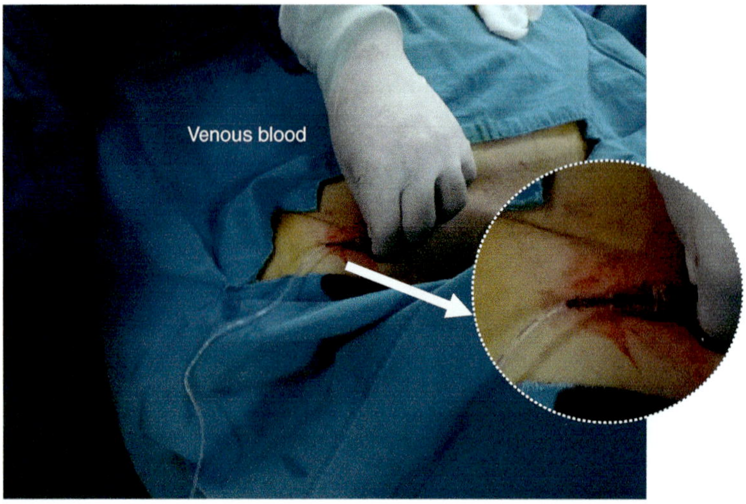

Fig. 5.4 Blood pressure was roughly estimated with an extension tube filled with natural solution and collected to the needle. Venous blood flowed out of the needle when the tube was dropped below the needle

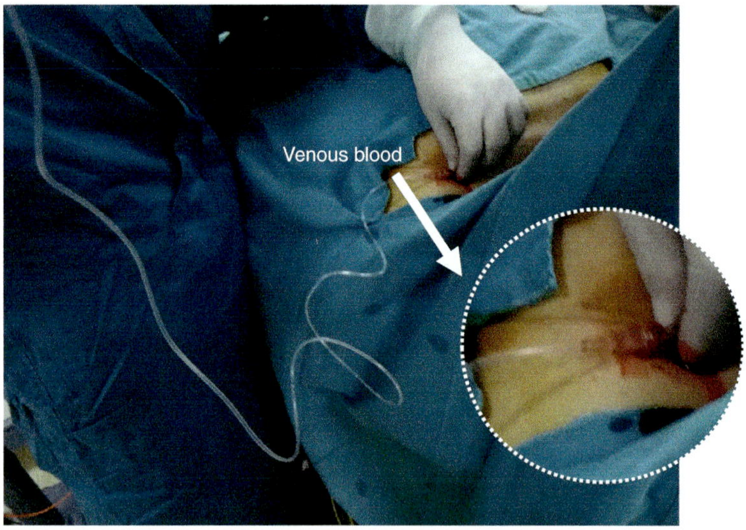

Fig. 5.5 Venous blood returned into the needle when the tube was raised above the needle

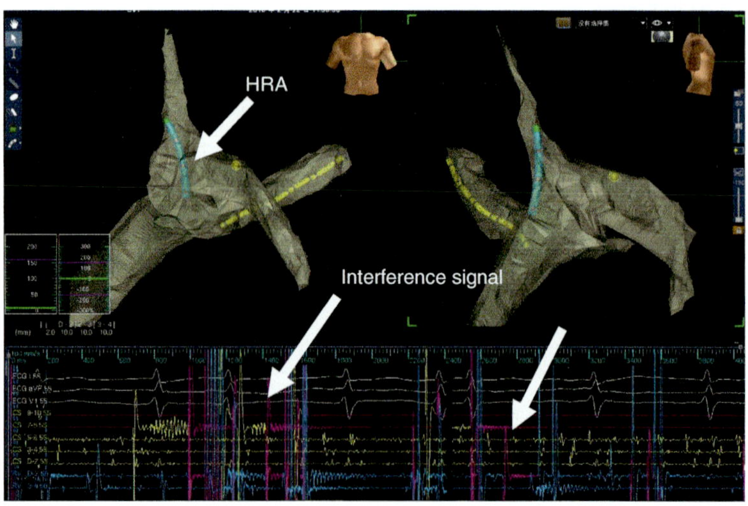

Fig. 5.6 Interference test is usually used for confirming the venous access of subclavian or internal jugular vein. The interference signal can be seen in the monitor by the entanglement of the catheter via a femoral vein with the J-shaped wire placed via subclavian or internal jugular vein

Monopolar Guide Wire

The tip of a special-designed monopolar guide wire can be exactly located by three-dimensional system. It can be inserted into the needle after a puncture and the metal conductive tail can be collected to a three-dimensional system using a clap-pin adaptor with cable.

Tips for Catheter Manipulation

Without fluoroscopic guidance, catheters can be efficiently placed according to the following tips:

1. Prefer a catheter with a soft tip except there is a special need.
2. A femoral vein access as well as a steerable catheter are preferred for coronary sinus catheterization, which will save the time for confirming a venous access and reduce the potential risk of pneumothorax or hemothorax.
3. The introducing sheath should be large enough to allow advancing or withdrawing catheters smoothly; the skin and local tissue should be cut and dilated appropriately if a long sheath is used for introducing catheters.
4. Important anatomic positions should be labeled and the length of the catheter should be roughly estimated before catheter placement; generally we place the tip of a catheter at about three fingers cranial to the xiphoid process, and observe the distance between the collector or handle of a catheter and the patient's heel (Figs. 5.7 and 5.8).
5. In order to reduce the friction force and improve the sense of resistance from the tip of catheters, all catheters should be bedewed with heparinized natural water immediately before and during catheter manipulation.
6. All the manipulations must be gentle; this is the case especially with zero-fluoroscopic technique. "Short-distance advancement and slightly hold" technique, instead of "large-distance advancement and tightly clench" technique, is preferred for catheter manipulation; insert 1–2 cm each time by more

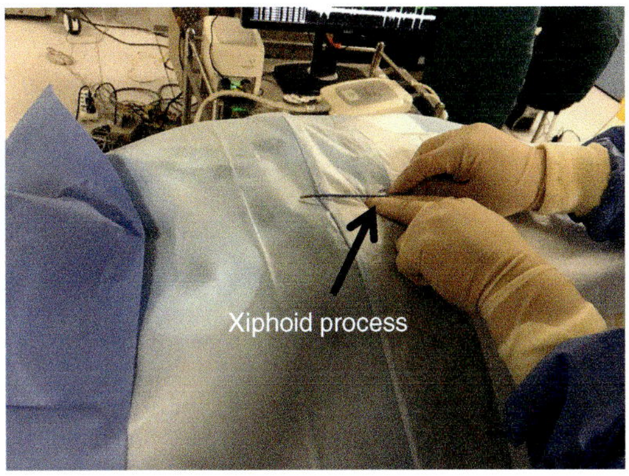

Fig. 5.7 The operator placed the tip of an ablation catheter three fingers cranial to the xiphoid process and marked with a blue dot on the monitor of the Carto system

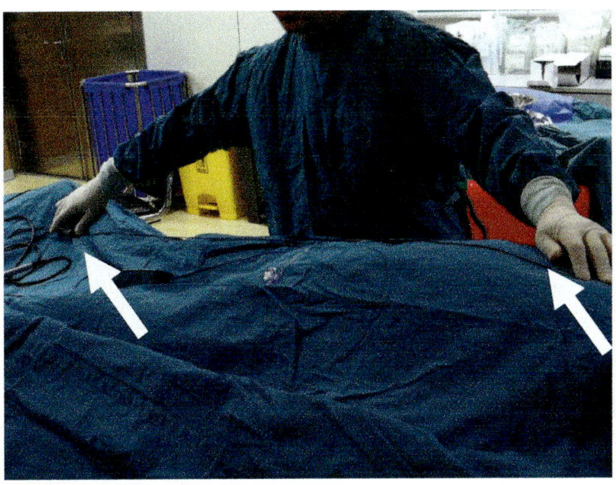

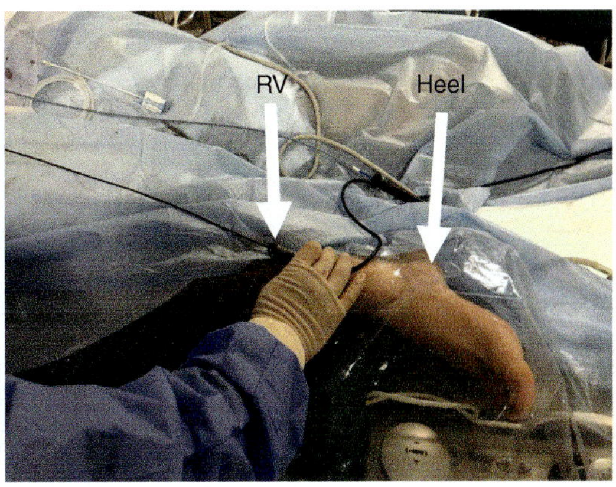

Fig. 5.8 The operator placed the tip of a right ventricular (RV) catheter near the xiphoid process and observed the distance between the catheter's tail and the patient's heel

times and hold the catheter with the slightest force using the thumb and index finger for catheter insertion, whereas 3–5 cm each time, less times, and tight clench with all the fingers are not recommended (Figs. 5.9 and 5.10).

7. Choose proper views for inserting catheters into particular structure; anterior-posterior (AP) view plus right lateral (RL) view is recommended for catheter insertion through venae cava since almost big venous bifurcations extend laterally. The two views are also recommended to place a catheter into a superior vena cava; as a RAA is located at the anterior and lateral part of a right atrium, the operator manipulates the catheter posteriorly and medially to avoid a likely perforation of the filmy right atrial appendage (RAA) (Fig. 5.11) [2, 8].
8. An operator should be particularly cautious in dealing with fragile structures such as coronary sinus, right atrial appendage, and left atrial appendage. Generally, strong structures

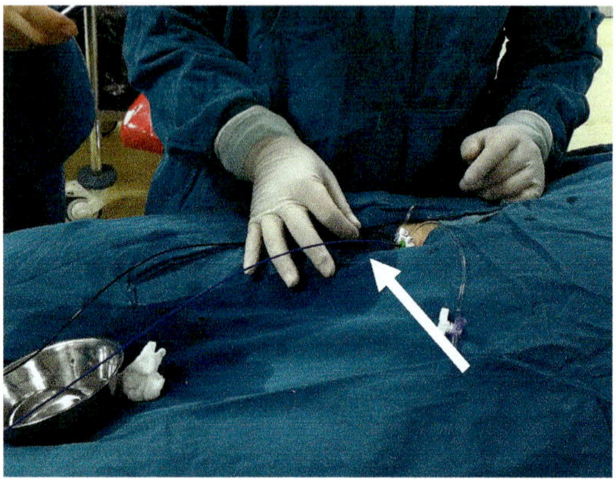

Fig. 5.9 "Short-distance advancement and slightly-hold" technique is preferred for placing catheters without fluoroscopic guidance. Using this technique, an operator holds a catheter slightly just with two fingers and advance the catheter only 1–2 cm each time, and the catheter is advanced to the target chamber by more times of manipulation

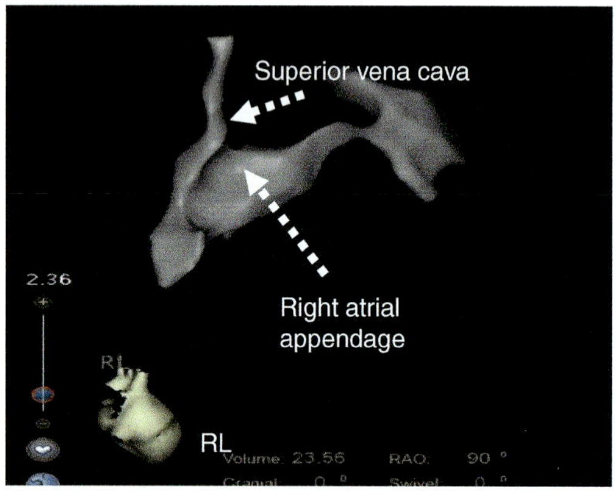

Fig. 5.11 To avoid the potential risk of perforation of right atrial appendage, right lateral view (RL) plus anterior-posterior (AP) view is recommended for placing electrodes through superior venae cava

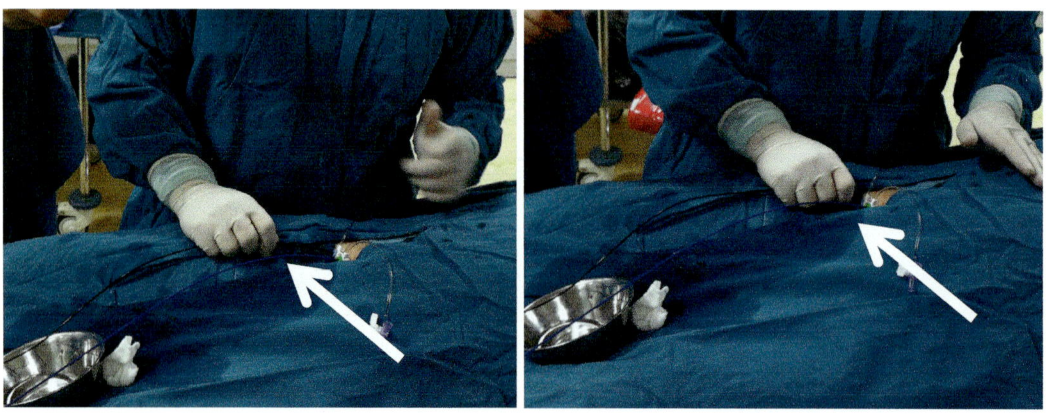

Fig. 5.10 Avoid to use "large-distance advancement and tightly-clench" technique for placing catheters without fluoroscopic guidance. Using this technique, the operator usually tightly clenches a catheter with all the fingers and advance the catheter 3–5 cm each time, and the catheter is advanced to the heart chamber by few times of manipulation

and relatively safe areas are firstly selected for catheter manipulation, model reconstruction, and revealing the anatomic location of those fragile structures.

9. Occasionally, a catheter may slip into left subphrenic venae and the electrogram recorded by the catheter presents an atrial wave plus a ventricular wave, but the amplitude is relatively small and the distal part of catheter is relatively fixed (Figs. 5.12 and 5.13).

Catheter Placement

Generally, anterior-posterior (AP) view plus right lateral (RL) view is recommended for guiding catheter insertion through vessels by three-dimensional navigation system.

Three-Dimensional Navigation System Based on Impedance Measurements

To place catheters using three-dimensional navigation system based on impedance measurements (e.g., EnSite NavX™), an operator can begin with any catheter since it is an open platform and compatible to all kinds of catheters.

Insert the catheters into the right atrium, then right ventricular apex, and the His bundle via a femoral vein, respectively. Place a catheter into the coronary sinus via a subclavian vein, a right internal jugular vein, or a femoral vein. A venous access needs to be confirmed if the coronary sinus catheter is placed by subclavian or jugular vein, which can be judged by the characteristic color of venous blood, the pressure measurement, and the interference signal of the J-shaped wire with a catheter placed in the middle of the right atrium via femoral vein [2].

It is better to advance several catheters with different curve to the heart chamber at one time and advance the catheter alternatively, which can improve the efficiency of catheter placement. An operator can change the insertion to the second catheter with a different curve, which may be helpful to find the correct vessel path when the first catheter meets obstacle somewhere in the vena cava.

Before the insertion, roughly evaluate the length required to be inserted into the sheath as follows: (1) place the tip of the catheter about three fingers cranial to the xiphoid process, which usually locates at the middle of right atrium; (2)

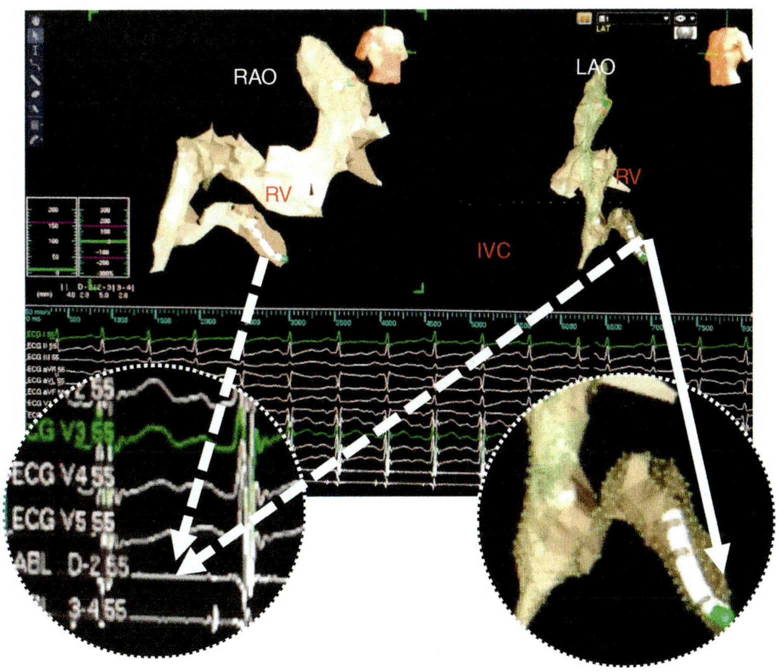

Fig. 5.12 An ablation catheter slipped into the left subphrenic venae and the catheter could not capture the ventricle. The local electrogram recorded by the catheter presented an atrial wave plus a ventricular wave, but the amplitude was small and the distal part of catheter was relatively fixed

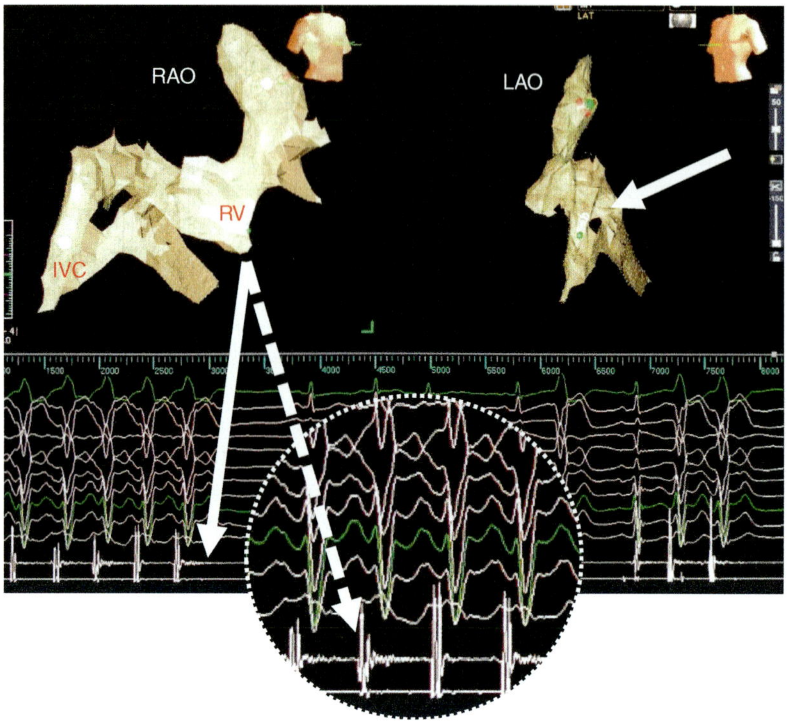

Fig. 5.13 The ablation catheter was advanced into the right ventricle and the catheter could capture the ventricle. The local electrogram also presented an atrial wave plus a ventricular wave; the amplitude was large and the distal part of catheter was free

observe and remember the distance between a catheter tail and the ankle and/or the heel of a patient (Figs. 5.7 and 5.8).

The length of all kinds of electrophysiological diagnostic catheters generally varies from 110 to 115 cm. The collector is usually about at the level of the patient's heel if the patient's stature is about 160–165 cm (Tables 5.1, 5.2, 5.3, 5.4, and 5.5).

RVA Catheter

We recommend that a catheter is inserted into the vena cava using "short-distance and slightly-hold" technique mentioned above. The operator needs to observe the moving track on the monitor and the intracardiac electrogram recorded by the catheter. Usually the track should go nearly straight to the heart chamber. Withdraw the catheter and change the direction in case of the following situations: (1) obvious resistance is still perceived with "short-distance and slightly-hold" technique; (2) the track shows a nearly right-angle turn; and (3) the anticipated intracardiac electrogram does not appear when the inserted part exceeds the length evaluated in vitro to reach the target place.

Slightly rotate the catheter when it reaches the lower part of a right atrium. Construct the model at the same time. Change the project views into RAO plus LAO view. The catheter then is advanced toward 12 o'clock in LAO view. A bigger ventricular wave and a smaller atrial wave are anticipated as the operator advances the catheter.

His Catheter

The "His" catheter can be advanced and placed similarly according to the method for placing RVA.

Coronary Sinus Catheter

Generally a coronary sinus (CS) catheter is recommended to be placed after the RVA catheter or His catheter. RAO view plus LAO view is preferred for placing CS catheter.

1. *Place CS catheter via inferior vena cava*

   Use a steerable CS catheter; place the catheter according to the following steps: (a) advance the catheter into the right atrium until catheter tip is horizontal to the tip of His catheter in cranial-caudal direction; (b) flex the tip

Table 5.1 Non-navigation ablation/diagnostic catheters of Biosense Webster Inc.

Brand and type	Catalog no.	Curve	Color	Diameter	Space (mm)	Length (cm)
Celsius® ablation (TC)						
4 mm Non-nav	D7TCAL252RT	A	Yellow	7F	2–5–2	115
4 mm Non-nav	D7TCBL252RT	B	Red	7F	2–5–2	115
4 mm Non-nav	D7TCCL252RT	C	Green	7F	2–5–2	115
4 mm Non-nav	D7TCDL252RT	D	Blue	7F	2–5–2	115
4 mm Non-nav	D7TCEL252RT	E	White	7F	2–5–2	115
4 mm Non-nav	D7TCFL252RT	F	Orange	7F	2–5–2	115
4 mm Non-nav braided tip	D8BTCDL252RT	D	Blue	8F	2–5–2	90
4 mm Non-nav braided tip	D8BTCEL252RT	E	White	8F	2–5–2	90
4 mm Non-nav braided tip	D8BTCFL252RT	F	Orange	8F	2–5–2	90
Avail® diagnostic						
Quad A curve (fixed curve)	F6QRA010RT	A	Yellow	6F	10	115
Quad F curve (fixed curve)	F6QRF010RT	F	Black	6F	10	115
Quad F curve (fixed curve)	F6QF002RT	F	Black	6F	1	115
Webster® diagnostic						
Deca (fixed curve)	F5ADP282RT	P	Gray	5F	2–8–2	60

TC thermocouple, *THR* thermistor. Biosense Webster Inc., Diamond Bar, CA, USA

Table 5.2 Three-dimensional navigation catheters of Biosense Webster Inc.

Brand and type	Catalog no.	Curve	Color	Diameter	Space (mm)	Length (cm)
Navistar® 4 mm (TC)						
4 mm Nav B curve	NS7TCBL174HS	B	Red	7F	1–7–4	115
4 mm Nav C curve	NS7TCCL174HS	C	Green	7F	1–7–4	115
4 mm Nav D curve	NS7TCDL174HS	D	Blue	7F	1–7–4	115
4 mm Nav E curve	NS7TCEL174HS	E	White	7F	1–7–4	115
4 mm Nav F curve	NS7TCFL174HS	F	Orange	7F	1–7–4	115
Navistar® ThermoCool®						
3.5 mm Nav TC B curve	NI75TCBH	B	Red	7.5F	2–5–2	115
3.5 mm Nav TC C curve	NI75TCCH	C	Green	7.5F	2–5–2	115
3.5 mm Nav TC D curve	NI75TCDH	D	Blue	7.5F	2–5–2	115
3.5 mm Nav TC F curve	NI75TCFH	F	Orange	7.5F	2–5–2	115
3.5 mm Nav TC J curve	NI75TCJH	J	Black	7.5F	2–5–2	115
ThermoCool® SmartTouch						
ST D curve	D133604IL	D	Blue	8F	1–6–2	115
ST F curve	D133605IL	F	Orange	8F	1–6–2	115
ST J curve	D133606IL	J	Black	8F	1–6–2	115
Lasso® NAV SAS						
D curve	DLN1215CT	D	Blue	7F	4.5	115
	(Ring diameter, 15 mm; annular tip diameter, 4.5F)					
PentaRay® D curve	D128211	D	Blue	7F	2–6–2	115
	(Branch tip diameter, 3F)					

TC thermocouple, *THR* thermistor. Biosense Webster Inc., Diamond Bar, CA, USA

of the CS catheter like a "7" and the tip of CS catheter is at 1–2 cm below the tip of His catheter; (c) the catheter tip is often on the line vertical to the junction of inferior vena cava with right atrium in RAO 45° view; (d) rotate the catheter clockwise and direct it toward the septum to catch the CS orifice in LAO view; (e) release the curve if the catheter tip slips into the orifice of coronary sinus; and (f) advance the CS catheter into the distal part of

Table 5.3 Ablation/diagnostic catheters of APT Medical Inc.

Brand and type	Catalog no.	Curve	Color	Diameter	Space (mm)	Length (cm)
Triguy™ ablation catheter						
Ablation 4 mm (TC)	902122	D	Blue	7F	2–5–2	85
Ablation 4 mm (THR)	902172	D	Blue	7F	2–5–2	85
Ablation 4 mm (TC)	902128	A	Yellow	7F	2–5–2	110
Ablation 4 mm (THR)	902178	A	Yellow	7F	2–5–2	110
Ablation 4 mm (TC)	902129	B	Red	7F	2–5–2	110
Ablation 4 mm (THR)	902179	B	Red	7F	2–5–2	110
Triguy™ diagnostic catheter						
Fixed curve-decapolar-CS	901533	CS	Blue	6F	2–8–2	65
Steerable decapolar-CS	901666	MPD-S	Blue	6F	2–5–2	110
Fixed curve-quadripolar-RV	901445	MPBe	Blue	6F	10	120
Fixed curve-quadripolar-RV	901446	MPA	Blue	6F	10	120
Fixed curve-quadripolar-His	901454	HIS	Blue	6F	5	120

TC thermocouple, *THR* thermistor. APT Medical Inc., Shenzhen, Guangdong, China

Table 5.4 Ablation/diagnostic catheters of St. Jude Medical

Brand and type	Catalog no.	Curve	Color	Diameter	Space (mm)	Length (cm)
Ablation (Thermocouple)						
Safire™ S–Curl	402821	Small		7F	2–5–2	115
Safire™ M–Curl	402822	Medium		7F	2–5–2	115
Safire™ L–Curl	402823	Large		7F	2–5–2	115
Therapy™ 4 mm tip	83432	Small		7F	2–5–2	110
Therapy™ 4 mm tip	83405	Medium		7F	2–5–2	110
Therapy™ 4 mm tip	83408	Large		7F	2–5–2	110
Therapy™ Cool Flex™ M	A088015	Medium		7F	0.5–5–2	110
Therapy™ Cool Flex™ L	A088016	Large		7F	0.5–5–2	110
Diagnostic catheter						
Supreme™ electrophysiology catheter	401436	NA		6F	10–10–10	120
Inquiry™ steerable diagnostic catheters	81102	NA		6F	2–5–2	110

St. Jude Medical, St. Paul, MN, USA

coronary sinus. In the second step, the position of His potential can be replaced with the peak of tricuspid annulus if the "His" potential is difficult to be recorded within 1 min. In the fifth step, adjust the catheter tip a little anteriorly or posteriorly in RAO view, or cranially or caudally in LAO view, if it cannot slip into the orifice (Figs. 5.14 and 5.15).

Occasionally, the span from CS orifice to inferior cava is relatively large and the curve of CS catheter is not long enough to reach the orifice. The operator needs to manually shape the curve so as to increase the curve size.

2. *Place CS catheter via superior vena cava*

A catheter of fixed curve can be placed into coronary sinus according to the following steps: (a) advance the catheter into the right atrium till the catheter tip is at 1–2 cm below the tip of His catheter; (b) rotate the catheter anticlockwise and direct it toward the septum in LAO view; (c) move the catheter tip a little anteriorly or posteriorly in RAO view, or cranially or caudally in LAO view, if it cannot slip into the orifice; and (d) advance the CS catheter into the distal part of coronary sinus.

HRA Catheter

Similarly, advance and place the HRA catheter according to the method for placing RVA.

Ablation Catheter

Advance the ablation catheter according to the following method: (1) preliminarily estimate the length required to reach the target site in vitro

Table 5.5 Transseptal sheath and needles

Sheath/needle	Catalog no.	Curve	Guide wire length	Guide wire diameter	Sheath/needle size	Dilator usable length	Sheath/needle usable length
1. Transseptal sheath							
HeartSpan™ fixed curve braided transseptal sheath[a]	FCL-160-02	55°	135 cm	0.035 in.	8.5F	65 cm	60 cm
Swartz™ braided SL transseptal guiding introducer sheath (SL1)[b]	406840	SL1	180 cm	0.032 in.	8F	67 cm	63 cm
Swartz™ braided SL transseptal guiding introducer sheath (SL1)[b]	406849	SL1	180 cm	0.032 in.	8.5F	67 cm	63 cm
FAST-CATH™ guiding introducer sheath (SR0)[b]	406844	SR0	145 cm	0.038 in.	8F	67 cm	63 cm
FAST-CATH™ guiding introducer sheath (SR0)[b]	406853	SR0	145 cm	0.038 in.	8.5F	67 cm	63 cm
Triguy™ transseptal access kit[c]	20150510	T0	150 cm	0.032 in.	8.5F	67 cm	62 cm
2. Transseptal needle							
HeartSpan™ needle[a]	FND-019-01	55°	NA	NA	21G	NA	71 cm
BRK™ needle	407200	50°	NA	NA	18G	NA	71 cm
Triguy™ needle[c]	20150510	50°	NA	NA	18G	NA	71 cm

[a]Merit Medical, South Jordan, UT, USA
[b]St. Jude Medical, St. Paul, MN, USA
[c]APT Medical Inc., Shenzhen, Guangdong, China

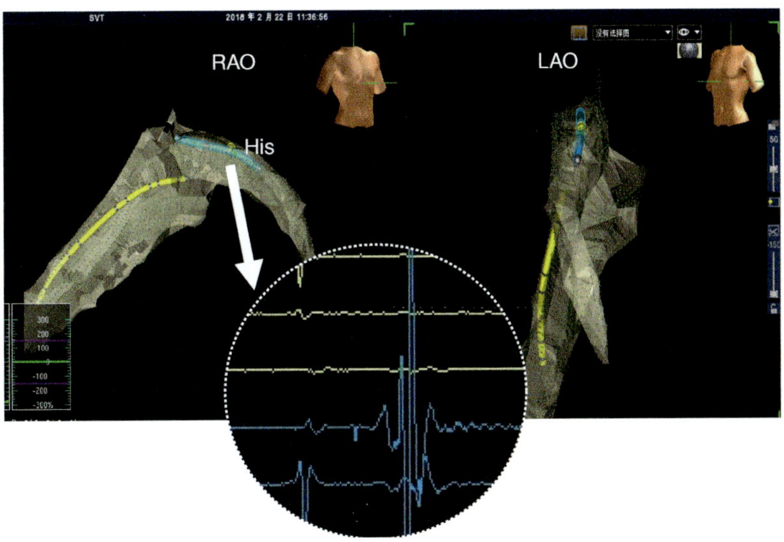

Fig. 5.14 Locate the position of His catheter or the peak of tricuspid annulus before placing coronary sinus catheter

(e.g., measuring the length from xiphoid process to the patient's heel with the ablation catheter); (2) observe the relationship between the handle of the ablation catheter and the patient's heel when the catheter tip is placed at xiphoid process in vitro; (3) slow down the advancement and observe if there is intracardiac electrogram recorded by the ablation catheter during insertion, especially when the catheter is close to the heart chamber; and (4) use the position of the collector of diagnostic catheter placed before as a reference to place an ablation catheter.

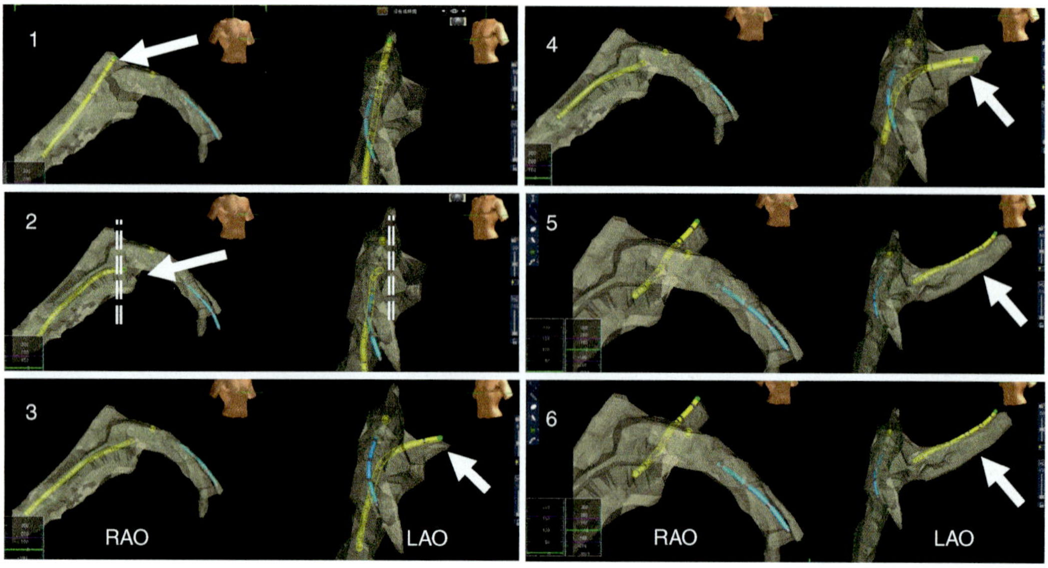

Fig. 5.15 Place coronary sinus catheter according to the following steps (1–6): flex the tip of the catheter like a "7" and place the tip of CS catheter at 1–2 cm below the tip of His catheter or the peak of tricuspid annulus; then rotate the catheter clockwise toward the septum to catch the orifice; release the curve and advance the catheter into distal part of coronary sinus

Determine the length required to be inserted into the lumen with the aid of the following tips: (1) the length of most diagnostic catheters usually varies from 110 to 115 cm; (2) the length of most ablation catheters is about 110–115 cm; (3) some ablation catheters, which are specially designed for right-sided ablation, is only 90 cm; (4) the tail of an electrophysiology catheter or a long ablation catheter (110 cm) is usually located at the patient's heel when the tip reaches the right atrium of the patient in medium stature; (5) the handle of a short ablation catheter (90 cm) is usually located at the patient's knees when the tip of ablation catheter reaches the right atrium of the patient in medium stature; and (6) usually the handle of an ablation catheter is parallel to the collector of a diagnostic catheter if they are almost the same in length (Fig. 5.16).

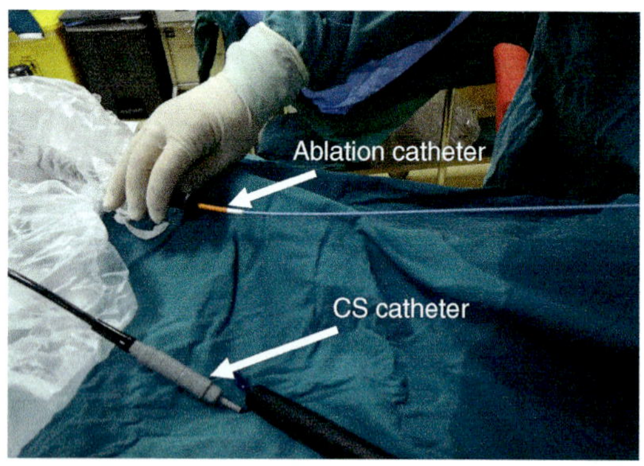

Fig. 5.16 The ablation catheter was 115 cm in length and coronary sinus catheter was 110 cm. The position of the ablation catheter could be used as a reference for judging the length of coronary catheter to be advanced

The shape of the moving track created on three-dimensional system usually looks like an inverted "U" in LAO view when a catheter is retrograde advanced through aortic arch via femoral artery. Withdraw the catheter if the shape looks like an "S" in LAO view (Fig. 5.17). Label the position with two or three white points when the ablation catheter reaches the lowest point in aortic root. Then the catheter can be inserted into the left ventricle as the conventional method under fluoroscopic guidance; be cautious to avoid possible injury to the aortic valve and to the coronary artery.

Long Sheath (e.g., SL1 Sheath)

A long sheath can be introduced according to the following three methods.

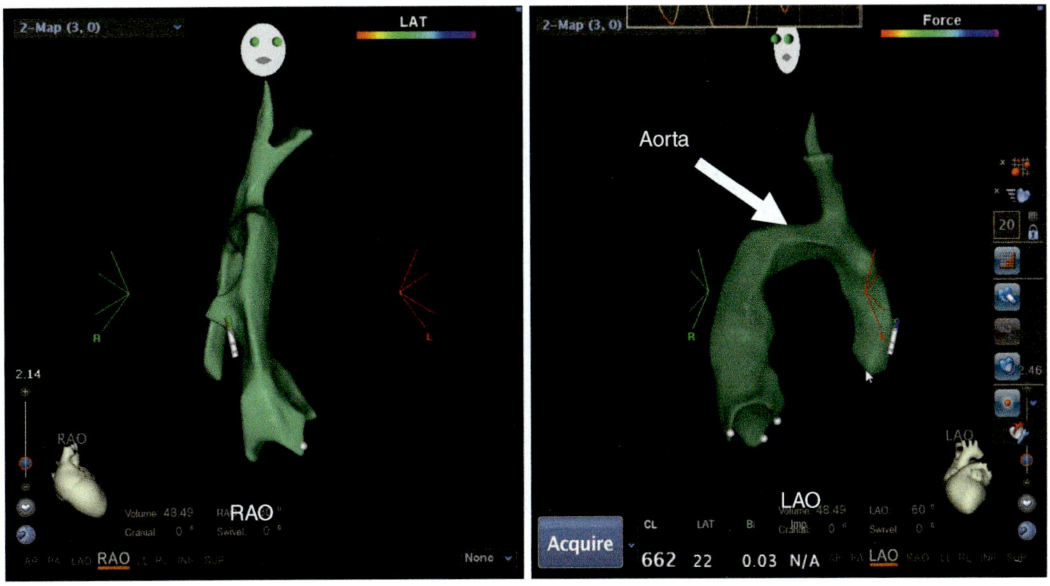

Fig. 5.17 Left anterior oblique view is recommended for advancing catheter placed via femoral artery. Aorta looks like an inverted "U" in this view

1. *Place a long sheath via an ablation catheter*
   (a) Gently insert the long guide wire, which is packed with the long sheath, the longer the better, at least 30 cm; and then advance the sheath-dilator assembly about 10–20 cm along the wire.
   (b) Withdraw the dilator and guide wire, insert an ablation catheter, and collect the catheter with three-dimensional navigation system.
   (c) Advance the ablation catheter through the long sheath till resistance is felt when the tip of ablation catheter reaches the distal curve of the long sheath.
   (d) Then hold the catheter shaft and withdraw the long sheath a little so as to display the tip of ablation catheter on the monitor of three-dimensional mapping system.
   (e) Advance the catheter to the right ventricle and flex the catheter to make a sharp curve (Fig. 5.18).
   (f) Advance the long sheath till obvious resistance is felt, which is resulted from the sharp curve.

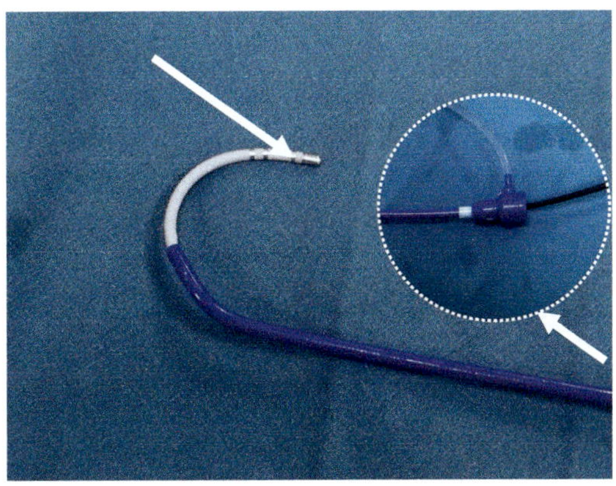

Fig. 5.18 Flex the ablation catheter to make a sharp curve in the right ventricle and then advance the sheath till obvious resistance is felt when a long sheath is guided via an ablation catheter without fluoroscopic guidance

The distance from the distal edge of the kneecap to groin is usually about 35–40 cm, which can be used a reference for estimation during catheter placement.

In order to guarantee a safe advancement and to identify the tip's position of the sheath, observe if there are the following manifestations: the intracardiac electrogram recorded by the proximal electrodes will disappear and the image of ablation catheter will become deformed when

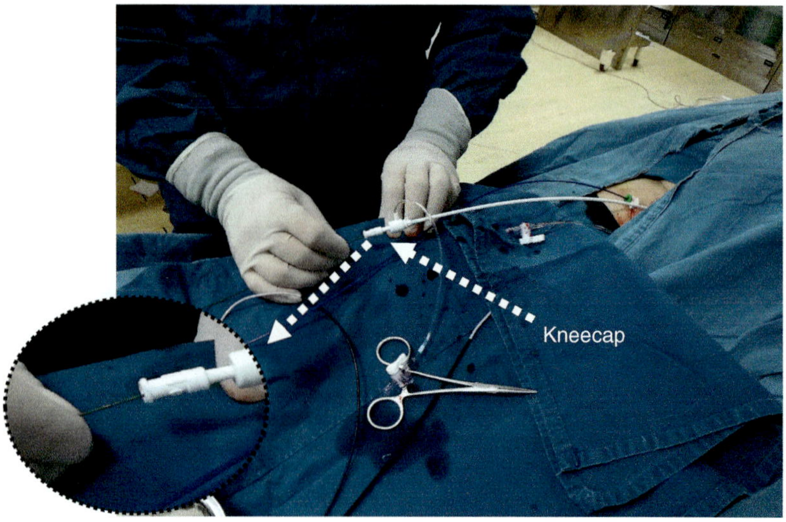

Fig. 5.19 A long sheath was placed via the packed guide wire, which is 135 cm in length. The long guide wire was advanced till the wire's tail was close to the patient's heel. Then the long sheath was advanced toward heart chamber but stopped when the sheath's end reached the distal edge of kneecap. The wire was then exchanged with an ablation catheter collected with the three-dimensional system

the tip of long sheath begins to shield the proximal electrodes.

2. *Place a long sheath via the packed guide wire*
   (a) Gently insert the long guide wire (e.g., 135 cm in length), which is packed with the long sheath, the longer the better, till the wire's tail is close to the patient's heel, and the wire's tip can almost reach the mandibular joint.
   (b) Advance dilator-sheath assembly till the tail of guide wire extends out the sheath and into the vessel about 10 cm.
   (c) Collect the tail of the guide wire with a cable, an alligator clip-to-pin cable, to the three-dimensional system.
   (d) Display the tip of the guide wire on the monitor and advance the tip of the guide wire to the heart chamber.
   (e) Advance the dilator-sheath assembly to the heart chamber and always keep the tip of the guide wire outside the assembly.

Avoid advancing the assembly straightly to the heart chamber if the heart chamber has not been reconstructed yet. An operator should estimate the length before insertion and insert the guide wire much deeper than the sheath so as to protect the tissue with the soft wire. Usually advance the long sheath toward heart chamber but slow down the advancement when the sheath's end is about at the distal edge of kneecap (Fig. 5.19).

As we all know, the usable length of most dilators is less than 67 cm, whereas the distance between the kneecap and the xiphoid process is about 70 cm in a patient in medium stature, which is about 160 cm high. Thus, the tip of the dilator is usually nearly at the orifice of inferior vena cava. Exchange the wire with an ablation catheter and advance the sheath into the heart guided by three-dimensional system.

3. *Place a long sheath via a monopolar guide wire*
   (a) Insert a monopolar guide wire into the vessel and collect the tail of monopolar wire with the three-dimensional system.
   (b) Advance the wire directly into the heart chamber till the tip of guide wire records a big atrial wave.
   (c) Advance sheath-dilator assembly to the heart chamber and always keep the tip of the guide wire outside the assembly.

The best method to introduce a long sheath is by monopolar guide wire. A common packed guide wire can be used for introducing the long sheath if there is no monopolar wire; an ablation catheter can also be used for introducing the long sheath unless obvious friction resistance is felt during the advancement.

Three-Dimensional Mapping System Based on Magnetic Location Technology

As for placing catheters guided by magnetic location technology (e.g., Carto™) and without fluoroscopy, a sensor-based catheter, which is usually an ablation catheter, needs to be used firstly for model reconstruction; choose an appropriate ablation catheter if the ablation target (e.g., AVNRT) is definite according to ECG characteristics; choose a medium catheter which is suitable for most kinds of situation if the ablation target is not definite.

In our center, the size of an ablation catheter is determined according to the following principles: (1) choose a big-curve catheter (e.g., F curve, 4 mm, Navistar) usually for the ablation of AVNRT; (2) choose a medium-curve catheter for unknown type of SVT and use a SL1 sheath for increasing the span if the final diagnosis is AVNRT or right-sided AVRT.

Locate the anatomic marks in vitro and label the position on three-dimensional model with two or three blue points before inserting the ablation catheter (e.g., xiphoid process, three-finger width over xiphoid process, presternum).

Advance the ablation catheter into the heart with the aid of three-dimensional navigation system and the marks mentioned above.

Again, label 2–3 key points on the model with the ablation catheter before the insertion of diagnostic catheters. Those points include (1) the His potential or the peak of tricuspid valve if the "His" potential is not easy to be detected within 10 s and (2) the lowest point of tricuspid valve.

The methods to place diagnostic catheters such as HRA, RVA, CS, and His are similar to the method using electric field navigation system. However, it is recommended to reconstruct coronary sinus with the ablation catheter first (Fig. 5.20). A soft ablation catheter (4 mm Navistar®, Biosense Webster Inc., Diamond Bar, CA, USA) is preferred for the reconstruction and further ablation in patients with SVT.

As we all know, the magnetic field is limited to the area nearby a heart chamber. As an operator places catheters without fluoroscopic guidance, the moving track cannot be displayed on the monitor if the catheters are below the umbilicus area. Hence, an operator must be

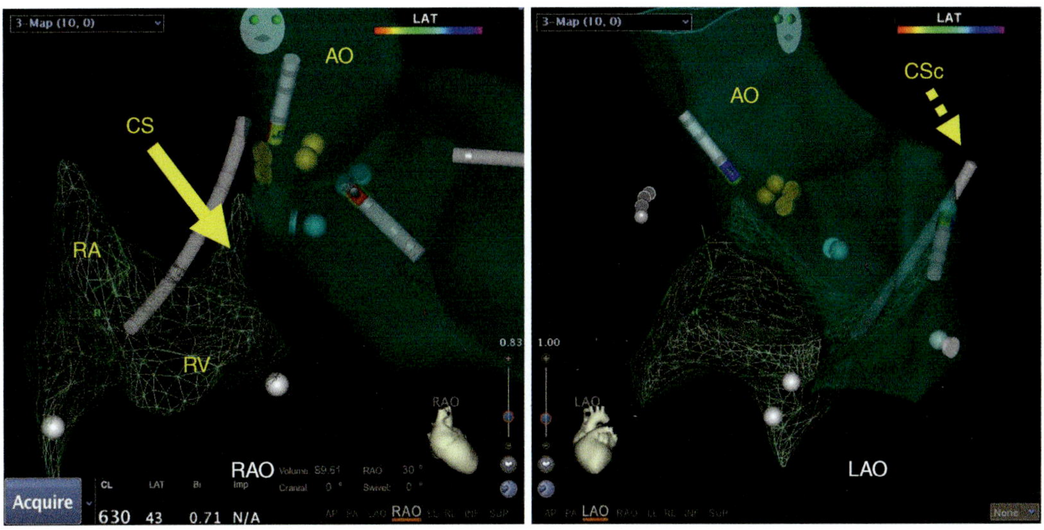

Fig. 5.20 The model was reconstructed during zero-fluoroscopic ablation of left accessory pathway using Carto™ system. Coronary sinus (CS) was reconstructed first with a soft ablation catheter. *CSc* coronary sinus catheter, *AO* aorta, *RA* right atrium, *RV* right ventricle, *RAO* right anterior oblique view, *LAO* left anterior oblique view

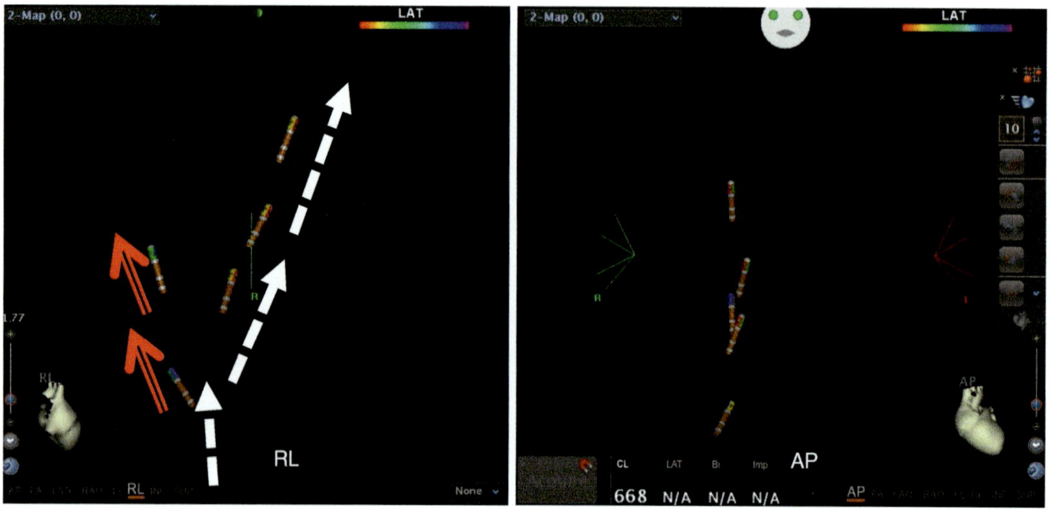

Fig. 5.21 Snapshot tool was used for guiding catheter placement. The red solid arrow showed a wrong direction and the dotted arrow indicated a correct direction in right later view when the catheter was about at the collection of two common iliac veins

particularly gentle and patient, and avoid rapid advancement before he/she can see the moving track of a catheter. However, as for a sensor-based ablation catheter, snapshot tool could help us adjust the direction in AP view plus RL views (Fig. 5.21).

At times, a catheter, especially RVA, will slip into vascular bifurcations if the insertion is guided by EnSite system. However, it is not the case if the insertion is guided by Carto system; the reason might be due to the first introduced ablation catheter, which can act as a sliding rail. Anyway, it needs more time and patience to insert catheters into heart chamber using magnetic field system than it does using electric field system.

Model Reconstruction

Preparation Before Model Reconstruction

Tell the patient to breathe smoothly and avoid body movement if the patient is conscious.

Remember to remove any metal guide wire inside the heart chamber before model reconstruction when electric field navigation system (e.g,. EnSite NavX™) is used.

System Reference and Positional Reference

EnSite System

1. System reference

   Traditionally, the system reference patch is placed on the patient's abdomen according to the default setting. However the patient's subscapularis is better for placing the patch if the patient is very obese and with vigorous respiration movements.

2. Positional reference

   Generally, external skin patch can be utilized as the reference during vessel puncture and right-sided mapping, whereas the coronary sinus (CS) catheter is recommended to be used as a reference during left-sided mapping if the position of CS catheter is stable [2]. Whatever you do, you need to be alert to the dislodgment of the positional reference, especially when intracardiac reference is used.

   It is better to leave a shadow of the coronary sinus catheter using system reference as positional reference; then leave the second shadow of the coronary sinus catheter using coronary sinus catheter as positional reference. These two shadows may help the operator to restore the original position of the CS catheter.

Carto System

There are three patches on the back and three others on the chest, which surround the heart. Positional reference usually utilizes the system reference.

Respiration Compensation

EnSite System

Perform an initial optimization and respiration compensation just before catheter placement. The second optimization and respiration compensation is recommended for model reconstruction after all the catheters are at position. Occasionally the third respiration compensation is required if the patient's respiration pattern changes obviously or an ablation site is at a high-risk area (e.g., near the His region). Operators should recheck the exact location of important markers such as the His bundle before power delivery.

Carto System

As for atrial fibrillation, reconstruct the left atrium and appendage with the respiratory gating technique (Accuresp algorithm, Biosense Webster, Diamond Bar, CA). During the training of respiration, talking with the patient may be helpful for achieving a successful training whereas intensified respiration is not recommended.

Model Reconstruction

Focus on the Targeted Area

Just reconstruct the virtual geometry of targeted areas. The targeted areas can be judged by electrophysiological analysis or after a rough mapping [2].

A relatively detailed reconstruction of right cardiac chamber is required if transseptal catheterization (TSP) is to be performed without fluoroscopic guidance. A retrograde approach via a femoral artery is recommended for arrhythmias originating in the left heart chamber. Although TSP can be performed without fluoroscopic guidance, it is a little time consuming and needs more expense for SVT ablation.

Usually, it is not necessary to reconstruct a full virtual geometry of the heart chamber. Just focus on the targeted area, and only relevant critical landmarks need to be labeled.

Selective geometry reconstruction focused on the targeted area will save procedure time and improve efficiency. Many novices and experienced operators have the tendency to reconstruct the whole cardiac chamber, including many unnecessary areas, when they begin to perform zero-fluoroscopic ablation [2].

Arrange Proper Reconstruction Sequence

As mentioned above, an operator should be particularly cautious in dealing with fragile structures such as coronary sinus, and right and left atrial appendage. Generally, stronger structures and safer areas are reconstructed firstly so as to reveal the anatomic location of those fragile structures. As for the reconstruction of left atrium: (1) reconstruct the inferior part firstly and then the superior part and (2) reconstruct the posterior wall firstly and then the anterior wall when it comes to superior part (Figs. 5.22 and 5.23).

The reconstruction sequence for an electrophysiological study or a right-sided cardiac mapping is recommended as follows: (1) inferior vena cava; (2) bottom of right atrium; (3) tricuspid annulus or His position; (4) right ventricle; (5) posterior part of high right atrium; and (6) superior vena cava (Fig. 5.24).

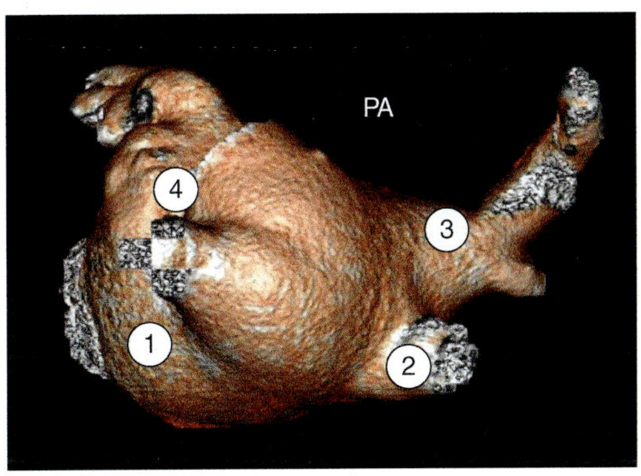

Fig. 5.22 The reconstruction sequence (1–4) of left atrium recommended for a novice was labeled in posterior-anterior (PA) view. Usually reconstruct the bottom area firstly and finally reconstruct the fragile atrial appendage

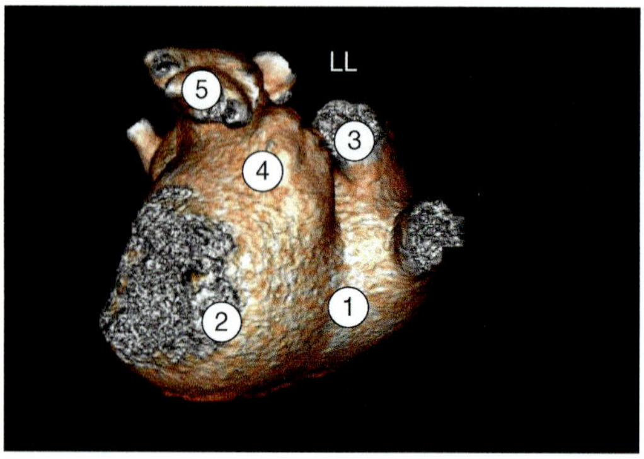

Fig. 5.23 The reconstruction sequence (1–5) of left atrium (LL) recommended for a novice was labeled in left lateral view. Reconstruct the bottom area firstly and finally reconstruct the fragile atrial appendage

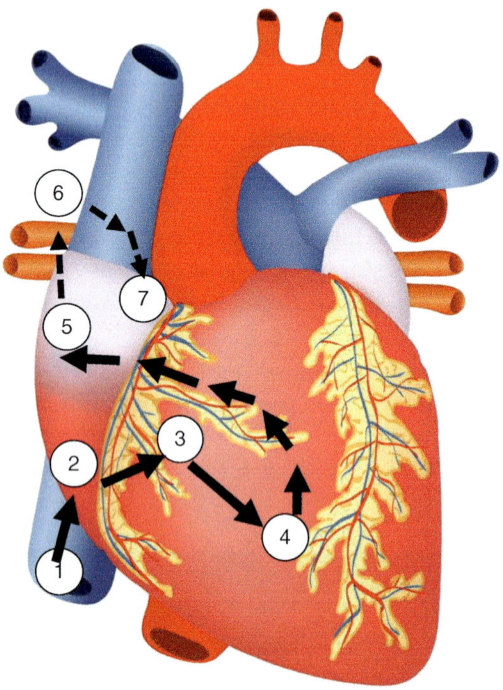

Fig. 5.24 As to an electrophysiological study or right-sided ablation, the reconstruction sequence (1–7) of the heart chamber for a novice was labeled in anterior-posterior view. The catheter was advanced and placed according to the following sequence: inferior vena cava, the tricuspid annulus, right ventricle, His bundle, high right atrium, superior vena cava, and atrial appendage if necessary

Keep Key Sites of Vessel Path

Delete the unimportant part of the track recorded during catheter insertion. Keep the key sites of the path, which will help to guide the following manipulation. Usually, keep those parts of the vena cava at where it is easy to slip into bifurcations during catheter insertion. Keep the aorta arch to avoid an unexpected insertion into the carotid artery.

Make Reconstruction by Stages

An operator needs to consider the procedure time, the patient's compliance and tolerance, and whether the patient is conscious or not before model reconstruction. Sometimes it is better to reconstruct the model by stages when the patient is conscious and cannot keep stationary in certain duration.

During the ablation of atrium fibrillation, just reconstruct a detailed model of the left pulmonary vein antrum (PVA) plus several points of right pulmonary vein for the ablation of left PVA; then reconstruct a detailed right PVA plus several points of left pulmonary vein for the ablation of right PVA.

Use a softer mapping catheter firstly (e.g., Lasso® or Pentaray®) and then a stiffer catheter.

Soft ablation catheter such as 4 mm Navistar® or Safire® can be considered for model reconstruction if an ablation catheter is used firstly.

Select Appropriate Project Views

Appropriate views may ease operators and save procedure time. The following project views are optional for zero-fluoroscopic ablation technique:

1. Catheter placement: anterior posterior (AP) plus right lateral (RL) views.
2. Atrial flutter: RAO plus LAO views, and turn over to reveal the inferior part of the model in LAO view, which facilitates to display the isthmus line better.
3. Right ventricular outflow tract (RVOT) arrhythmias: RAO plus LAO views.
4. Supraventricular tachycardia (SVT): RAO plus LAO views.
5. Atrial fibrillation: (a) left pulmonary vein antrum, AP or anterior posterior (PA) plus left lateral (LL) views; (b) right pulmonary vein antrum, AP or PA plus right lateral (RL) views.

Set Proper Display Pattern

A proper display pattern of a model can improve procedural efficiency.

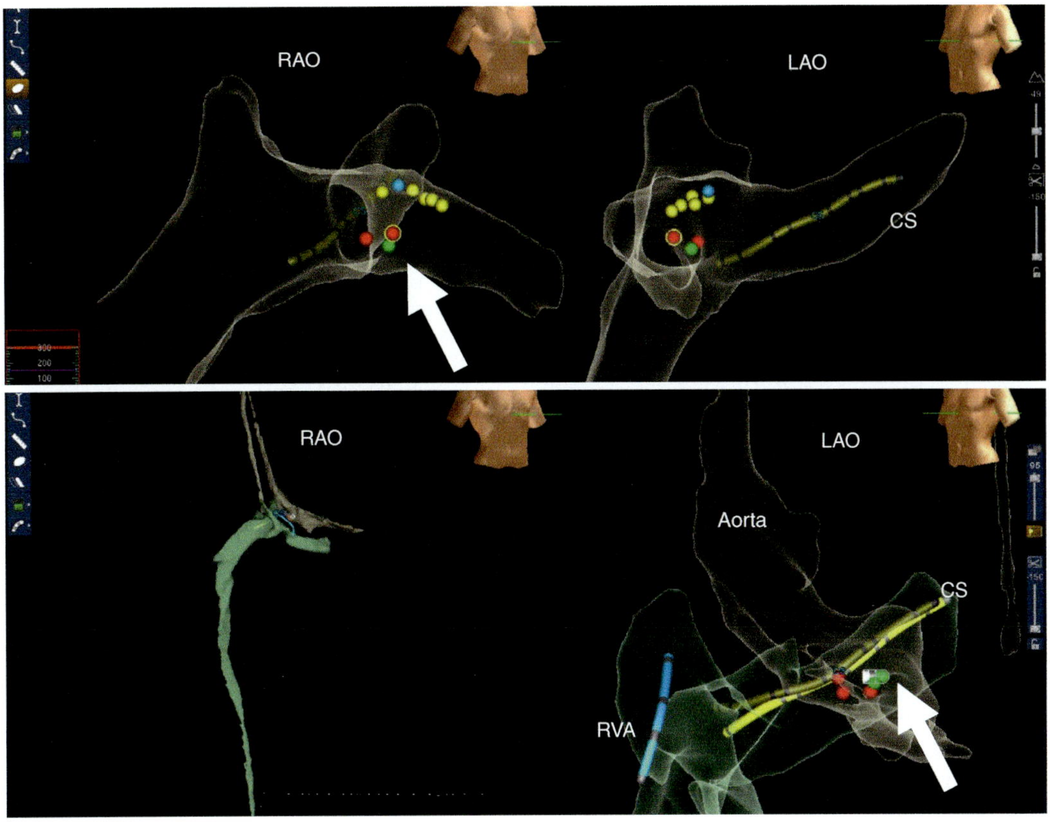

Fig. 5.25 The model was set in edge enhancement and surface translucency, which was easy for the operator to see the catheter's shadows and the labeled dots

Set the model in mesh pattern for the ablation of right ventricular outflow tract (RVOT) arrhythmias, which will be convenient to observe the distance between the tip of ablation catheter and the site of earliest activation.

Display the model in semitransparency when an operator performs the first antrum ablation in atrial fibrillation. Close the semi-transparent pattern when the operator performs the second antrum ablation. Usually semi-transparent pattern helps an operator to see the ablation points clearer during the first antrum ablation whereas the marked points in the first antrum interfere the display of second antrum in semitransparency.

Set the model in edge enhancement and surface translucency at the maximum, which will make the model look like a sketch, during the ablation of SVT when EnSite NavX™ is used (Fig. 5.25) [2].

Mark the Key Points by Default Setting

Mark the key points during model reconstruction. It is better to mark different anatomic structures with a set of colors by default in a lab. We generally mark the annulus, the bottom of aortic root, with white dots, His area with yellow dots, the largest His potential with blue dot, appendage with light red color, ideal target with green dots, and ablation points with maroon dots [2].

References

1. Calkins H, et al. Radiation exposure during radiofrequency catheter ablation of accessory atrioventricular connections. Circulation. 1991;84:2376–82.
2. Wang Y, et al. Ablation of idiopathic ventricular arrhythmia using zero-fluoroscopy approach with equivalent efficacy and less fatigue: a multicenter comparative study. Medicine (Baltimore). 2017;96:e6080. https://doi.org/10.1097/MD.0000000000006080.

3. Ruiz-Granell R, et al. Implantation of single-lead atrioventricular permanent pacemakers guided by electroanatomic navigation without the use of fluoroscopy. Europace. 2008;10:1048–51. https://doi.org/10.1093/europace/eun139eun139.
4. Casella M, et al. "Near-zero" fluoroscopic exposure in supraventricular arrhythmia ablation using the EnSite NavX mapping system: personal experience and review of the literature. J Interv Card Electrophysiol. 2011;31:109–18. https://doi.org/10.1007/s10840-011-9553-5.
5. Gist K, Tigges C, Smith G, Clark J. Learning curve for zero-fluoroscopy catheter ablation of AVNRT: early versus late experience. Pacing Clin Electrophysiol. 2011;34:264–8. https://doi.org/10.1111/j.1540-8159.2010.02952.x.
6. Bulava A, Hanis J, Eisenberger M. Catheter ablation of atrial fibrillation using zero-fluoroscopy technique: a randomized trial. Pacing Clin Electrophysiol. 2015;38:797–806. https://doi.org/10.1111/pace.12634.
7. Scaglione M, et al. Zero-fluoroscopy ablation of accessory pathways in children and adolescents: CARTO3 electroanatomic mapping combined with RF and cryoenergy. Pacing Clin Electrophysiol. 2015;38:675–81. https://doi.org/10.1111/pace.12619.
8. Chen G, et al. Zero-fluoroscopy catheter ablation of severe drug-resistant arrhythmia guided by EnSite NavX system during pregnancy: two case reports and literature review. Medicine (Baltimore). 2016;95:e4487. https://doi.org/10.1097/MD.0000000000004487.
9. Gaita F, Guerra PG, Battaglia A, Anselmino M. The dream of near-zero X-rays ablation comes true. Eur Heart J. 2016;37:2749–55. https://doi.org/10.1093/eurheartj/ehw223, pii: ehw223.
10. Yang L, et al. Meta-analysis of zero or near-zero fluoroscopy use during ablation of cardiac arrhythmias. Am J Cardiol. 2016;118:1511–8. https://doi.org/10.1016/j.amjcard.2016.08.014, pii: S0002-9149(16)31374-1.
11. Fernandez-Gomez JM, et al. Exclusion of fluoroscopy use in catheter ablation procedures: six years of experience at a single center. J Cardiovasc Electrophysiol. 2014;25:638–44. https://doi.org/10.1111/jce.12385.

Learning Curve of Zero Fluoroscopy

6

Amee M. Bigelow and John M. Clark

Introduction

Nonfluoroscopic three-dimensional mapping for arrhythmia ablation: tool or toy?

That was the title of a manuscript published in 2000 [1]. Time and experience have proven that three-dimensional mapping is a powerful tool in the world of electrophysiology. This chapter reviews the learning curve through which the profession has evolved since that time.

First, let's consider why one might want to endure the learning curve. The most apparent reason is to decrease radiation exposure to the patient. According to the National Council on Radiation Protection and Measurement, between 1981 and 2006 there was a 730% increase in medical radiation exposure in the United States [2]. Prior to 1980 medical radiation accounted for only a small fraction of the average annual radiation exposure. By 2006, medical radiation exposure had become the number one source of radiation for Americans. Because of that, the as low as reasonably achievable (ALARA) radiation dose principle is being aggressively pursued. Radiation carries both deterministic and stochastic risks. Deterministic risks are those side effects that are predictable at discrete doses of radiation, such as radiation dermatitis. Stochastic effects have no minimal threshold. These effects are primarily related to the long-term risk of malignancy and birth defects. Stochastic effects are the risks which the ALARA principle is intended to minimize. Other, less apparent, reasons to pursue minimal fluoroscopy include decreased radiation to the medical staff, the ability to perform ablation in the pregnant female, and the ability to make the procedure portable.

Decreasing radiation exposure to the patient has the secondary benefit of decreasing radiation exposure to the staff. We try not to dwell on the fact that our chosen profession has inherent risks, but they are real. A busy interventional cardiologist can have a lifetime risk of occupationally induced cancer as high as 4% [3]. A 2013 publication noted that 85% of head and neck tumors are left sided in physicians who work primarily with fluoroscopy [4]. Eliminating fluoroscopy will eliminate those occupational risks. But eliminating fluoroscopy will also eliminate the need for radiation protective equipment, such as lead aprons, thyroid shields, and lead goggles. Multiple studies have outlined the orthopedic problems related to long-term usage of such equipment [5–7]. Some electrophysiology

A. M. Bigelow
Division of Cardiology, Department of Pediatrics, Heart Institute at Cincinnati Children's Hospital Medical Center, Cincinnati, OH, USA
e-mail: amee.bigelow@cchmc.org

J. M. Clark (✉)
Division of Cardiology, Department of Pediatrics, Heart Center at Akron Children's Hospital, Akron, OH, USA
e-mail: jclark@akronchildrens.org

R. Proietti et al. (eds.), *Cardiac Electrophysiology Without Fluoroscopy*,
https://doi.org/10.1007/978-3-030-16992-3_6

(EP) labs have already achieved such a level of experience with fluoroless procedures that lead aprons are not worn for the majority of cases. The improved staff comfort associated with this is an appealing reason EP labs will be willing to undergo the learning curve.

Pregnancy is an uncommon situation among patients undergoing ablation, but one in which a zero fluoroscopy approach is of great benefit. While a pregnant patient with medical refractory arrhythmias is uncommon, a pregnant staff member is a situation that every lab will deal with over time. There is benefit here also, because the staff member can continue performing her job in the EP lab if it is fluoroscopy free.

Tachycardia-induced cardiomyopathy is a rare situation. These patients will sometimes require ECMO support. In that setting it would be feasible to do the ablation in the ICU rather than transporting the patient to the interventional lab, if fluoroscopy is not needed. For any or all of the above reasons, one may wish to pursue more robust radiation reduction measures in the EP lab. This chapter may help smooth the path and expedite the process as one goes through the learning curve.

History of Fluoroless Technology

To understand the evolution of three-dimensional mapping one must also understand the history of the tools available. There are four three-dimensional navigation systems currently available. These include the EnSite system (Abbott), the CARTO system (Biosense Webster), Mediguide (Abbott), and the Rhythmia system (Boston Scientific). Only two of these systems, the CARTO system and the EnSite system, have played a significant role in shaping the current state of the profession, and will, therefore, be the main points of discussion.

The CARTO system was first released in 1995 as a navigation and ablation tool. It was adopted by most of the major academic institutions and it was found to play a useful role in mapping of complex arrhythmia substrates. The system's function was dependent on magnetic fields. The patient was positioned lying on a pad containing several magnets. A magnetic detector within the tip of a proprietary catheter could then localize the position of the tip of that catheter three-dimensionally in space. Because the magnetic fields did not change during the case there was a high degree of accuracy and reproducibility regarding the location of the catheter tip [8].

The EnSite system was released in 1999. Its functionality is based on electrical impedances rather than magnetic fields. The system requires placement of six electrode patches on the patient's torso, setting up three orthogonal electrical fields. By measuring impedances within the three fields, the computer can localize the catheter electrode three-dimensionally within the body relative to a reference electrode. The EnSite system had the benefit of a broader field of view of catheters within the body. However, because lung volume and fluid volume both impacted electrical impedances, the system was more prone to geometrical shift.

In 2002 Drago et al. reported the first ever series of patients undergoing an ablation without fluoroscopy [9]. Their series consisted of 21 children with symptomatic WPW and right-sided accessory pathways. They were able to use the CARTO system to successfully ablate 20 of the 21 pathways. In nine patients no fluoroscopy was used. This sentinel report remains a major milestone in the evolution of electrophysiology.

However, there were no other reports published on this topic for 5 years after Drago's initial findings. The reason for this long delay can be understood upon closer inspection of what Drago's group had accomplished.

The CARTO system employed in that first report was the first generation. The only catheter that could be localized on that system was the radiofrequency catheter available through Biosense Webster. No mapping catheters and no other radiofrequency or cryoablation catheters could be visualized. So, as a tool for performing zero-fluoroscopy ablation, the original CARTO system was only useful for right-sided manifest accessory pathways. The system was also hindered by a narrow field of view and cumbersome geometry creation. The magnetic fields could not detect the catheter outside of the patient's thorax and therefore the catheter needed to be advanced from the femoral vein to the heart without any visual data. Creating a three-dimensional geometry required point-by-point three-dimensional marks. This was a slow process and yielded geometry with little correlation to the actual anatomy. Figures 6.1 and 6.2 give examples of the quality of image that could be created using the first version (Fig. 6.1) of CARTO compared to the most current version (Fig. 6.2).

In 2007 additional studies were reported. Tuzcu reported his experience of 28 patients with right-sided tachycardia mechanisms undergoing ablation [10]. Twenty-four of the 28 underwent ablation with zero fluoroscopy. Of the four patients requiring fluoroscopy, two were infants, one had typical and atypical atrioventricular nodal reentry tachycardia (AVNRT), and one had a parahisian pathway. Among the zero-fluoroscopy group, 15 had AVNRT and 9 had accessory pathways. He reported a 92% acute success rate and no complications. That same year, Clark and colleagues reported their experience with a minimal fluoroscopy approach [11]. Their series had 30 patients undergoing ablation for supraventricular tachycardia (SVT). Twenty-four of the procedures were performed without fluoroscopy. Of the six patients requiring fluoroscopy, five of them needed it only to perform transseptal puncture. Compared to age- and rhythm-matched controls, they noted a 95% reduction in radiation exposure.

What the two studies from 2007 shared in common was the use of the EnSite system for catheter navigation. At the time, EnSite had several advantages over CARTO for use as a zero-fluoroscopy tool. Being impedance based, it is not restricted to proprietary catheters. It is able to localize any electrode on any mapping or ablation catheter. Also cardiac geometry creation is a faster process with the ability to obtain an appropriate amount of detail needed for an ablation in minutes (Fig. 6.3). In addition, the electrodes can be localized from the moment they exit the sheath into the femoral vein and, therefore, visual guidance of the catheter up the IVC is possible (Fig. 6.4).

From those two studies, it now appeared that electrophysiologists had a tool that could significantly decrease radiation exposure without significant additional work.

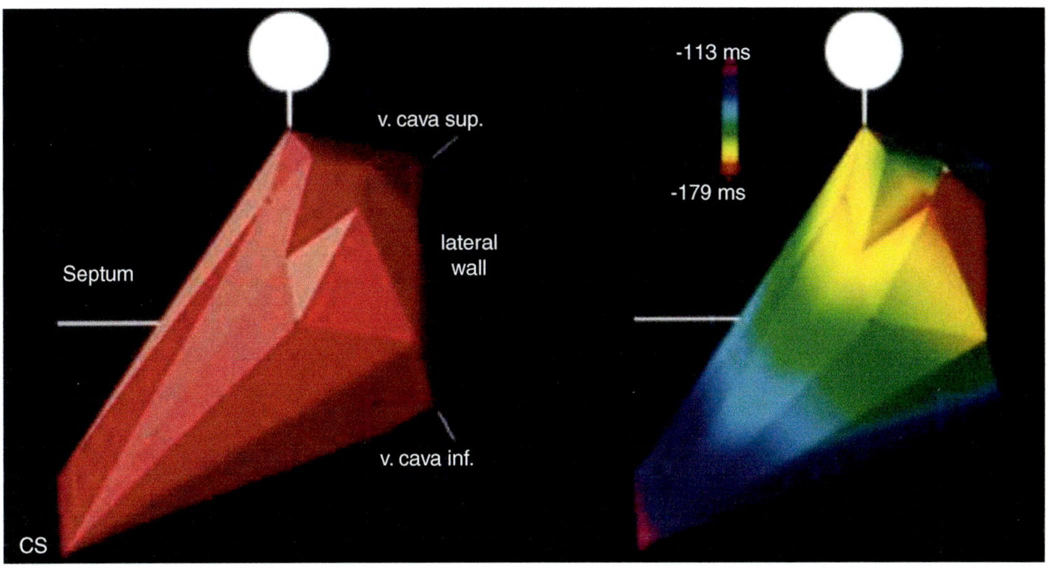

Fig. 6.1 CARTO map with posterior-anterior (PA) view of the right atrium during sinus rhythm. Anatomy reconstruction (left side) and color-coded physiological activation sequence (right side). The sinus node and the physiological activation focus during sinus rhythm are clearly seen in red. *CS* coronary sinus

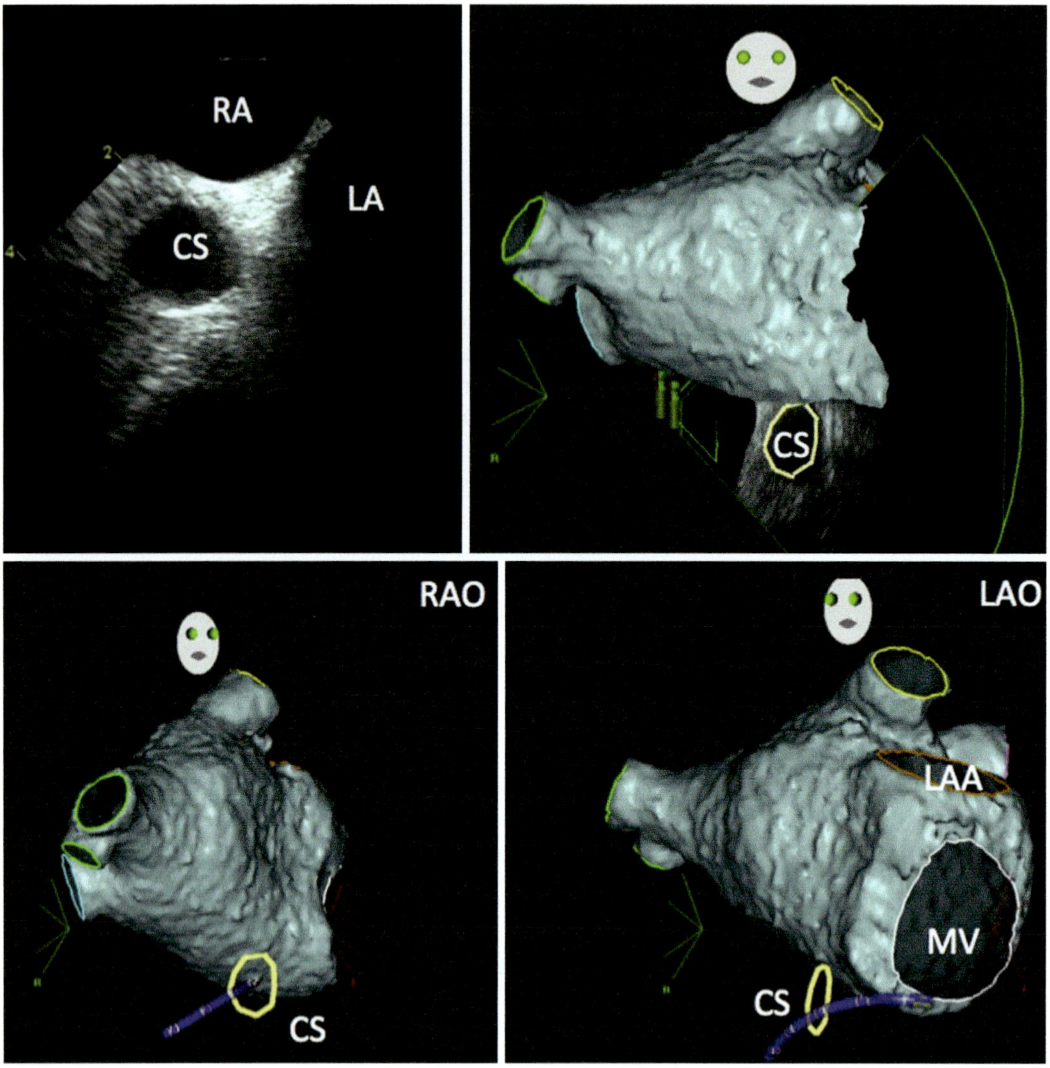

Fig. 6.2 Current image quality available with CARTO 3

Early experience brought to light the fact that transseptal puncture was one of the most common reasons for fluoroscopy use when pursuing a minimal-fluoro procedure. Clark et al. reported the use of transesophageal echocardiography for transseptal puncture [12] and Ferguson reported his group's use of intracardiac echo to accomplish the same goal [13]. The ability to cross the septum without fluoroscopy paved the way for all arrhythmias to potentially be approached with a zero-fluoroscopy procedure. From 2007 until 2013, all published series of zero-fluoroscopy ablation utilized the EnSite system. This included reports by Pachon et al. [14] addressing atrial flutter, Ferguson et al. [13] and Reddy et al. [15] addressing atrial fibrillation, Miyamoto et al. [16] and Von Bergen et al. [17] looking at ventricular tachycardia, and Casella et al. [18] looking at SVT. There were other publications in addition to these [11, 19–25].

As experience was rapidly increasing in no-fluoroscopy ablation with the EnSite system, CARTO was less effective in this specific characteristic. That fact was unfortunate because it created a large disparity in the availability of a nonfluoroscopic approach, based solely on the mapping system available at each institution. Since the majority of large academic centers uti-

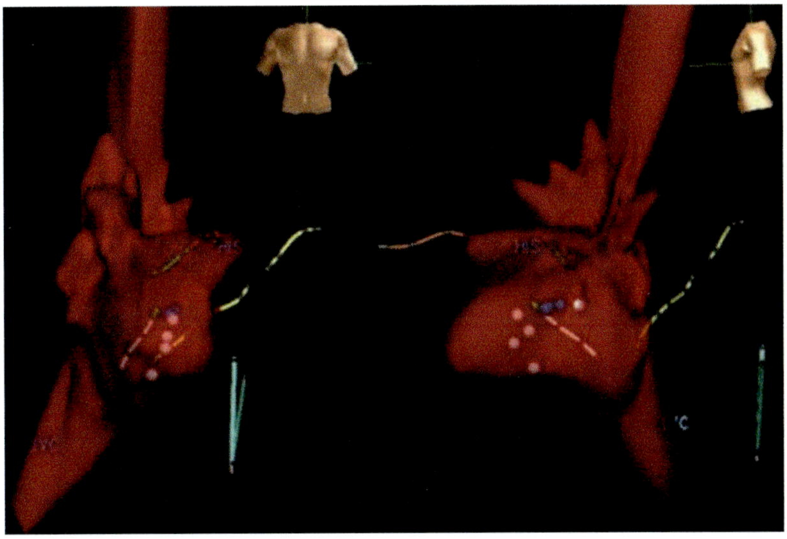

Fig. 6.3 Image detail from Tuzcu's first report of fluoroless ablation using Ensite

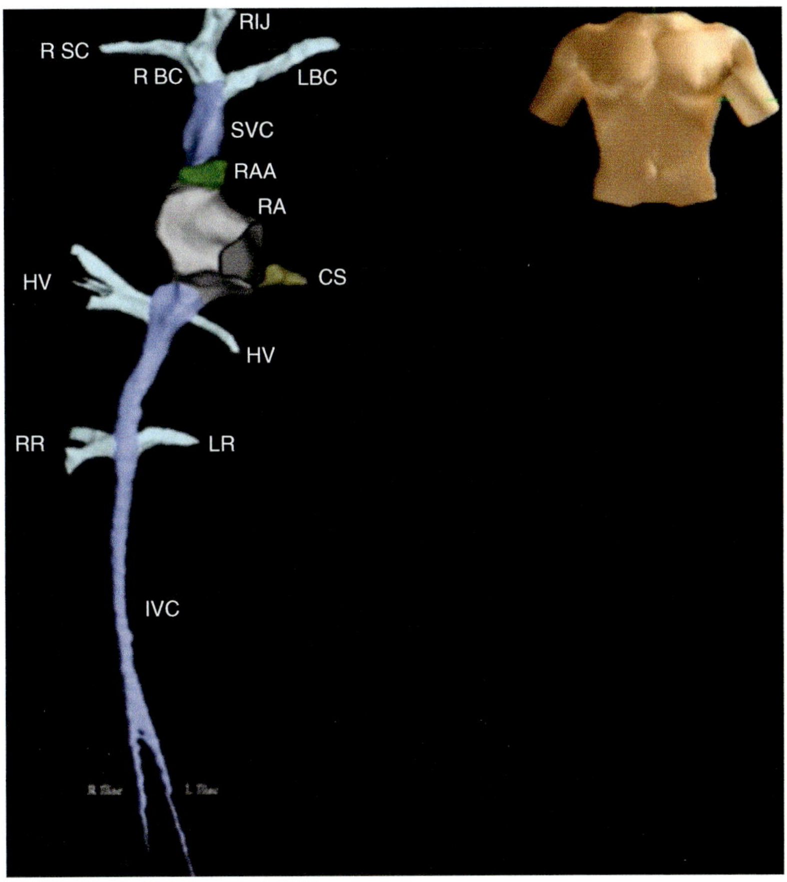

Fig. 6.4 Field of view using Ensite. Catheter can be imaged from femoral sheath to heart

lized the CARTO system, the organizations that were typically leaders and innovators within the profession found themselves handicapped by technology. They had to wait for the availability of CARTO 3 before they could begin the learning process in earnest.

While only a minority of hospitals were utilizing EnSite for fluoroless procedures, many more hospitals and patients benefited from the experience. The attention being paid to fluoroless procedures with EnSite attracted a new interest in ways to minimize radiation exposure. Those institutions that did not use EnSite began to look at ways to decrease fluoroscopy time and minimize exposure by other means, like altering frame rates, shielding, filtering, and angling of fluoroscopy. Pass et al. were able to decrease radiation exposure by adjusting the fluoro frame rate and consciously being aware of how long the fluoro pedal was activated [26].

In 2009, CARTO 3 was released. It took several years for many centers to transition to the newer system and gain familiarity with its functions. The two major benefits of CARTO 3 were the ability of the system to track nonproprietary catheter electrodes, and to rapidly create a more realistic geometry. Pass' group was one of the first to embrace the new system. They had done much to minimize radiation exposure and raise awareness of radiation doses during the years when their system did not allow a routine fluoroless procedure. In 2014 they published data of procedures with CARTO 3 and were now leading the field in experience with this system [27]. From 2014 through 2017 there was a steady increase in fluoroless procedures with CARTO 3 [28–44]. Fifteen years after Drago's first publication, institutions now had more access to functional three-dimensional mapping tools, and the era of fully fluoroless procedures can now advance more rapidly.

Learning Curve of the Physician

Just as there was an evolution in the technology of three-dimensional mapping, there will also be an evolution in the performing physician's technical skills. Knowledge of the experiences of other physicians can accelerate the pace at which one becomes proficient in these new procedures.

If one has little or no experience with 3D mapping systems, then the first step will be to gain familiarity with how the data is acquired and presented. Fluoroscopy allows for very little image control. The image is always in black and white. There are a few levels of magnification available. There is a broad, but not unlimited, range of angles to view from. And there is only minimal control over image quality. Imaging is not continuous, but rather requires activating the fluoro pedal when catheters need to be seen. With 3D mapping, there is far greater flexibility in data presentation. The images are always in color. The color palate is extensive, and broadly programmable to the operator's taste.

The amount of information represented on the screen is entirely of the operator's choosing, from sparse to exquisitely detailed. On one extreme, some labs will mark a catheter at the His location and then in the coronary sinus, and use that as their entire geometry for ablation of AVNRT. While quite minimalistic, it does provide adequate location information, and takes only seconds to generate the image. At the other end of the spectrum, one can import 3D MRI or CT images and "fuse" the images with the 3D mapping system data, thereby creating a minutely detailed geometry. Most EP labs fall somewhere in between the extremes. Our own typical approach is to draw SVC, IVC, right atrium, tricuspid valve, and coronary sinus. That is sufficient for the majority of cases, but more can be added to it if needed.

The geometry and catheters can be viewed from infinite angles and infinite range of magnification. The walls of the geometry can be displayed as transparent, translucent, or opaque. The walls can be "peeled" back to view inside a chamber. Areas of special interest can be marked for later reference. Areas of low voltage, representing scar tissue, can be drawn in. All of the imaging data is visible continuously, in real time, without the need to step on a fluoroscopy pedal. There are some limitations with certain important structures with no visibility on 3D mapping, like implanted pacing or defibrillator leads, and artificial valves. Also, the shaft of the catheter is not visible, only the location of the electrodes. How much geometrical information is acquired is user dependent. The length of time to draw that geometry will depend on experience. To draw our typical amount of geometry mentioned above, it takes an average of 11 min from the time of the first sheath placement until geometry is complete. In our first 30 patients without fluoro, it took an average of 31 min, so we have trimmed off 20 min, but we had over 2 years' experience with the 3D system before we started doing procedures without fluoro. One should expect that geometry creation will be clumsy at first, but usually within a few months it will be a fairly seamless process.

Once a comfort level has been established with drawing basic geometry and manipulating catheters within it, approximately 70% of SVT cases will be ablatable without fluoroscopy. Atrial flutter, AVNRT, and right-sided accessory pathways can all be addressed with that amount of anatomic detail. Ablating typical atrial flutter involves placing a multipole catheter from the coronary sinus across the tricuspid isthmus, creating a line of lesions through the isthmus, and documenting bidirectional block across the isthmus. All of that is easily done with fluoroscopy. Once one is comfortable with the 3D mapping system, they will be equally comfortable to perform the same tasks without fluoroscopy. A report by Macias et al. compared EnSite and CARTO 3 for this ablation procedure [29]. The group was already accustomed to using EnSite for fluoroless ablation of atrial flutter before they began trialing CARTO 3. In their report, they compared their first 20 EnSite atrial flutter ablations with their most recent 20 EnSite atrial flutter ablations, and then compared their first 20 CARTO 3 atrial flutter ablations. They demonstrated their learning curve with EnSite, noting that the procedure times and fluoro times improved from early cases to late cases. Also, the number of procedures requiring any fluoroscopy improved with time. In their early experience, 85% of cases were completed without fluoro. In their later experience, 95% of cases were fluoroless. Interestingly, their experience from their first 20 cases using CARTO 3 was very similar to their later experience with EnSite. The procedure times and fluoro times were better than their initial experience using EnSite. This suggests that a large part of the learning curve for fluoroless procedures will translate between systems (Table 6.1). Once an EP lab has gained a comfort level of avoiding fluoroscopy with one system, the learning curve for another system will likely be accelerated.

Supraventricular tachycardia due to AVNRT is another rhythm that should be easily ablated

Table 6.1 Catheter ablation procedure

	Group A CARTO® 3	Group B Initial EnSite-NavX™	Group C Late EnSite-NavX™	*P*
Initial AFI, *n* (%)	9 (45)	7 (35)	10 (50)	0.62
AF, *n* (%)	4 (20)	9 (45)	7 (35)	0.24
Two DC, *n* (%)	2 (10)	8 (40)	0 (0)	0.002
3D RA, *n* (%)	18 (90)	18 (90)	0 (0)	<0.001
Activation map, *n* (%)	10 (50)	0 (0)	0 (0)	<0.001
Success, *n* (%)	19 (95)	20 (100)	20 (100)	0.36
Complications, *n* (%)	0 (0)	1 (5)	0	0.36
Fluoroscopy, *n* (%)	2 (10)	3 (15)	1 (5)	0.57
Procedure times, min				
Fluoroscopy	0.33 ± 1.3	4.1 ± 12.5	0.08 ± 0.35	ns
RF	13.7 ± 10	15.5 ± 16	19.4 ± 14.3	ns
Total duration	158 ± 54	147 ± 46	123 ± 37[a]	
Diagnostic	89 ± 35	82 ± 31	50 ± 23[b]	
Ablation	66 ± 27	65 ± 32	73 ± 32	ns
Recurrence, *n* (%)	1 (5.2)	0 (0)	1 (5)	0.57

AF atrial fibrillation, *AFL* atrial flutter, *DC* diagnostic catheters, *3D RA* three-dimensional reconstruction of right atrium, *RF* radiofrequency

[a] $P = 0.05$ Group C versus Group A

[b] $P < 0.01$ Group C versus Groups A and B

Table 6.2 Procedural and follow-up data of the different arrhythmias' ablations over the three periods

	Period 1	Period 2	Period 3	*P*
AVNRT				
Fluoroscopy time (min)	13 ± 7	3 ± 4	1 ± 2	<0.001
Complications	0%	0.5%	0%	ns
2-year recurrence	3%	2%	2%	ns
WPW/AVRT				
Fluoroscopy time (min)	18 ± 11	11 ± 8	4 ± 4	<0.001
Complications	1%	0%	0%	ns
2-year recurrence	0%	1%	1%	ns
AT				
Fluoroscopy time (min)	8 ± 5	6 ± 4	2 ± 2	<0.001
Complications	1%	0%	1%	ns
2-year recurrence	7%	12%	9%	ns
FLU				
Fluoroscopy time (min)	9 ± 6	8 ± 6	1 ± 2	<0.001
Complications	0%	0%	1%	ns
2-year recurrence	12%	8%	11%	ns
AF				
Fluoroscopy time (min)	31 ± 17	19 ± 14	9 ± 9	<0.001
Complications	7%	4%	3%	0.03
2-year recurrence	42%	39%	37%	ns

without fluoroscopy. Koch's triangle is readily defined without fluoroscopy. The His electrogram can be recorded and labeled. The coronary sinus can be cannulated, and the tricuspid annulus can be identified. Whether one uses radiofrequency (RF) energy or cryoenergy, the approach is simple. However, the CARTO system still does not allow for simple use of cryoenergy due to proprietary catheter issues. There are ways to work around it [28] and Pass' group defined a way to "trick" CARTO to allow for cryoablation [38]. But, if your EP lab is one that primarily uses cryoenergy when ablating on the atrial septum, you would be best served by the EnSite system. One of the benefits of either 3D mapping system is that the catheter can be seen continuously. This is of great value when working close to the AV node or His bundle. Solimene et al. reported their fluoroscopy use from a 6-year period. In that timeframe, they performed 433 ablations for AVNRT. They divided the period into three segments of 2 years each. They compared fluoroscopy times for each period. They used CARTO as the primary tool, but also used EnSite at times. Their fluoroscopy time averaged 13 ± 7 min in the early period, and 1 ± 2 min in the late period ($P < 0.001$). They found similar results for all of the arrhythmias studied (Table 6.2) [33].

Clark and colleagues published results of the use of EnSite and cryoablation for AVNRT ablation in a pediatric lab [20]. There were 27 patients in the early and 35 patients in the late period. There was no fluoro used for either group. Success and complications did not differ between groups. There was a 20% decrease in procedure time between early and late groups ($P < 0.01$). Both of these studies demonstrate a learning curve with fluoroless procedures. Solimene concludes: "One of the most important factors implied in the fluoroscopy reduction is probably the operator experience. In our series all operators showed a significant reduction in the use of fluoroscopy, regardless their skill level, experience, learning curve, and preference."

In addition to right-sided tachycardia mechanisms, left-sided accessory pathways with a PFO can be ablated without further geometry creation. However, left-sided pathways without a PFO will require further anatomic detail to address. The options are retrograde arterial, or transseptal puncture. Retrograde arterial is a fairly straightforward process, and is essentially the same as with fluoroscopy. Transseptal puncture, however, will require additional tools to accomplish. This could be either intracardiac echo (ICE) or transesophageal echo (TEE). Ferguson et al. were the first to report the use of ICE to eliminate fluoroscopy during transseptal puncture [13]. They used rotational ICE through a deflectable sheath to perform double-transseptal puncture. In 19 of 21 patients they were able to complete the ablation without fluoroscopy. There were no procedure-related complications. Reddy et al. reported similar results using nonrotational ICE and single-transseptal puncture [15]. In 20/20 patients, they completed the procedure without fluoroscopy. Figure 6.5 shows the imaging detail related to that procedure. There were no complications. ICE imaging does not require a second operator, and therefore is more time efficient. However, in smaller patients, vascular access can be an issue. For that reason, we have adopted an approach of TEE for transseptal puncture. That process is described in more detail in the pediatric chapter of this textbook, or in the original manuscript [12]. As a means of expediting the procedure, we have added to the TEE the use of the VisionWire guidewire (Biotronik, Inc.). This allows positioning of the transseptal sheath and dilator within the fossa, without the use of TEE.

Once an operator becomes proficient at drawing geometry and performing transseptal puncture

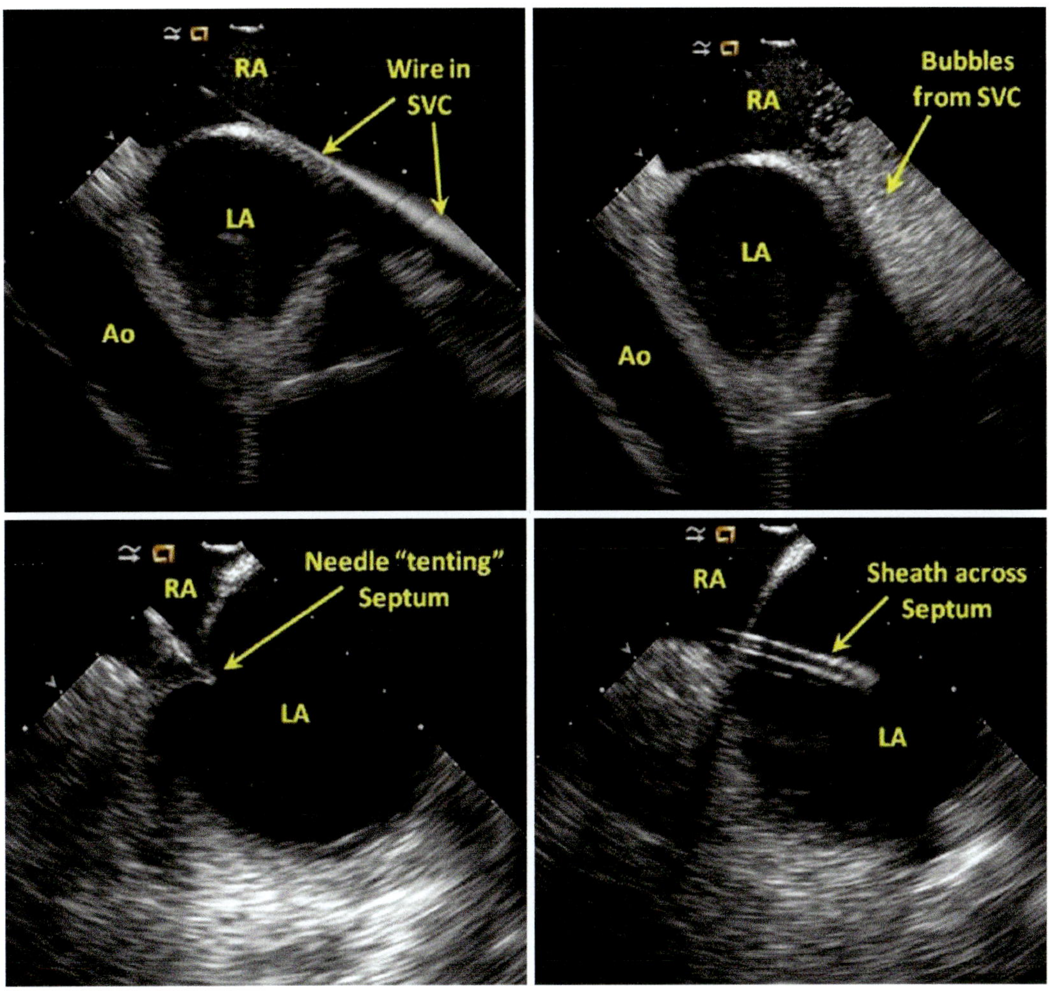

Fig. 6.5 Echo images for transseptal puncture, obtained with ICE

without fluoro, the majority of arrhythmias can be treated without radiation exposure. The hurdles remaining beyond that will likely be related to ablation of atrial fibrillation, and ventricular tachycardia. Atrial fibrillation requires transseptal puncture, but also requires more detailed anatomy of the left atrium. It is possible to spend the time drawing the left atrial anatomy with the 3D mapping system, but the systems also allow integration with other imaging modalities. Three-dimensional MRI or CT images can be imported into the system and linked via identifying fiducial points during geometry creation. This allows extremely detailed left atrial geometry without an exhaustive amount of time to create it. CARTOSound can also help with creating extensive anatomy by incorporating ICE images (Fig. 6.6).

Finally, VT ablation is burdened by the fact that long sheaths are often needed for the procedure, but not visible on 3D mapping systems. As discussed in the pediatric chapter of this textbook, electrode distortion can be used as a surrogate to identify the location of the tip of a sheath. This technique can often allow completion of a procedure without fluoroscopy. If all of the abovementioned techniques are employed, fluoroscopy is rarely needed, either in children [45] or adults [46–48]. Razminia published his group's experience of a completely no-fluoro approach to all arrhythmias [49]. In 500 consecutive patients, they performed ablation for 186 atrial fibrillation, 188 atrial flutter, 79 AVNRT, 111 focal atrial tachycardia, 30 ventricular ectopy, and 31 accessory pathways. Despite the variety of arrhythmias presenting for treatment, they used fluoroscopy only once in the 500 patients. This study represents the extreme of what can be accomplished with the current technology. However, the technology is still in its infancy. Many improvements can be made to optimize utilization of the technology. As those technological improvements emanate, results like Razminia's will become the routine, instead of the extreme.

Committed electrophysiologists and staff are essential to endure the learning curve to minimize radiation exposure and perform consistently fluoroless ablations. As more labs become comfortable with the procedure, more tools will become available to make the process easier. Eventually, fluoroscopy will be phased out. Figure 6.7 shows a graphic trend of the author's radiation badge readings over a 10-year period surrounding the transition to a fluoroless approach.

There have been tremendous advances in fluoroless ablation over the last 15 years, both in physician skill and technological improvements. As the tools available continue to improve, and physicians

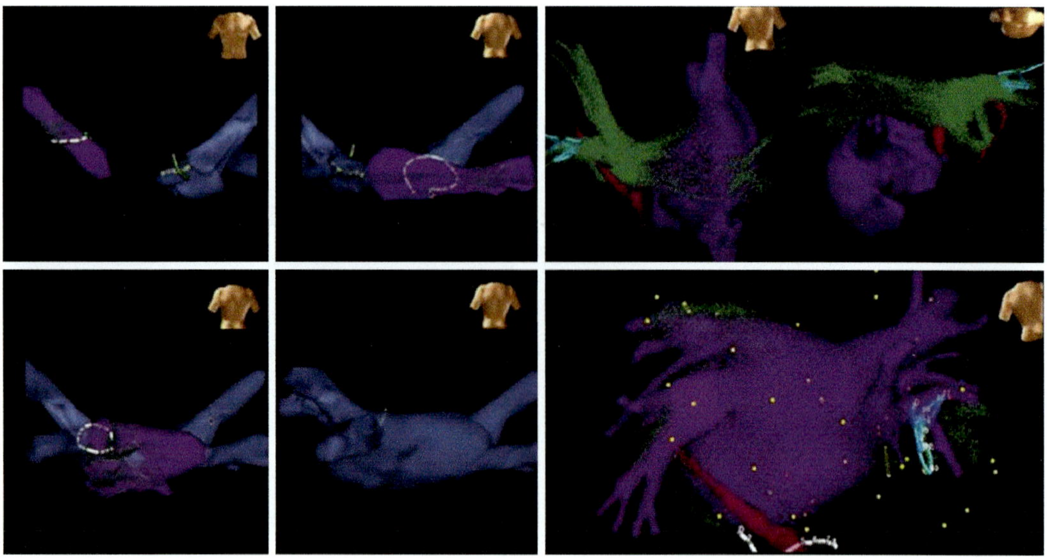

Fig. 6.6 Left atrial geometry created by fusing 3D CT image with Ensite

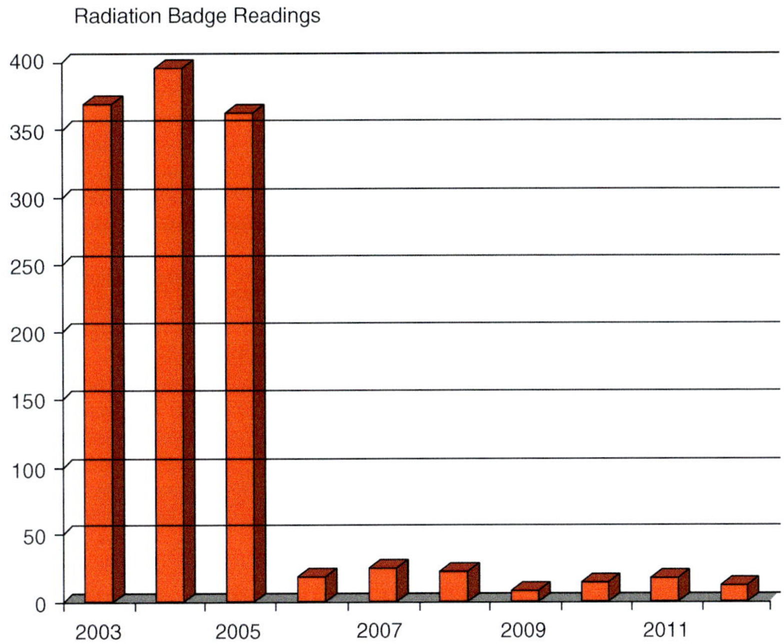

Fig. 6.7 Graphic display of author's radiation badge readings over 10-year period encompassing transition time from fluoroscopy to 3D mapping

continue to gain experience, there will be less need for radiation. By the year 2030, fluoroscopy use for catheter ablation will be mostly of historical interest. By then, the traditional, fluoroscopically based EP lab may also have become obsolete [50].

References

1. Khongphatthanayothin A, Kosar E, Nademanee K. Nonfluoroscopic three-dimensional mapping for arrhythmia ablation: tool or toy? J Cardiovasc Electrophysiol. 2000;11(3):239–43.
2. Schauer DA, Linton OW. NCRP report no. 160, ionizing radiation exposure of the population of the United States, medical exposure—are we doing less with more, and is there a role for health physicists? Health Phys. 2009;97(1):1–5.
3. Limacher MC, Douglas PS, Germano G, et al. ACC expert consensus document. Radiation safety in the practice of cardiology. American College of Cardiology. J Am Coll Cardiol. 1998;31(4):892–913.
4. Roguin A, Goldstein J, Bar O, Goldstein JA. Brain and neck tumors among physicians performing interventional procedures. Am J Cardiol. 2013;111(9):1368–72.
5. Goldstein JA, Balter S, Cowley M, Hodgson J, Klein LW. Interventional Committee of the Society of Cardiovascular Interventions. Occupational hazards of interventional cardiologists: prevalence of orthopedic health problems in contemporary practice. Catheter Cardiovasc Interv. 2004;63(4):407–11.
6. Smilowitz NR, Balter S, Weisz G. Occupational hazards of interventional cardiology. Cardiovasc Revasc Med. 2013;14(4):223–8.
7. Klein LW, Tra Y, Garratt KN, et al. Occupational health hazards of interventional cardiologists in the current decade: results of the 2014 SCAI membership survey. Catheter Cardiovasc Interv. 2015;86(5):913–24.
8. Worley SJ. Use of a real-time three-dimensional magnetic navigation system for radiofrequency ablation of accessory pathways. Pacing Clin Electrophysiol. 1998;21(8):1636–45.
9. Drago F, Silvetti MS, Di Pino A, Grutter G, Bevilacqua M, Leibovich S. Exclusion of fluoroscopy during ablation treatment of right accessory pathway in children. J Cardiovasc Electrophysiol. 2002;13(8):778–82.
10. Tuzcu V. A nonfluoroscopic approach for electrophysiology and catheter ablation procedures using a three-dimensional navigation system. Pacing Clin Electrophysiol. 2007;30(4):519–25.
11. Smith G, Clark JM. Elimination of fluoroscopy use in a pediatric electrophysiology laboratory utilizing three-dimensional mapping. Pacing Clin Electrophysiol. 2007;30(4):510–8.
12. Clark J, Bockoven JR, Lane J, Patel CR, Smith G. Use of three-dimensional catheter guidance and transesophageal echocardiography to eliminate fluoroscopy in catheter ablation of left-sided accessory pathways. Pacing Clin Electrophysiol. 2008;31(3):283–9.
13. Ferguson JD, Helms A, Mangrum JM, et al. Catheter ablation of atrial fibrillation without fluoroscopy using intracardiac echocardiography and electroanatomic mapping. Circ Arrhythm Electrophysiol. 2009;2(6):611–9.

14. Pachon M, Arias MA, Castellanos E, Puchol A. No fluoroscopy for cavotricuspid isthmus-dependent right atrial flutter ablation. Heart Rhythm. 2009;6(3):433–4.
15. Reddy VY, Morales G, Ahmed H, et al. Catheter ablation of atrial fibrillation without the use of fluoroscopy. Heart Rhythm. 2010;7(11):1644–53.
16. Miyamoto K, Tsuchiya T, Narita S, et al. Radiofrequency catheter ablation of ventricular tachyarrhythmia under navigation using EnSite array. Circ J. 2010;74(7):1322–31.
17. Von Bergen NH, Bansal S, Gingerich J, Law IH. Nonfluoroscopic and radiation-limited ablation of ventricular arrhythmias in children and young adults: a case series. Pediatr Cardiol. 2011;32(6):743–7.
18. Casella M, Pelargonio G, Dello Russo A, et al. "Near-zero" fluoroscopic exposure in supraventricular arrhythmia ablation using the EnSite NavX mapping system: personal experience and review of the literature. J Interv Card Electrophysiol. 2011;31(2):109–18.
19. Alvarez M, Tercedor L, Almansa I, et al. Safety and feasibility of catheter ablation for atrioventricular nodal re-entrant tachycardia without fluoroscopic guidance. Heart Rhythm. 2009;6(12):1714–20.
20. Gist K, Tigges C, Smith G, Clark J. Learning curve for zero-fluoroscopy catheter ablation of AVNRT: early versus late experience. Pacing Clin Electrophysiol. 2011;34(3):264–8.
21. Giaccardi M, Chiodi L, Del Rosso A, Colella A. 'Zero' fluoroscopic exposure for ventricular tachycardia ablation in a patient with situs viscerum inversus totalis. Europace. 2012;14(3):449–50.
22. Wan G, Shannon KM, Moore JP. Factors associated with fluoroscopy exposure during pediatric catheter ablation utilizing electroanatomical mapping. J Interv Card Electrophysiol. 2012;35(2):235–42.
23. Tuzcu V. Significant reduction of fluoroscopy in pediatric catheter ablation procedures: long-term experience from a single center. Pacing Clin Electrophysiol. 2012;35(9):1067–73.
24. Razminia M, Manankil MF, Eryazici PL, et al. Nonfluoroscopic catheter ablation of cardiac arrhythmias in adults: feasibility, safety, and efficacy. J Cardiovasc Electrophysiol. 2012;23(10):1078–86.
25. Ergul Y, Tola HT, Kiplapinar N, Akdeniz C, Saygi M, Tuzcu V. Cryoablation of anteroseptal accessory pathways in children with limited fluoroscopy exposure. Pediatr Cardiol. 2013;34(4):802–8.
26. Gellis LA, Ceresnak SR, Gates GJ, Nappo L, Pass RH. Reducing patient radiation dosage during pediatric SVT ablations using an "ALARA" radiation reduction protocol in the modern fluoroscopic era. Pacing Clin Electrophysiol. 2013;36(6):688–94.
27. Pass RH, Gates GG, Gellis LA, Nappo L, Ceresnak SR. Reducing patient radiation exposure during paediatric SVT ablations: use of CARTO(R) 3 in concert with "ALARA" principles profoundly lowers total dose. Cardiol Young. 2015;25(5):963–8.
28. Scaglione M, Ebrille E, Caponi D, et al. Single center experience of fluoroless AVNRT ablation guided by electroanatomic reconstruction in children and adolescents. Pacing Clin Electrophysiol. 2013;36(12):1460–7.
29. Macias R, Uribe I, Tercedor L, Jimenez-Jaimez J, Barrio T, Alvarez M. A zero-fluoroscopy approach to cavotricuspid isthmus catheter ablation: comparative analysis of two electroanatomical mapping systems. Pacing Clin Electrophysiol. 2014;37(8):1029–37.
30. Christoph M, Wunderlich C, Moebius S, et al. Fluoroscopy integrated 3D mapping significantly reduces radiation exposure during ablation for a wide spectrum of cardiac arrhythmias. Europace. 2015;17(6):928–37.
31. Scaglione M, Ebrille E, Caponi D, et al. Zero-fluoroscopy ablation of accessory pathways in children and adolescents: CARTO3 electroanatomic mapping combined with RF and cryoenergy. Pacing Clin Electrophysiol. 2015;38(6):675–81.
32. Bulava A, Hanis J, Eisenberger M. Catheter ablation of atrial fibrillation using zero-fluoroscopy technique: a randomized trial. Pacing Clin Electrophysiol. 2015;38(7):797–806.
33. Solimene F, Donnici G, Shopova G, et al. Trends in fluoroscopy time during radiofrequency catheter ablation of supraventricular tachycardias. Int J Cardiol. 2016;202:124–5.
34. Huo Y, Christoph M, Forkmann M, et al. Reduction of radiation exposure during atrial fibrillation ablation using a novel fluoroscopy image integrated 3-dimensional electroanatomic mapping system: a prospective, randomized, single-blind, and controlled study. Heart Rhythm. 2015;12(9):1945–55.
35. Montgomery JAEC. Zero-fluoroscopy intracardiac echocardiography-guided ablation of atrial fibrillation using a single-catheter technique. J Innov Card Rhythm Manag. 2015;6:2209–15.
36. Ceresnak SR, Nappo L, Janson CM, Pass RH. Tricking CARTO: cryoablation of supraventricular tachycardia in children with minimal radiation exposure using the CARTO3 system. Pacing Clin Electrophysiol. 2016;39(1):36–41.
37. Raju H, Whitaker J, Taylor C, Wright M. Electroanatomic mapping and transoesophageal echocardiography for near zero fluoroscopy during complex left atrial ablation. Heart Lung Circ. 2016;25(7):652–60.
38. Clark BC, Sumihara K, McCarter R, Berul CI, Moak JP. Getting to zero: impact of electroanatomical mapping on fluoroscopy use in pediatric catheter ablation. J Interv Card Electrophysiol. 2016;46(2):183–9.
39. Kuhne M, Knecht S, Muhl A, et al. Fluoroscopy-free pulmonary vein isolation in patients with atrial fibrillation and a patent foramen ovale using solely an electroanatomic mapping system. PLoS One. 2016;11(1):e0148059.
40. Nagaraju L, Menon D, Aziz PF. Use of 3D electroanatomical navigation (CARTO-3) to minimize or eliminate fluoroscopy use in the ablation of pediatric supraventricular tachyarrhythmias. Pacing Clin Electrophysiol. 2016;39(6):574–80.

41. Cano O, Andres A, Osca J, et al. Safety and feasibility of a minimally fluoroscopic approach for ventricular tachycardia ablation in patients with structural heart disease: Influence of the ventricular tachycardia substrate. Circ Arrhythm Electrophysiol. 2016;9(2):e003706.
42. Lerman BB, Markowitz SM, Liu CF, Thomas G, Ip JE, Cheung JW. Fluoroless catheter ablation of atrial fibrillation. Heart Rhythm. 2017;14(6):928–34.
43. McCauley MD, Patel N, Greenberg SJ, Molina-Razavi JE, Safavi-Naeini P, Razavi M. Fluoroscopy-free atrial transseptal puncture. Eur J Arrhthymia Electrophysiol. 2016;2(2):57–61.
44. Clark BC, Sumihara K, Berul CI, Moak JP. Off the pedal: fluoroless transseptal puncture in pediatric supraventricular tachycardia ablation. Pacing Clin Electrophysiol. 2017;40(11):1254–9.
45. Jan M, Zizek D, Rupar K, et al. Fluoroless catheter ablation of various right and left sided supraventricular tachycardias in children and adolescents. Int J Cardiovasc Imaging. 2016;32(11):1609–16.
46. Fernandez-Gomez JM, Morina-Vazquez P, Morales Edel R, Venegas-Gamero J, Barba-Pichardo R, Carranza MH. Exclusion of fluoroscopy use in catheter ablation procedures: six years of experience at a single center. J Cardiovasc Electrophysiol. 2014;25(6):638–44.
47. Seizer P, Bucher V, Frische C, et al. Efficacy and safety of zero-fluoroscopy ablation for supraventricular tachycardias. use of optional contact force measurement for zero-fluoroscopy ablation in a clinical routine setting. Herz. 2016;41(3):241–5.
48. Sanchez JM, Yanics MA, Wilson P, Doshi A, Kurian T, Pieper S. Fluoroless catheter ablation in adults: a single center experience. J Interv Card Electrophysiol. 2016;45(2):199–207.
49. Razminia M, Willoughby MC, Demo H, et al. Fluoroless catheter ablation of cardiac arrhythmias: a 5-year experience. Pacing Clin Electrophysiol. 2017;40(4):425–33.
50. Bigelow AM, Smith PC, Timberlake DT, et al. Procedural outcomes of fluoroless catheter ablation outside the traditional catheterization lab. Europace. 2017;19(8):1378–84.

7 AV Nodal Reentrant Tachycardia Ablation Without Fluoroscopy

Miguel Alvarez Lopez, María Emilce Trucco, and Félix Ayala-Paredes

Introduction

The AV node is a complex structure, where in normal AV nodal physiology each electrical impulse coming from the sinus node is conducted with decremental properties, using the anterior (or superior) aspect of the AV node, the so-called fast pathway (FP) which translates in a surface normal PR interval between 120 and 200 ms, whereas during typical AVNRT it is necessary another arm to complete the circuit, the so-called slow pathway (SP), located for most of the patients, at the posterior (inferior) aspect of the AV node, near the ostium of the coronary sinus; the normal sequence is then inverted, downward conduction proceeds by the SP (long PR) as the FP is usually blocked by an atrial premature beat (more premature than the FP's effective refractory period—ERP), and if the SP conducts slowly enough to allow the recovery of the FP, the impulsion can at the same time, continue to the ventricle, and return to the atrium by the recovered FP to start the reentry.

AVNRT is the most frequent paroxysmal supraventricular tachycardias, and usually starts between 20 and 40 years old and is more prevalent in women. In order to prevent the AVNRT initiation, it is necessary to eliminate or at least modify one of the reentry arms, usually the SP.

Anatomy, Normal and Abnormal Physiology

The AV node is an endocardial structure, localized in the right interatrial septum at the anterosuperior portion of the Koch's triangle. In the majority of the cases the right coronary artery irrigates this structure. We can associate the FP close to the His recording, as the bundle of His is the only structure we can identify with our catheters, and usually a catheter placed in that region is used as a marker to prevent the damage of the His bundle (and the AV node backward and downward close by). However, the first retrograde activation during typical AVNRT does not occur at the His level but a halfway between the His and the roof of the coronary sinus: in the right anterior oblique (RAO) incidence, posterior to the tendon of Todaro (electrical barrier)

M. A. Lopez
Cardiology Service, Arrhythmia Unit, Hospital Universitario Virgen de las Nieves, Granada, Spain
e-mail: Miguel.alvarez.sspa@juntadeadalucia.es

M. E. Trucco
Department of Cardiology, Arrhythmia Unit, Hospital Universitari Dr. Josep Trueta, Girona, Spain
e-mail: metrucco.girona.ics@gencat.cat

F. Ayala-Paredes (✉)
Division of Cardiology, Centre Hospitalier Universitaire de Sherbrooke, Sherbrooke, Canada
e-mail: felix.ayala-paredes@usherbrooke.ca

R. Proietti et al. (eds.), *Cardiac Electrophysiology Without Fluoroscopy*,
https://doi.org/10.1007/978-3-030-16992-3_7

and in left anterior oblique (LAO) more in the left side of the septum. The SP shows rarely a signal (with the standard 5 mm bipole spacing in most catheters) as clear as the His signal (which is almost always easy to find), the reason why an anatomical-only approach is very frequently used to ablate the SP. If there is only one FP, there could be many SP locations to target, and to maximize security visualization of catheters in many incidences and ideally at all times is a must, when ablation of the SP is decided.

This chapter is not intended to explain electrical properties of the AV node, neither to list all the maneuvers to arrive at the diagnosis of an AVNRT; please refer to excellent EP books or articles for these details. We want to explain how to navigate and ablate without fluoroscopy only, but some few considerations before entering in our matter.

AV nodal response to extra stimuli was described many years ago; the presence of dual physiology is demonstrated by the application of a decremental stimulus after a train of fixed stimuli (for refractory period homogenization). Normal response is when each stimulus increases in the conduction velocity through AV node in a decremental way. When the interval between the stimuli decreases and the AV node response is abrupt (an increment of more than 50 ms), the refractory period of the FP is obtained and the ventricles are depolarized through the SP [1].

Dual physiology is common in as much as half the population, but two other conditions are necessary to start an AVNRT: first, refractory periods of both pathways should be different enough to allow reentry (at the AV node level, both pathways get "slower and old" with age), but the SP in some patients gets older—rarely before the age of 40-, aging faster than the FP, that allows a marked difference of refractory periods, and conduction back through the SP once the FP blocks (refractory periods vary also a lot depending on autonomic influences, but the longer the "window" of refractory periods between the FP and the SP, the easier to start a reentry); second, a premature beat is needed, as premature as able to block in the FP to start reentry using downward conduction over the SP and come back to the atrium by the recovered FP, which, as it conducts faster than the SP, makes the upward conduction so fast that ventricles and atria are activated almost at the same time (this first beat of reentry, when a retrograde P wave is visualized very close to the QRS, is called echo beat); after this first upward beat, the impulse arrives at the SP going downward again at the posterior (inferior) aspect of the AV node, the reentry is established, and the AVNRT starts.

Anatomic and physiologic relationships mentioned above are related to the typical slow-fast AVNRT (FP ERP reached, downward conduction using the SP and upward reentry using the already recovered FP), which accounts for 90% of all AVNRTs encountered in clinical practice; but in some cases this circuit could be inverted: "fast-slow" AVNRT, with the first upward activation arriving at different levels in the coronary sinus before reaching back the atrium; and also some even more rare forms with similar ERPs between both arms (type "slow-slow") and very similar times turning up and down.

In some patients the induction is only found with a medication that alters the refractory periods (usually isoproterenol to accelerate, or beta-blockers [2] or calcium channel blockers to slow it at a point to allow reentry); or after the SP has been damaged by first attempts of ablation; or with a progressive increment of AV conduction times without a clear "jump" (either during progressively shorter S1 train—to test the Wenckebach point—or with mini "jumps" not reaching the 50 ms cutoff); but even in these cases, the ablation in the "slow" pathway region eliminates the AVNRT, confirming that sometimes smaller differences in refractory periods of both arms are enough to sustain the arrhythmia.

In the AVNRT the only necessary element is the AV node (and the perinodal tissue); the atrium and the ventricles may be absent and they are not needed to sustain the arrhythmia. The conduction during tachycardia is concentric (the earliest activation site is central and therefore the coronary sinus activates usually from proximal to distal).

Even if it is not needed, some patients arriving at the emergency room with AVNRT have a troponin measurement, sometimes in the abnormal ranges; as coronary artery disease is rare in young patients, this is just explained by the stretch caused by very fast heart rates: supraventricular tachycardia faster than 190 bpm is more frequently associated with troponin rise [3].

Invasive Treatment of the AVNRT

For acute termination of the arrhythmia carotid sinus massage or Valsalva maneuver [4, 5] is useful. If not responding, in hospital settings IV adenosine is the drug of preference to stop an AVNRT [6].

In our days, most physicians agreed that the only curative treatment to AVNRT is ablation, targeting usually the SP, with over 95% acute success rates, less than 10% recurrences rate, and a low complication rate—complete AV block—ranging from 0% to 1% depending on the type of energy used for ablation.

If drugs are still used to prevent recurrences (beta- or calcium channel blockers), they are merely palliative; most of the young patients would rarely accept a medication for life, and older patients sometimes have a paradoxical response with more frequent episodes (if a SP is slowed too much, the "window" widens for any premature beat to start the arrhythmia [2]) once medication is started.

Ablation is now an easy technique; it has evolved in very few years from surgical ablation [7–9] to direct DC shocks destroying SP and FP at the same time [10–14], radiofrequency ablation [15], selective SP ablation [16–19], and cryoablation [20, 21].

EP Study in Patients with AVNRT

Even with very low complications rate, a good preparation includes discussion of all the options available, and at least 2 or 3 days of all AV-blocking agent discontinuation before the procedure (or 5 half-lives whichever is longer).

As in any medical activity there are multiple ways to approach this type of ablation; usually the more catheters used the more simultaneous information is available, which helps especially at the beginning of a practice; then, when the physician has more experience, less catheters are necessary to obtain the same information, and even if not suggested all of the EP study and ablation for the AVNRT could be done with only one catheter.

Surface EKG helps also to decide how many catheters are needed, as sometimes the diagnosis is so clear that less information is necessary to obtain at the EP study. In the most complete setting four diagnostic catheters are used, one for the right high atrium, one for the His, one for the ventricle, and one for the coronary sinus; all catheters can be inserted using both femoral accesses, but if the coronary sinus is hard to find a superior (jugular, subclavian, or brachial) access could be used. Usually a CS catheter inserted from below allows mapping the roof of the CS, while a catheter inserted from above is useful to map the floor of the CS. Mild sedation is widely used, but for AVNRT the rule is as less as possible, as too much would render the arrhythmia noninducible.

Catheter Positioning Without Fluoroscopy

The most difficult part of all the procedure is catheter positioning, not because of intrinsic difficulty, but just because of a new paradigm needed: to navigate using new tools, intracardiac electrograms (EGMs) at the beginning, then a virtual anatomy created while dragging catheters on the chamber of interest, or even just EGMs and catheter visualization for more advanced users. Please refer to the chapter on catheter placement for details; briefly, the first catheter is advanced gently from the groin through the inferior vena cava (IVC) until atrial EGMs are detected; if advanced too fast the catheter would pass to the superior vena cava (SVC); at the beginning of the experience, measuring the distance from the groin to the chest with the catheter on the outside could help to give an idea on how much the catheter needs to be advanced until the atrium is reached; if IVC valves prevent atrial access, a softer and smaller quadripolar catheter could be used and advanced until atrial signals are seen, and then stiffer catheters' advance becomes easier as valves are now open; in the very beginning, we can leave some "marks" while the first catheter advances, to show the road through the atrium (Fig. 7.1). Once the roving catheter is on the atrium, IVC and SVC are "drawn" rotating the catheter with a gentle curve, followed by the right atrium; since the beginning, simultaneous RAO and LAO views help to orientate the movement of the roving catheter. Tricuspid valve is easily depicted once annotated on places where there are simultaneous atrial and ventricular signals. His bundle is located (and marked) at its usual position, also guided by EGMs; the catheter is then flexed posteriorly and advanced anteriorly to obtain big ventricular signals; then a gentle retraction, clockwise torque, and freeing simultaneously the curve allow the access to the coronary sinus ostium, and the catheter is then advanced to create CS virtual anatomy as far as possible. The other catheters needed are advanced in the same way as described before; depending on the system used, the reference catheter can be switched to the decapolar catheter placed in the CS, if needed. We are ready to start the EP study to prove dual physiology, absence of other mechanisms or substrates, and SVT induction in a standard fashion (Fig. 7.2).

EP Study

Once the catheters are placed and basal measurements are done, we start with decremental atrial—and then ventricular—stimulation (to find the AV and VA Wenckebach point). This simple maneuver sometimes shows a dual-pathway physiology when the AH (PR) prolongs enough to see the P waves coming from the S1 train inscribed before

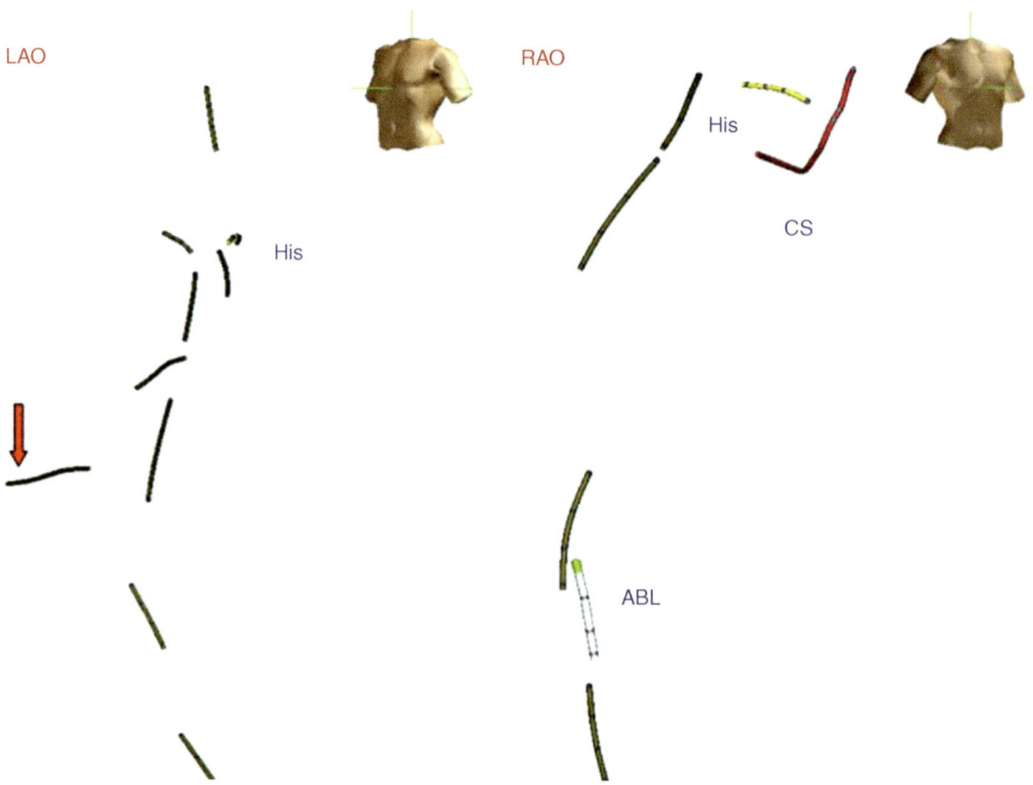

Fig. 7.1 NavX system. On LAO and RAO some "marks" on the pathway on the first catheter introduced are left that allow the other catheters to be placed following the marked "road"; in LAO a right subhepatic vein is marked with the red arrow, to prevent the ablation (ABL) catheter to follow that path. Coronary sinus (CS) is placed from the left brachial vein from above

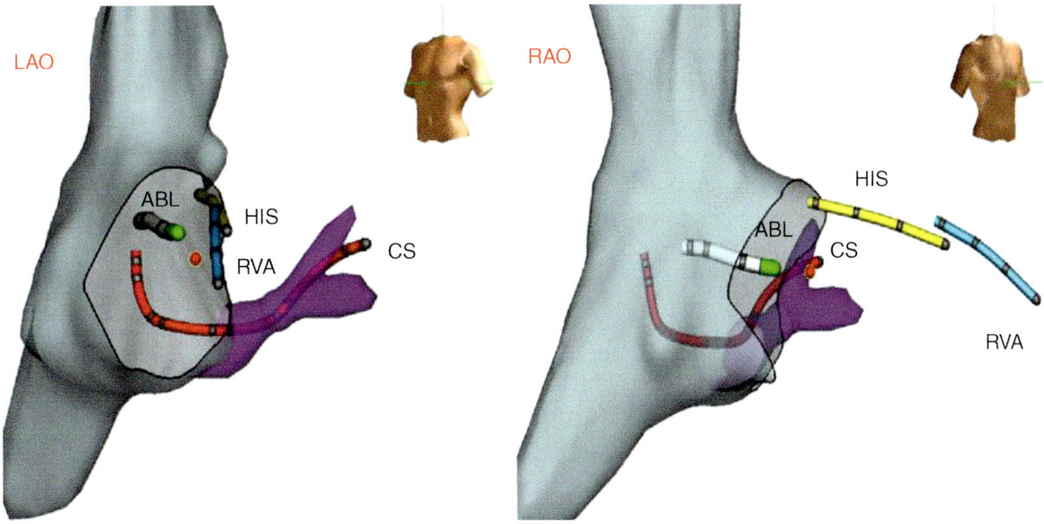

Fig. 7.2 Standard LAO and RAO views in NavX system, showing four catheters: coronary sinus (CS, coming from above, left brachial vein), His, right ventricular apex (RVA), and ablation (ABL) while navigating near the tricuspid valve

the previous QRS; this phenomenon tends to occur just prior to find the Wenckebach point, and in some cases the arrhythmia starts only in this way.

Ventricular programmed stimulation would exclude an accessory pathway if a VA dissociation is observed, or at least the presence of a left-sided accessory pathway when the retrograde conduction is concentric (first atrial activity seen in the His catheter by opposition to the distal coronary sinus recordings). Accessory pathways seldom have decremental properties, so decremental retrograde conduction (with P waves seen later and later) makes an accessory pathway less likely in the differential diagnosis.

Atrial (or ventricular) programmed stimulation (fixed S1 and progressive 10 ms decrement in S2) is highly effective to prove the dual-AV node physiology, when a "jump" of at least 50 ms is found. Conventional S1 trains are used at 600 and 400 ms, but different options could be used: slower if the Wenckebach point is found before 400 ms or faster if isoproterenol is utilized.

If the arrhythmia has not been found yet we can either:

- Revert sedation.
- Increase the number of extra stimuli (S1–S2–S3, etc.) until the atrial ERP is reached before the AV nodal refractory period.
- Use IV isoproterenol (to increase at least 10% in the heart rate) and redo all the atrial and ventricular programmed stimulation protocol.
- Stop isoproterenol and continue induction maneuvers during the "washout" of the drug.
- Change stimulation site (coronary sinus, low atrium).
- Use short-lived beta-blockers (to vary refractory periods and conduction properties in one arm more than in the other).
- If premenopausal female, try to repeat the EP study 2 weeks later in another phase of the hormonal cycle.

Ideally we should be able to induce the AVNRT in a reproducible manner, as to abolish an easily induced arrhythmia is the best success target.

Differential Diagnosis

Very rarely an arrhythmia mechanism is confirmed only with one maneuver; in most of the cases different pieces of information add to a puzzle to confirm or exclude a putative mechanism; even when clear, we should never rely on only one piece of evidence as we can only see what we are expecting to find, and if in our head we have excluded some mechanisms it is very difficult sometimes to then see a clear evidence that the arrhythmia has a different origin from what we expected. Dual-AV nodal physiology and a "jump" seen during programmed stimulation are highly related to the AVNRT, but sometimes for example an accessory pathway (AP) is also needed to conduct upwards and have the arrhythmia sustained. The diagnosis of AVNRT is the sum of exclusion of other possible mechanisms of arrhythmia.

There are simple maneuvers to exclude other mechanisms [22]:

- If during arrhythmia there is no one-to-one relationship between atria and ventricles, an AP is excluded.
- Typical AVNRT conducts with a concentric fashion, with a short HA (VA less than 70 ms), while other forms have a VA superior to 100 ms.
- If we can dissociate (without entrainment) the arrhythmia with brief faster atrial or ventricular trains, we can also eliminate an AP as a mechanism.
- With ventricular stimulation, a short train faster than the arrhythmia with entrainment would show two different patterns: AAV or AV type, the former in atrial tachycardia cases, and the latter in reentrant arrhythmias (AVNRT and AVRT).
- During sinus rhythm, ventricular extra stimuli with progressive shorter intervals provoke a decremental VA conduction, excluding accessory pathways.
- In parahisian pacing without His capture VA increases.
- Difference between VA during ventricular stimulation and VA during tachycardia is >85 ms.
- Ventricular postpacing interval is >115 ms.
- HA during tachycardia is less than HA during ventricular stimulation.
- Finally, in arrhythmia, applying ventricular extra stimuli during refractory His, with advancement of the A signal, proves that an AP is present; and if the arrhythmia stops without an A it proves that the AP participates in the arrhythmia.

Once we have eliminated other mechanisms we can safely start the ablation, as again AVNRT is the diagnosis once other mechanisms have been excluded. When a limited number of catheters are used, we should also change the position of our catheters during the arrhythmia, to confirm that the activation sequence is always septal first (for example, if only a His and a coronary sinus recording are used, we can miss a right atrial tachycardia if one of the catheters is not moved to the right atrium during the arrhythmia, to find finally that right atrium was activated before the His catheter). "Weird" electrophysiological characteristics are in most of the cases a signature that the AV node (AVNRT) is part of the mechanism of the arrhythmia.

Radiofrequency Ablation of the AVNRT Without Fluoroscopy

One of the advantages of using 3D mapping systems is the simultaneous RAO and LAO views; other, multiple and infinite angulations are also possible; catheters are also visualized at all times, increasing safety.

In RAO, we advance the ablation catheter into the ventricle to have more V than A, near and initially downward the coronary ostium region. Even if we have the His catheter showing the FP region (that we should avoid), we recommend, before starting RF, to carefully look for His signals in the ablation catheter, to prevent FP damage and AV block. As the RF catheter tends to move with heartbeats and respiration, we start with RF application as far as possible from the His (FP) region as heat tends to travel wider than the catheter contact region.

Once the area is targeted we give a small clockwise torque to put it as close as possible to the septal area (confirmed by the LAO view) and we can start ablation as inferior as possible (and posterior or caudal/dorsal in the anatomic plane), looking for a big ventricular EGM and a small (and if possible fractionated, approximately relation 1:4 between atrium and ventricle) atrial EGM (if the atrial signal is too big, we can enter in the coronary sinus, and simultaneous LAO confirms this impression; we can then start ablation (20–40 W—using a nonirrigated 4 mm catheter and 15–20 s for each application waiting for a junctional rhythm to appear, which confirms that we are irritating the SP; if so we can continue for another 30–60 s; if not we can advance or retract the catheter by small movements, looking for better EGMs; and if there is no junctional rhythm, we can start moving upward, toward the His catheter (FP), until we consider we are too close (usually less than 1 cm is too close) to the His to safely apply RF). Once a junctional rhythm is obtained we can follow in that region until complete abolition of that automatic rhythm, usually 1–2 min; in each position and before each application we should confirm that the catheter has not displaced to the coronary sinus. Incidences never imagined using fluoroscopy are easily achieved, just rotating our virtual anatomy (Fig. 7.3).

Non-fluoro ablation using 3D mapping systems has multiple benefits to help achieving SP ablation: not only catheters are seen at all times, but also His recordings can be annotated in the virtual anatomy to prevent the ablation catheter to move close (if a big inspiration displaces the catheter too much we can safely stop RF soon); coronary sinus is usually marked with a different color in the virtual anatomy, to help better ascertain when the RF catheter bounces between tricuspid valve and coronary sinus ostium at the time of ablation. We use a light caudal tilt on LAO virtual incidence to allow us better visualize the ablation catheter when ablating in the SP region, and we mark promptly with a different color code the sites with good junctional rhythm. When ablation is applied on the roof of the coronary sinus ostium, we tilt in the opposite direction (cephalic tilt) to be able to visualize the RF catheter and prevent it from approaching to the posterior side of the His region (this image is also helpful when

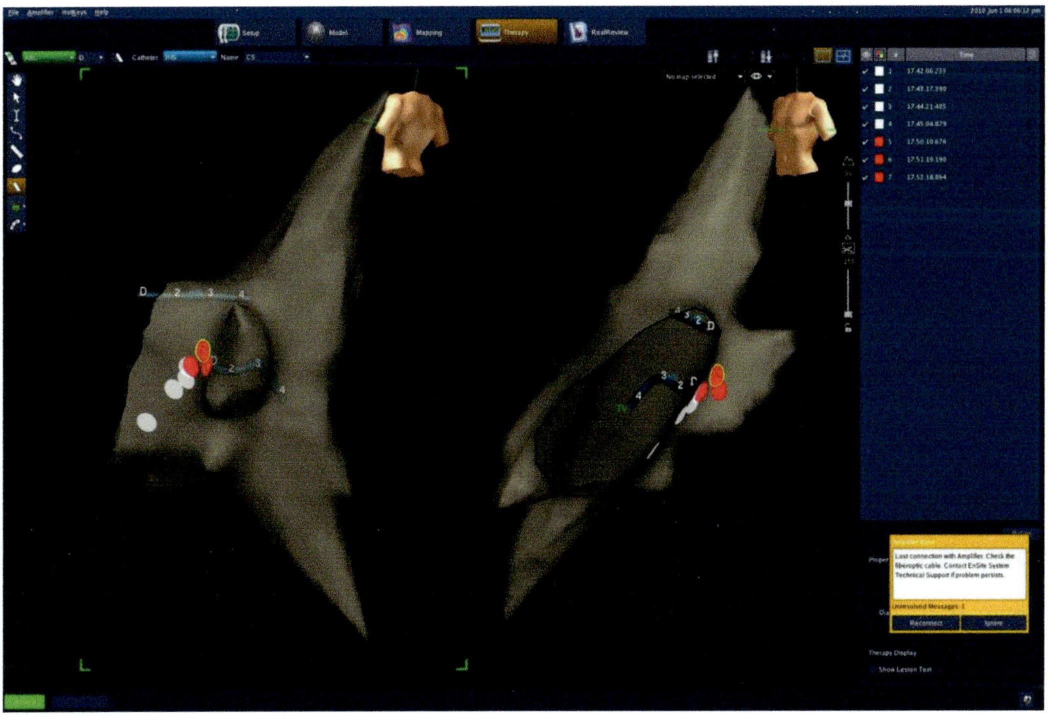

Fig. 7.3 NavX system. Posterior (left panel) and standard LAO incidence (right panel) are used to confirm posterior direction (left panel, near the anterior aspect of the coronary sinus ostium), and septal contact (right panel) while still far from the His catheter (upper catheter)

cryoablation is needed as this is usually the successful area to ablate) [23].

It is important to confirm during RF applications that there is a stable AV relationship (one P followed by one QRS); any single P or QRS should prompt RF immediate cessation. We can also, and once the junctional rhythm has appeared, start pacing the atrium, to monitor 1:1 conduction over the ventricles, especially if we are approaching the His (FP) region.

Once we have obtained a lesion with good junctional rhythm, we should test the result trying to restart the arrhythmia. Once the arrhythmia is no longer inducible we can stop the procedure; minimal endpoint is to prevent the arrhythmia from starting; a better result is obtained if the SP physiology ("jump") persists, but with no or single "echo"; best result is achieved if the SP is completely abolished and no more "jump" is found. Focal lesions are preferred, but with time and experience minimal movements are allowed without stopping RF in order to find the junctional rhythm.

After the effective lesion, it is used (without any evidence found) to wait for a variable time frame (30–60 min) in order to see if the SP "recovers."

Some patients have a giant coronary sinus ostium, with the catheter displacing always into the coronary sinus; this characteristic, as in older patients in whom the "shrinking" of the tendon of Todaro with the age displaces the AV node-His closer to the coronary sinus ostium, diminishes the area available for ablation; and in these cases some applications can be done in the first 2 cm of the coronary sinus (with lower energy 20–30 W settings) in order to find the SP region.

Unfortunately how close we should apply RF near the His is not an exact science either; it depends on age at the time of ablation, severity of symptoms, and energy used, and all these could be summarized as that it comes with experience, and unfortunately experience comes only after having been too close and finished with some AV blocks in some few patients. In order to prevent a complete AV block, we should always try first to target the other putative slow pathways, located always far into the coronary sinus, instead of approaching further and further close to the compact AV node and the His. Rarely SP is found only in the left side and transseptal approach is needed to find them (same considerations, big "V" and small and

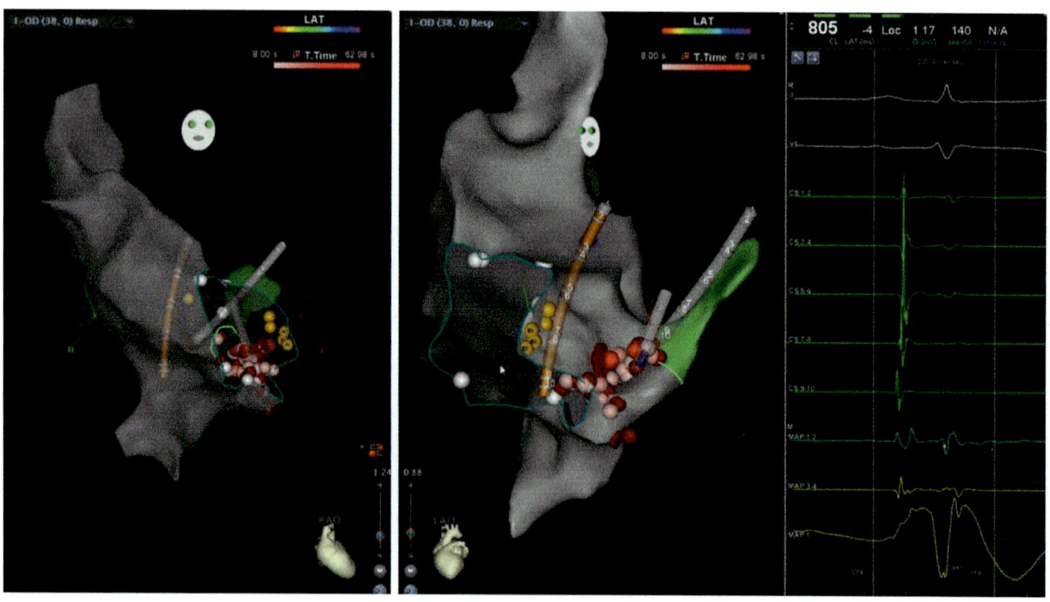

Fig. 7.4 Carto 3 system. RAO (left panel) and LAO (right panel) views; after some applications on the right side (including in the first centimeters of the coronary sinus), and having AVNRT still inducible, a patent foramen ovale (PFO) allows access to the left atrium, where successful site is found in the posteroseptal mitral annulus

fractionated "A" signals in the posterior aspect of the mitral valve) (Fig. 7.4).

Very rarely, a complete AV block is obtained with RF when we ablate into or very near the posterior aspect of coronary sinus ostium (far from the His region and with no His potentials); the mechanism invoked is the mechanical damage of the AV node artery, with an ischemic AV block, as wherever the origin of this artery there is no dual irrigation of the AV node and if this terminal artery is occluded an AV block could follow; the other possibility is the downward displacement of the compact AV node, as it occurs in aging patients.

To help the non-fluoroscopic ablation, we did a small study using the Biosense Carto-3 in 39 patients where we tagged all His potentials found in the virtual anatomy; in all patients His signals were recorded in more than a single area, with a mean His area of 1.44 cm^2; mean distances from the closer effective RF ablation lesion to caudal and cephalic His recordings were 15.9 and 25.5 mm (range for caudal to RF of 4.7–31.5 mm and for cephalic to RF 10.9–39.9 mm). We had one complete intraprocedural AV block, a patient with incessant AVNRT (after first RF applications); as we applied going higher, we did not realize that the closest RF lesion was delivered at 6 mm from the most caudal His, but at 26.9 mm from the upper His recording (the usual position of a single quadripolar catheter). This case depicted sometimes how close FP can be found to the places judged "safe" for fluoroscopy. No transient or complete AV block was found in lesions applied at least 10 mm far (caudal) from the lowest His recording in more than 200 patients done to date; so we can say that 10 mm far from the lowest His recorded is probably a safe window to apply RF, but that lower or caudal His is impossible to be marked in a fluoroscopy environment system, another advantage of using 3D mapping systems (Fig. 7.5a, b) [24].

We should also keep in mind that usually, going upwards (approaching the His catheter) even if it is the most tempting idea (especially when we obtain good junctional rhythms all the way up—which is easy to understand as there is slow pathway all the way up) once a good junctional rhythm is obtained in a lower position,

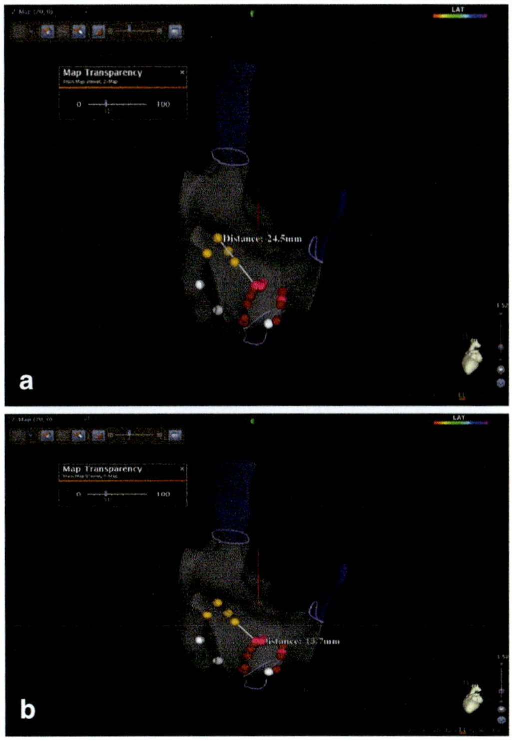

Fig. 7.5 Carto 3 system. LAO for both figures. (**a**) Shows the distance between successful ablation sites and the highest His recorded (usually where a His catheter sits, a comfortable 24.5 mm); (**b**) shows that His signals can be recorded far down, and that the real distance was 13.7 mm from the successful RF site and lowest His recorded

that SP is already eliminated, and if there is still AVRNT induced it uses another SP, and then it is rewarding to try to go into the coronary sinus or to the left side, to try to safely ablate the SP responsible of the tachycardia. Yes we can destroy those other SP also burning up in the septum, as they should to close the circuit, to arrive to the compact AV node, but the price to pay is sometimes AV block; going leftwards is time consuming but safe (Fig. 7.4).

A controversial point (for experienced users) is the utility of a 3D reconstruction of the right atrium and coronary sinus. We are already used to work (in a fluoroscopy environment) without any clear image but shadows of those structures, and there is no randomized studies proving that 3D reconstruction increases ablation safety or success. A case–control study done in Granada showed that 3D geometry just adds extra time to

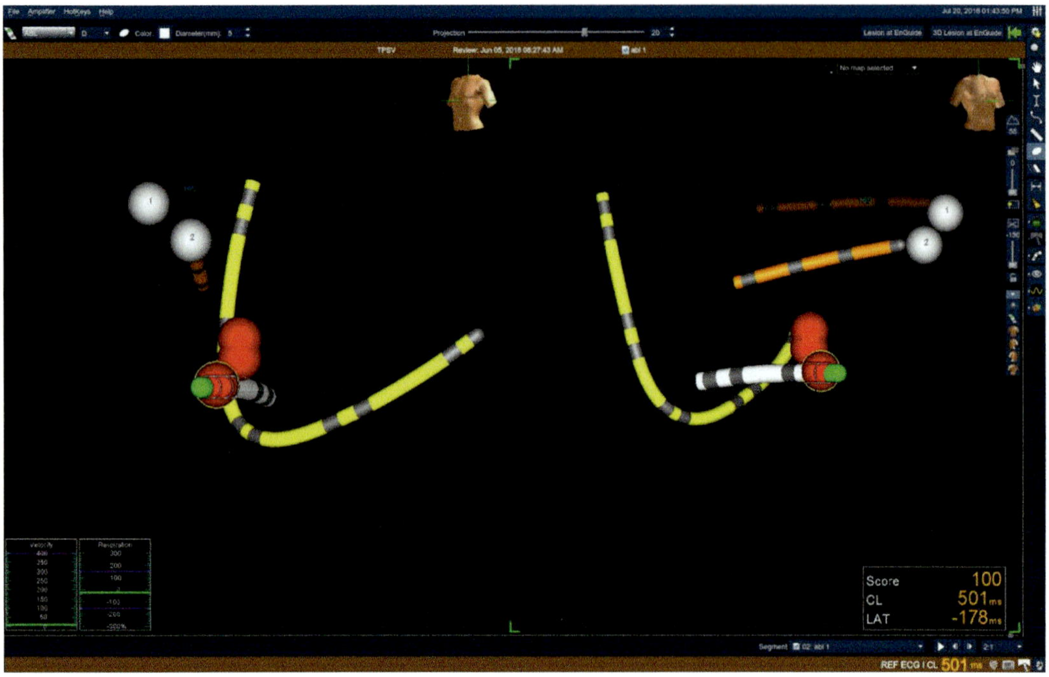

Fig. 7.6 AVNRT ablation using 3D systems to visualize only catheters, without any 3D reconstruction; visualizing catheters at all times and intracardiac signal provides enough information to perform ablation

the procedure, without any other advantage. At the beginning, however, 3D reconstruction helps to understand better this new environment and to increase confidence in catheter positioning and navigation without X-rays. In Granada we have stopped creating 3D reconstructions, and ablation is performed based on signals and just catheter visualization (Fig. 7.6).

Finally when a too close position is no longer safe to test RF, we can either try other sources of energy (cryoablation) or accept some possible effects of nonsuccessful RF lesions to modify at long-term SP physiology.

In cases of documented arrhythmia but no induction at the procedure (and sometimes even not clear-cut 50 ms "jump" to prove dual-AV node physiology), we can try to eliminate the SP if no other mechanisms are found, with the same previous considerations. 3D mapping systems could also help in this condition; a recent report using voltage and activation maps in sinus rhythm (NavX and Carto) showed that successful RF sites (in the triangle of Koch) were found in the closer vicinity (3–5 mm) of voltage transition zones, achieving junctional rhythm in 95% of patients when ablation was applied at latest activation site [25]. We replicate the experience using hyperdensity maps obtained with the Rhythmia system with SP signals recorded also in the close vicinity in most of the patients, with AVNRT abolished when the latest activation area in sinus rhythm was targeted for ablation (Fig. 7.7).

Cryoablation of the AVNRT Without Fluoroscopy

If in most cases RF ablation is a safe and successful source of energy, in some patients the even far low risk of 1% to damage permanently the AV conduction is too high; or once RF is used, the arrhythmia is still inducible and to apply RF close to the FP is judged too risky, we can use this technique developed at the end of the century in Montreal.

Any catheter can be used with Abbot NavX or Boston Rhythmia systems, and a cryocatheter can be used with no restriction depending on the age the operator judges is too young to accept an

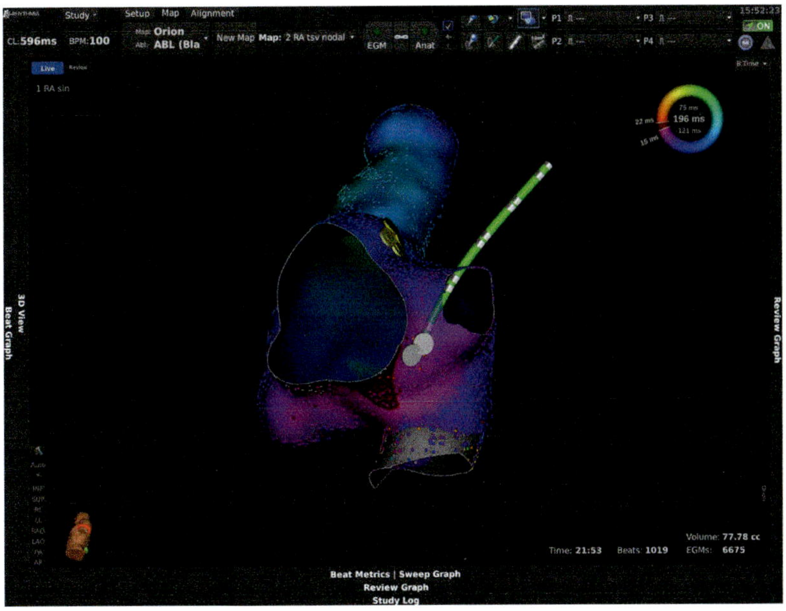

Fig. 7.7 Rhythmia activation map in sinus rhythm; latest activation site depicted in dark red (at 5 h on the tricuspid annulus); His in yellow dots, and SP signals in gray dots. Cryoablation was successfully applied in this latest activation area, after many other cryoablation applications failed elsewhere

AV block (at our center, in 2017, we decided that younger than 50 years old merits a cryocatheter when ablation is needed near the AV node).

Carto system needs some "tricks" to prevent cost escalation; we start the day scheduling the patients that will need for sure ablation (i.e., flutter or AP-AVRT cases), and then for the next case, where arrhythmia is unclear (EP study) or a cryocatheter will be used for ablation, the previous patient ablation catheter is placed in a bag beneath the thoracic region (usually under the mattress) of the new case, as a NAV catheter should be on the "matrix" area to be able to create a virtual anatomy; then a decaNav catheter is used to create the virtual anatomy, and the cryocatheter could be then visualized as any other catheter and used for ablation (however, no ablation points can be automatically acquired).

All the anatomic and physiologic considerations are the same at the time to search for the right spot to find the SP; however we can lower to 0% the risk of inadvertent complete AV node damage. This is due to multiple factors, as the cryoadhesion (the catheter sticks to the tissue once the cooling starts), allowing smaller lesions, more superficial and with sharper borders. We describe the principal concepts related to cryoablation:

- Safer technique does not mean that a complete AV block is not possible; however, we can apply closer to the FP, as all the surroundings have a higher temperature and the freezing is applied only to the contact surface between the catheter and the tissue; even more, we can use the cryomapping (to test safety at −30 °C) and even a complete AV block at −30° will be reverted if the cryomap is stopped, or continued to freeze at −70° to −80° to obtain a permanent lesion (SP persistence should be tested after 30 s of freezing, to avoid long unsuccessful applications).
- Each full application for cryoenergy takes between 4 and 5 min, and we should monitor the A–H times, as prolongation will preclude AV node damage.
- In contrast to RF ablation, a junctional rhythm is rarely or never seen during cryoablation.
- As small lesion volume allows to apply closer to the His region, to decrease recurrences, and once SP is abolished, after 4 min of freezing is done at successful site, and just when temperature starts to come back to zero (the catheter is no longer adhering to the tissue), it is suggested to start a new "security" application.

There are no available guidelines to decide when to mandatorily use cryoablation, but depending on resources it should be used at least when a RF procedure was complicated by a transient AV block, and the arrhythmia is still inducible, or a more flexible indication is when 1% of risk is deemed too high, as newer cryocatheters show a similar efficacy profile, with a lesser risk [26].

Results

AVNRT ablation without fluoroscopy has the same results as in cases done with conventional technology. Security is not compromised and success does not differ. Most of the reports available are produced in single centers (and in most of the cases by single operators in those centers). There is information arriving slowly from multicenter initiatives on supraventricular tachycardia ablation: a Spanish registry using EnSite NavX [27] and Italian registry with Carto [28]. Procedural acute success was 96.4% and 100%, respectively; complication rates were also low: 0.8% and 0.3% only. In the Spanish registry 86.7% of cases were done without fluoroscopy (mostly right-sided procedures) and in the Italian registry 67.2% of cases were also fluoroscopy free, and operator and patient ages were predictors to achieve complete fluoroscopy-free procedures. Even if not all patients were treated in a complete fluoroscopy-free environment, the exposition to radiation was so reduced to predict a significant reduction in future expected cancer incidence [29].

How many procedures are needed to be able to do most of the procedures without fluoroscopy? There is no absolute answer, as it depends on many different aspects, mostly related to personal appreciation and habits; usually the older the electrophysiologist, the more reluctant to change, while fellows exposed to these techniques during their training and female electrophysiologist are faster embracing fluoroscopy-free environments while in practice. In the Italian registry, welcoming all substrate and all supraventricular arrhythmias, after 30 cases most operators were confident enough to do procedures without fluoroscopy; other authors report that 17 procedures are enough [30]. In our opinion, once the operator firmly believes that the system used reflects well the position of the catheters, he or she will start the case without lead aprons since the beginning, and try to develop other ways to solve the problem if some difficulties arise, while if lead protection is in place it is tempting to come back to what we better know and what we have trusted for longer time. Usually, the greater the experience the lesser the situations where we need to wear back a lead apron, but, in any situation, patient security must prevail, and fluoroscopy is welcomed if we judge it is needed.

Conclusion

The non-fluoroscopic approach is a feasible and safe alternative to fluoroscopy for AVNRT ablation. This method ensures low complication rates, high acute procedural success rates, and comparable long-term outcomes. Anatomy and physiology are needed when an AVNRT is targeted to ablation. Usually both fast and slow pathways are well differentiated to let the RF catheter safely eliminate the slow pathway; but the AV node and its surroundings are a complex structure to navigate, and a good sense of this 3D space plus a good dose of respect are needed if we want to cure AVNRT. Fluoroscopy-free environments (or at least ALARA procedures) should be part of training for AVNRT and other arrhythmia substrates.

References

1. Moe GK, Preston JB, Burlington H. Physiologic evidence for dual A-V transmission system. Circ Res. 1956;4:357–75.
2. Wu D, Denes P, Dhingra R, Khan A, Rosen KM. The effects of propranolol on induction of AV nodal reentrant paroxysmal tachycardia. Circulation. 1974;50:665–77.
3. Ben Yedder N, Roux JF, Ayala Paredes F. Troponin elevation in supraventricular tachycardia: primary dependence on heart rate. Can J Cardiol. 2011;27:105–9.
4. Lim SH, Anantharaman V, Teo WS, Goh PP, Tan AT. Comparison of treatment of supraventricular tachycardia by Valsalva manoeuvre and carotid sinus massage. Ann Emerg Med. 1998;31:30–5.

5. Walker S, Cutting P. Impact of a modified Valsalva manoeuvre in the termination of paroxysmal supraventricular tachycardia. Emerg Med J. 2010;27:287–91.
6. DiMarco JP, Sellers TD, Berne RM, West GA, Belardinelli L. Adenosine: electrophysiologic effects and therapeutic use for terminating paroxysmal supraventricular tachycardia. Circulation. 1983;68:1254–63.
7. Pritchett LC, Anderson RR, Benditt DG, Kasell J, Harrison L, Wallace AG, Sealy WC, Gallagher JJ. Reentry within the atrioventricular node: surgical cure with preservation of atrioventricular conduction. Circulation. 1979;60:440–6.
8. Ross DL, Johnson DC, Denniss AR, Cooper MJ, Richards DA, Uther JB. Curative surgery for atrioventricular junctional ("AV nodal") reentrant tachycardia. J Am Coll Cardiol. 1985;6:1383–92.
9. Cox JL, Holman WL, Cain ME. Cryosurgical treatment of atrioventricular node reentrant tachycardia. Circulation. 1987;76:1329–36.
10. Scheinman M, Morady F, Hess DS, Gonzalez R. Catheter-induced ablation of the atrioventricular junction to control refractory supraventricular arrhythmias. JAMA. 1982;248:851–5.
11. Gallagher JJ, Svenson RH, Kasell JH, et al. Catheter technique for closed-chest ablation of the atrioventricular conduction system: a therapeutic alternative for the treatment of refractory supraventricular tachycardia. N Engl J Med. 1982;306:194–200.
12. Haissaguerre M, Warin JF, Lemetayer P, Saoudi N, Guillem JP, Blanchot P. Closed-chest ablation of retrograde conduction in patients with atrioventricular nodal reentrant tachycardia. N Engl J Med. 1989;320:426–33.
13. Epstein L, Scheinman M, Langberg J, Chilson D, Goldberg HR, Griffin JC. Percutaneous catheter modification of the atrioventricular node. Circulation. 1989;80:757–68.
14. Goy JJ, Fromer M, Schlaepfer J, et al. Clinical efficacy of radiofrequency current in the treatment of patients with atrioventricular node reentrant tachycardia. J Am Coll Cardiol. 1990;6:418–23.
15. Lee MA, Morady F, Kadish A, Schamp DJ, Chin MC, Scheinman MM, Griffin JC, Lesh MD, Pederson D, Goldberfer J, Calkins H, deBuitleir M, Kou WH, Rosenheck S, Sousa J, Langberg JJ. Catheter modification of the atrioventricular junction with radiofrequency energy for control of atrioventricular nodal reentry tachycardia. Circulation. 1991;83:827–35.
16. Haissaguerre M, Gaita F, Fischer B, Commenges D, Montserrat P, d'Ivernois C, Le Metayer P, Warin JF. Elimination of atrioventricular nodal reentrant tachycardia using discrete slow potentials to guide application of radiofrequency energy. Circulation. 1992;85:2162–75.
17. Jackman WM, Beckman KJ, McClelland JH, Wang X, Friday KJ, Roman CA, Moulton KP, Twidale N, Hazlitt A, Prior MI, Oren J, Overholt ED, Lazzara R. Treatment of supraventricular tachycardia due to atrioventricular nodal reentry by radiofrequency catheter ablation of slow-pathway conduction. N Engl J Med. 1992;327:313–8.
18. Jazayeri MR, Hempe SL, Sra JS, Hempe SL, Dhala AA, Blanck Z, Deshpande SS, Avitall B, Krum DP, Gilbert CI, Akhtar M. Selective transcatheter ablation of the fast and slow pathways using radiofrequency energy in patients with atrioventricular nodal reentrant tachycardia. Circulation. 1992;85:1318–28.
19. Akhtar M, Jazayeri MR, Sra J, Blanck Z, Desphande S, Dhala A. Atrioventricular nodal re-entry: clinical, electrophysiological, and therapeutic considerations. Circulation. 1993;88:282–95.
20. Friedman PL, Dubuc M, Green MS, Jackman WM, Keane DT, Marinchak RA, Nazari J, Packer DL, Skanes A, Steiberg JS, Stevenson WG, Tchou PJ, Wilber DJ, Worley SJ. Catheter cryoablation of supraventricular tachycardia: results of the multicenter prospective "frosty" trial. Heart Rhythm. 2004;1:129–38.
21. Rivard L, Dubuc GP, Novak P, Roy D, Macle L, Thibault B, Talajic M, Khairy P. Cryoablation outcomes for AV nodal re-entrant tachycardia comparing 4-mm versus 6-mm electrode-tip catheters. Heart Rhythm. 2008;5(2):230–4.
22. Knight BP, Ebinger M, Oral H, Kim MH, Sticherling C, Pelosi F, Michaud GF, Strickberger SA, Morady F. Diagnostic value of tachycardia features and pacing maneuvers during paroxysmal supraventricular tachycardia. J Am Coll Cardiol. 2000;36:574–82.
23. Alvarez M, Tercedor L, Almansa I, Ros N, Galdeano RS, Burillo F, Santiago P, Penas R. Safety and feasibility of catheter ablation of atrioventricular nodal re-entrant tachycardia without fluoroscopic guidance. Heart Rhythm. 2009;6(12):1714–20.
24. Chaumont J, Al Baridi E, Roux J-F, Badra M, Arseneau F, Ayala-Paredes F. His area is closer than expected to RF ablation lesions in AVNR Tachycardia. Abstract 612. CCS Congress. October 30, 2012. Toronto. Canada. Can J Cardiol. 2012;28(5):S327.
25. Kurian T, Abney LE, Gonogunta A, et al. Ablation of latest site(s) of activation within voltages bridges, voltage transition zones, and adjacent low voltage areas in the triangle of Koch to guide ablation for AVNRT. HRS May 11, 2018. Boston USA. Heart Rhythm. 2018;(5 Suppl) B-PO05-065 S515.
26. Wells P, Dubuc M, Klein GJ, Dan D, Roux JF, et al. Intracardiac ablation for atrioventricular nodal reentry tachycardia using a 6 mm distal electrode cryoablation catheter: prospective, multicenter, North American study (ICY-AVNRT). J Cardiovasc Electrophysiol. 2018;29(1):167–76.
27. Álvarez M, Bertomeu-González V, Arcocha MF, Moriña P, Tercedor L, Ferrero de Loma Á, Pachón M, García A, Pardo M, Datino T, Alonso C, Osca J, Investigators of the Spanish Multicenter Registry of Fluoroscopy-free Ablation. Nonfluoroscopic catheter ablation. Results from a prospective multicenter registry. Rev Esp Cardiol. 2017;70:699–705.
28. Pani A, Giuseppina B, Bonanno C, Bongiorni MG, et al. Predictors of zero X-ray ablation for supra-

ventricular tachycardias in a nationwide multi-center experience. Circ Arrhythm Electrophysiol. 2018;11(3):e005529.
29. Casella M, Dello Russo A, Pelargonio G, et al. Near zerO fluoroscopic exPosure during catheter ablAtion of supRavenTricular arrhYthmias: the NO-PARTY multi-center randomized trial. Europace. 2016;18:1565–72.
30. Raziminia M, Willoughby MC, Demo H, et al. Fluoroless catheter ablation of cardiac arrhythmias: a 5-year experience. Pacing Clin Electrophysiol. 2017;40(4):425–33.

8 Non-fluoroscopic Catheter Ablation of Accessory Pathways

Santiago Horacio Rivera
and José Luis Merino Llorens

Introduction

Catheter ablation of accessory pathway (AP)-mediated tachycardia is the treatment of choice for many patients with clinical supraventricular tachycardia (SVT) and has been traditionally performed under fluoroscopy guidance [1]. Fluoroscopy is certainly a highly effective way to navigate catheters and to monitor their location. However, the use of fluoroscopy requires the administration of ionizing radiation and exposes patients to potential harmful effects, including an increased risk of carcinogenesis [2]. Prolonged radiation exposure is associated with a higher incidence of dermatitis, cataracts, malignancies, and congenital defects [3]. There is no lower threshold to prevent malignancy appearance with radiation [4]. Even low doses can be harmful, and no completely safe dose exists. Children have a higher risk of malignancies due to their higher radiation sensitivity and longer life expectancy. Arrhythmia invasive treatment without fluoroscopy is extremely important in pregnant women and children, who represent the population most vulnerable to radiation. More important, less radiation exposure is beneficial not only for patients, but also for the operator and EP team health during a long interventional career [5].

Conventional fluoroscopic catheter mapping has limited spatial resolution and involves fluoroscopy and ionizing radiation doses to patients and staff. The introduction of electroanatomic mapping systems (EAMS) has provided the possibility to perform simple and complex electrophysiological procedures avoiding or limiting the use of radiation [6]. Compared to conventional radiofrequency ablation, non-fluoroscopic ablation significantly reduces fluoroscopy, ablation time, and radiation dose, without significant differences in procedure duration, success rate, long-term success rate, complication rates, and recurrence rates [5]. Radiation can be significantly reduced without compromising efficacy and safety. For this reason, patients and physicians should be aware of the risk of radiation exposure and the benefits of the imaging/procedure balanced by the required radiation exposure. Performing a non-fluoroscopic (or near-zero) catheter ablation procedure should therefore represent an aim for all electrophysiology labs.

In this chapter, we revise briefly general concepts of accessory pathways and then the current situation regarding non-fluoroscopic catheter ablation of APs.

S. H. Rivera (✉)
Cardiac Electrophisiology Department, Buenos Aires Cardiovascular Institute (ICBA), Buenos Aires, Argentina

J. L. M. Llorens
Cardiology Service, La Paz University Hospital, Madrid, Spain
e-mail: jlmerino@arritmias.net

R. Proietti et al. (eds.), *Cardiac Electrophysiology Without Fluoroscopy*,
https://doi.org/10.1007/978-3-030-16992-3_8

Relevant Anatomy

Left free wall (FW) APs usually exhibit a discrete atrial insertion near the mitral annulus. It then skirts on its epicardial aspect and may cross the annulus at variable depths [7]. The ventricular insertion usually branches into multiple connections, towards the apex. The typical AP length is 5–10 mm, with a maximal diameter of 0.1–7 mm [8]. The left epicardial AV groove contains the left circumflex artery and the coronary sinus (CS), which runs an average of 10–14 mm on the atrial side of the true annulus [9]. The anterior limit of the left free wall is well demarcated by the aorto-mitral continuity, which rarely contains AP connections. The tricuspid valve annulus is less well formed and discontinuous [10]. The right atrial and ventricular myocardium tend to overlap or fold over one another, as they insert on the annulus [11]. Right free wall APs may cross discontinuities or skirt the epicardial aspect of the annulus. These anatomical aspects contribute to catheter instability during ablation [12].

The anatomy of the posteroseptal or inferoseptal region is complex, as this area includes the pyramidal space (Fig. 8.1). It represents the confluence of all four cardiac chambers and the CS, with the central fibrous body as the superior boundary of this space [13]. The anterior aspect is the interventricular septum and the posterior wall is formed by the convergence of both atriums. The tricuspid annulus is displaced 5–10 mm forward and inferiorly with respect to the mitral annulus [14]. This displays a gap in which lies the right atrium-left ventricular sulcus, which is the junction between the inferomedial right atrium and the posterosuperior process of the left ventricle. Most of the AP connections at this region are believed to run from the right atrium to left ventricle, from the paraseptal left atrium to the left ventricle and from the paraseptal right atrium to the right ventricle. In up to 20% of PS APs, the AV circuit results from CS musculature connections between the ventricle and the left atrium, and 21% of these connections occur in association with a CS diverticulum [15].

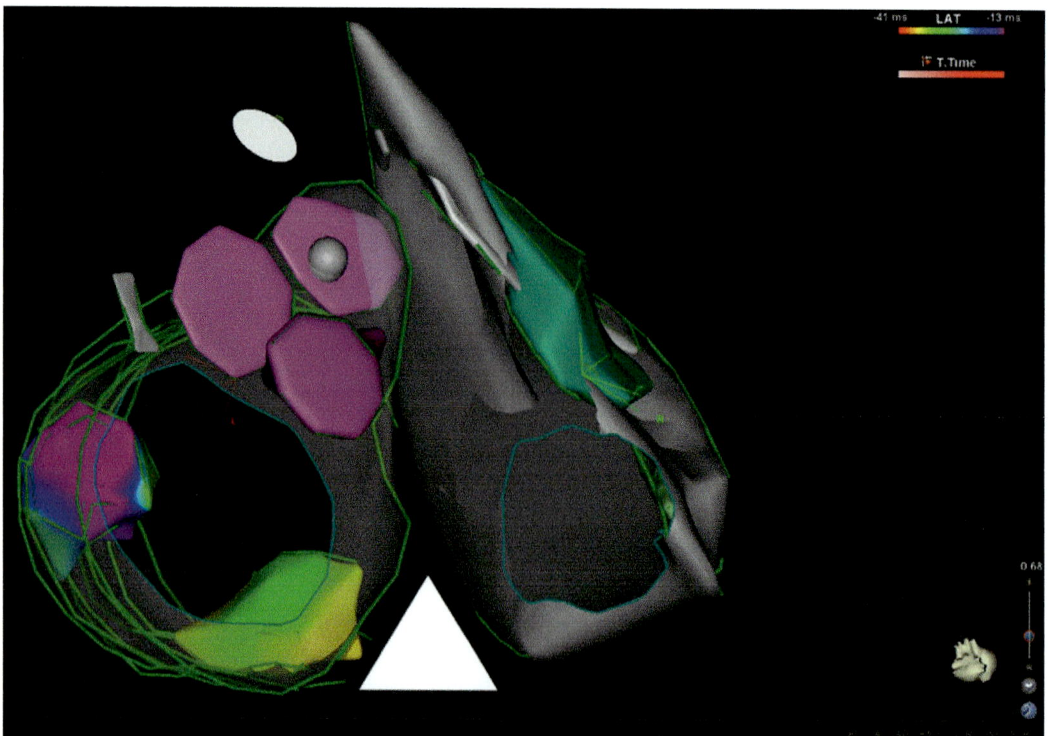

Fig. 8.1 Posterior view of the base of the heart. The pyramidal space is marked by a white triangle

Anteroseptal APs are located at the apex of the triangle of Koch. This region is also referred to as superoparaseptal, considering that there is no atrial septum anterior to the His recording location as the atrial walls are separated here by the aortic root. On the other hand, PS APs are also referred to as posterior paraseptal, because the CS itself is posterior (inferior) to the true atrial septum (thin rim of atrial tissue surrounding the fossa ovalis). Both AS and PS APs can be considered free wall APs as there is no true atrial septum at both locations. True septal or midseptal APs are located in the floor of the triangle of Koch, between the His bundle and the anterior region of the CS ostium [16].

Characteristics of Accessory Pathways and Atrioventricular Reentrant Tachycardia

Reciprocating atrioventricular reentry tachycardia (AVRT) is maintained by the presence of an accessory pathway (AP) [17, 18]. The most common location of APs is at the free wall (FW) [19]. Left and right APs account for 50–60% and 10–20%, respectively [19]. The second most common location is posteroseptal (PS), accounting for 25–30% of APs [19, 20]; these connections have been associated with longer procedure times, greater radiation exposure, and radiofrequency doses than any other location [21]. Midseptal APs account for <5% of all APs, of which 85% show antegrade conduction, 15% present retrograde conduction exclusively, and 4% antegrade only [22]. Compared with septal and left free wall location, right FW APs are less likely to demonstrate retrograde conduction, participate in reciprocating tachycardia, and be associated with inducible atrial fibrillation [23]. Pathways in the right FW are more likely to demonstrate decremental antegrade conduction, while left FW APs are more likely to demonstrate decremental retrograde conduction and have longer retrograde refractory periods [24]. The retrograde atrial activation sequence during SVT involving septal APs may look concentric, unlike FW APs in which atrial activation is eccentric [25].

Regarding ECG characteristics, all left FW APs should demonstrate a positive delta wave in lead V1 or V2, and a negative delta wave in lead I, aVL, or V6 which usually confirms location. As the pathway location moves from posterior to lateral to anterior, the delta wave in the inferior leads, specially aVF and lead III, changes from negative to isoelectric to positive in polarity [26]. Confusion may arise in the interpretation of a positive delta wave in lead V1, as possible diagnosis of left free wall AP; this finding is diagnostic of a left free wall AP only if R > S. A positive delta wave in lead V1 with a R < S in V1 is consistent with a right FW AP or a minimally preexisted left FW AP. A negative delta wave in V1 is consistent with a septal AP. As the pathway position moves from right superior to right middle and right inferior free wall, the delta wave in inferior leads aVF and II changes from positive to isoelectric to negative [27].

A negative P wave during orthodromic reciprocating tachycardia (ORT) in lead I is highly suggestive of a left FW AP, while a negative P wave in V1 is highly suggestive of a right-sided AP. A positive P wave in lead I during ORT is highly suggestive of a right FW AP. The presence of negative P waves and positive P waves during ORT in inferior leads is representative of inferior or superior locations, respectively. Isoelectric or biphasic P waves in any inferior lead suggest a middle FW location [28].

The pathways associated with permanent junctional reciprocating tachycardia (PJRT) are most commonly found at the posteroseptal location. These APs are usually concealed and exhibit slow decremental retrograde conduction properties that result in incessant tachycardia. For those pathways considered to be right sided, the delta wave in V1 is negative or isoelectric, with an abrupt R > S transition in lead V2 (75% of cases) [25–28].

Para-hisian pacing can distinguish retrograde conduction over an AP from over the AV node. At low pacing outputs, ventricular capture occurs, whereas at higher outputs, His capture will also occur resulting in a shorter paced QRS. If an AP is present, the stimulus to atrial interval will be identical at different pacing outputs, as the AP typically conducts more rapidly than the AV node. In the absence of an AP, the stimulus to atrial interval will be longer during ventricular-only capture [29]. Para-hisian pacing techniques consistently indicate the presence of retrograde conduction over a right free wall AP, while in 25% of cases of left free wall APs para-hisian pacing may be consistent with retrograde AV node conduction, or a paradoxical shortening of the V-to-A time due to more rapid activation of the left FW through the His-Purkinje system [29]. The comparison of the stimulus to atrial intervals observed with right ventricular apical versus basal pacing can also demonstrate the presence of an AP. The apex is closer to the His-Purkinje system, allowing for a shorter stimulus to atrial interval during apical pacing, in comparison to basal pacing.

Orthodromic (ORT) and Antidromic (ART) Reentrant Tachycardia Diagnosis

Demonstration of 1:1 atrial and ventricular conduction is obligatory. Electrophysiologic diagnostic criteria of ORT is suggested by the demonstration of a QRS-to-atrium time greater than or equal to 60 ms; constant ventricle-to-atrium intervals despite changes in the tachycardia cycle length (TCL); and the ability to advance atrial activation by PVC delivery during His bundle refractoriness (indicated by the presence of an AP but does not prove participation in the circuit) and reset the tachycardia (proves participation in the circuit) [24]. A preexcitation index (difference between TCL and the longest coupling interval of a right ventricular apical premature stimulus that advances the atrium) >70 ms is consistent with a left lateral AP [30]. A prolongation of the His/QRS-to-atrium interval of >35–40 ms during ORT with ipsilateral bundle branch block is diagnostic of a free wall AP [31]. If the VA interval is prolonged by less than 10 ms, the AP is likely to be truly septal in location. If the VA interval increases by 10–30 ms with right or left bundle branch block, the pathway is considered to have, respectively, a right or left ventricular insertion [31]. Another diagnostic criterion is the reproducible termination of the tachycardia by premature ventricular stimuli during His refractoriness without conduction to atrium.

ORT must be differentiated from atrial tachycardia (AT), which is best achieved by dissociating the ventricles from the atria during tachycardia. The demonstration of a V-A-A-V response after termination of ventricular pacing that entrains the atrium excludes ORT. If AVNRT is present, the stimulus to atrial interval during ventricular pacing will exceed the QRS to atrial interval by >85 ms, and the ventricular post-pacing interval will exceed the TCL by >115 ms [32].

Preexcited reciprocating tachycardia may use the AV node or a second AP as the antegrade limb. Antidromic tachycardia (ART) should be suspected whenever obligatory 1:1 AV relationship exists; when the QRS during tachycardia shares a same morphology as the QRS during maximal preexcitation or when the QRS morphology is reproduced by atrial pacing near the pathway insertion; with the advance of ventricular activation by atrial extra-stimuli near insertion with concomitant advance of the subsequent His and atrial activation (reset) [24]. Exclusion of ventricular tachycardia and bystander AP participation, specially AVNRT (His-to-A time in tachycardia <70 ms, consistent with AVNRT), is mandatory.

Mahaim Fibers

The term “Mahaim physiology” is used to describe APs with slow, decremental, and exclusively anterograde conduction [22]. The initial description by Mahaim and colleagues in 1938 included the nodofascicular, nodoventricular, and atriofascicular/atrioventricular APs [33, 34]. The later APs are mostly situated at the right side of the heart. The proximal insertion is at the atrial margin of the free wall tricuspid annulus, while the distal insertion can be either at the right bundle branch (atriofascicular) or directly into the apical ventricular myocardium (atrioventricular) [35]. The atrial component of the pathway has

AV nodal like properties and is responsible for exhibiting decremental conduction [36].

Atriofascicular APs demonstrate only minimal preexcitation during sinus rhythm, antegrade and decremental conduction (fixed AP-to-V interval), and long basal conduction times, with transient block response to adenosine [37]. Prolongation of the PR and AH interval associated with shortening of the HV interval is observed in response to atrial pacing. These APs are typically right sided, with rare exceptions. They directly participate in antidromic reciprocating tachycardia only, as conduction travels antegrade down the AP to the right bundle branch and retrograde back up to the His bundle, AV node, and then atrium [38, 39]. During tachycardia, advance of the V (presence of an AP) and subsequent A (reset) with PAC during AV node refractoriness can be observed. RBB activation precedes the His bundle activation during significant preexcitation. In antidromic tachycardia, there is a typically short HV and ventriculo-atrial intervals, as retrograde atrial activation begins near the end of the QRS [28]. The earliest ventricular activation and shortest post-pacing intervals are found at the right ventricular apex. Other diagnostic criteria include the differences in VH and HA intervals during spontaneous SVT and RV pacing (VH in SVT < VH with RV pacing; HA in SVT = HA during RV pacing) [28].

Non-fluoroscopic Ablation Approach

After gaining femoral access (please refer to the chapter on catheter placement for further details), which can be guided by vascular ultrasound, a single multipole catheter is placed from the right femoral vein, using the EAMS. The catheter is then advanced up to the inferior vena cava (IVC) until atrial electrograms are registered. An anatomical map of the right atrium is then created, dragging the catheter all around and using RAO and LAO incidences to guide catheter movements, including the superior (SVC) and inferior (IVC) vena cava, and tricuspid valve (Fig. 8.2). The tricuspid annulus serves as a landmark to position the coronary sinus (CS) catheter in the left anterior oblique projection of the EAMS.

The catheter is positioned in the right atrium and with a simultaneous downward deflection

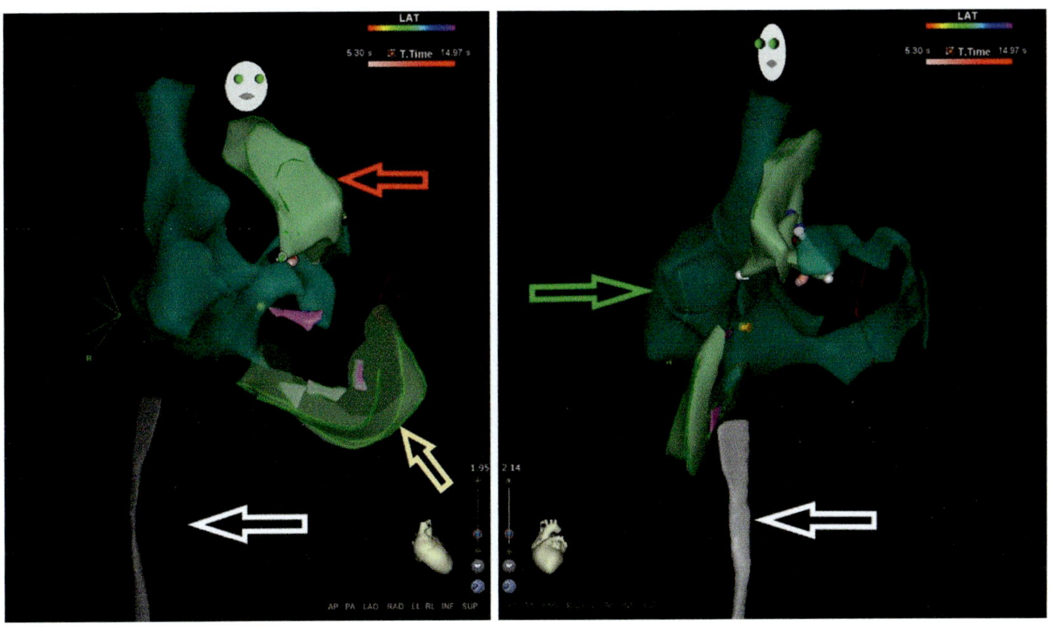

Fig. 8.2 White arrow: IVC; red arrow: aortic root; yellow arrow: RV apex; green arrow: right atrium and coronary sinus system

the tip is placed across the tricuspid valve into the right ventricle. The catheter is then pulled down to contact the inferior margin of the tricuspid valve and providing a clockwise rotation the tip moves back across the tricuspid valve and gets in contact with the lower atrial septum. Further clockwise rotation will engage the tip of the catheter into the CS ostium, and after releasing the torque the catheter will then extend into the CS. The CS anatomy can then be created.

For patients with manifest pathways, pathway location is mapped by localizing shortest atrioventricular (A-V) intervals in sinus rhythm. For patients with concealed pathways, location can be mapped by the earliest retrograde activation during SVT or during ventricular pacing. In these patients, a second mapping catheter is inserted via the right or left femoral vein and positioned in the right ventricular apex, first positioned to record the His electrogram and then given a downward deflection so that the curve of the catheter contacts the right ventricular outflow tract and deflects the tip towards the right ventricular apex. The flexion is then released to allow the catheter tip to contact the myocardium. If a left-sided pathway is confirmed, the mapping catheter can be used to probe for a patent foramen ovale (PFO). If no PFO is found, a transseptal puncture can be performed, guided by intracardiac (ICE) or transesophageal (TEE) echocardiography (Fig. 8.3; please refer to the chapter on transseptal puncture without fluoroscopy for further details). In brief, an ICE catheter is advanced from the left femoral vein to the right atrium (RA), guided by direct ultrasound visualization. From the right femoral vein, a guide wire is advanced into the SVC, which can be confirmed by ICE. A transseptal sheath and dilator are advanced over the wire into the SVC and the guide wire is removed for the transseptal needle to be inserted. The sheath, dilator, and needle are then pulled back as a unit from the SVC into the right atrium to position the tip of the dilator in the fossa ovalis. When the dilator tip is visualized tenting the fossa and aiming posterior to the aortic root, then the transseptal needle can be advanced out of the dilator, in order to puncture the fossa towards the left atrium. At this

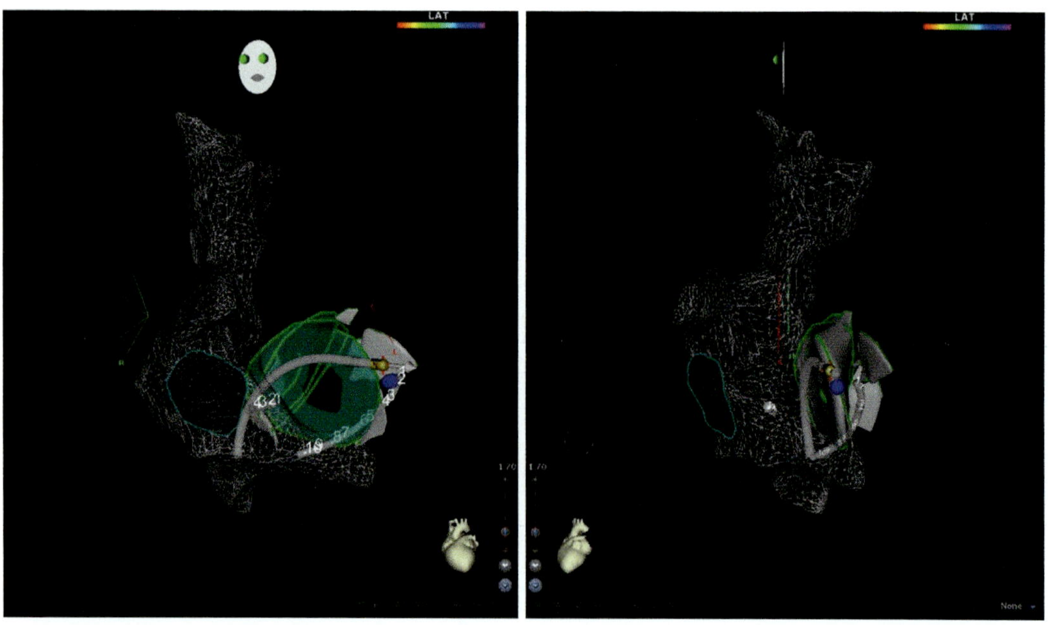

Fig. 8.3 Intracardiac echo-facilitated 3D electroanatomical map of both atriums (mesh = right atrium/right: left lateral view/left: LAO view). The ablation catheter is placed at the effective lesion site at the atrial insertion site of a left lateral AP (blue dot), through a transseptal approach

point, saline contrast can be injected to show left atrial filling and confirm the left atrial location of the needle tip. The dilator and sheath are carefully advanced over the needle and once the sheath is in good position, the needle and dilator are withdrawn. This whole transseptal approach depends on direct ICE or TEE visualization at each step.

Another way to perform transseptal puncture is to advance a J-wire through the femoral vein until its location in the RA is confirmed by ICE. Next, a transseptal sheath-dilator assembly is then advanced over the wire approximately, so that the tip is estimated to be in the mid-IVC region. The dilator and J-wire are then withdrawn, and the ablation catheter is advanced through the sheath. The ablation catheter's location could be tracked on the EAMS system once the distal electrodes exited the sheath, thus confirming the catheter/sheath location in the IVC. The ablation catheter is advanced into the SVC guided by the previously created anatomical map. The sheath is then advanced over the ablation catheter until an artifact is noted on its tip, as a result of an impedance change created as the sheath passes over the electrode. This provides confirmation that the sheath has reached the SVC. The ablation catheter is then removed and the J-wire and dilator are advanced through the sheath so that the J-wire tip is in advance of the dilator tip. Once the dilator is fully advanced and locked, the guide wire is removed. The transseptal needle is inserted into the sheath/dilator and then pulled down until the distal tip of the assembly abutted the interatrial septum as visualized by ICE. To avoid inadvertent puncture of the aorta or the left atrial posterior wall, the puncture performed under ICE guidance should place a view that allows for simultaneous imaging of the tenting fossa ovalis and the two left-sided pulmonary veins, to confirm that the puncture point is neither too anterior nor too posterior. Atrial pressure monitoring should be performed simultaneously, as the absence of blunting of the LA pressure waveform serves as confirmation that the posterior wall of the LA was not engaged.

Electroanatomical Mapping Systems, Intracardiac Echocardiography, and Intracardiac Echo-Facilitated 3D Electroanatomical Mapping Systems

Electroanatomical mapping systems have been shown to dramatically reduce fluoroscopic exposure [40], as the operator has the capacity to draw the venous system from the puncture site up to the heart entrance, providing anatomical landmarks, not clearly observed through fluoroscopy. Furthermore, navigation capabilities allow the operator to precisely return to the point of interest [41]. This is a true advantage over fluoroscopy, as the 3D electroanatomic system overcomes some of the difficulties as the disappearance of preexcitation after the initial radiofrequency pulses, and it makes it easier to accurately relocate the accessory pathway (AP), thus avoiding time- and radiation-consuming electrophysiological maneuvers [42]. This is of interest in unstable positions. Even the ablation of a para-hisian AP is feasible non-fluoroscopically since a cryoablation catheter can also be used with the EAMS [43].

Intracardiac echo has a measurable effect of reducing radiation and was generally deemed to be useful in cases requiring transseptal puncture [44]. Intracardiac echo-facilitated 3D EAMS provides a tool capable of recreating the cardiac anatomy without contact, just with the ICE proof (Fig. 8.4). In contrast to standard EAMS, it allows to demarcate solid anatomical structures such as papillary muscles, and even the coronary vessels. Carto-Sound has proven to reduce total X-ray time via a reduction in both mapping and remaining procedure X-ray time. Left atrial access time is also reduced using ultrasound-assisted 3D mapping compared to standard EAM [45].

EAM can also facilitate access to the left ventricle while performing a retrograde aortic approach. Most of the patients needing the ablation of an AP are young, so no vascular issues are expected; after femoral arterial puncture, the catheter is advanced to the aortic root and then an anatomical map of the aorta is created (in some para-hisian APs the atrial insertion could

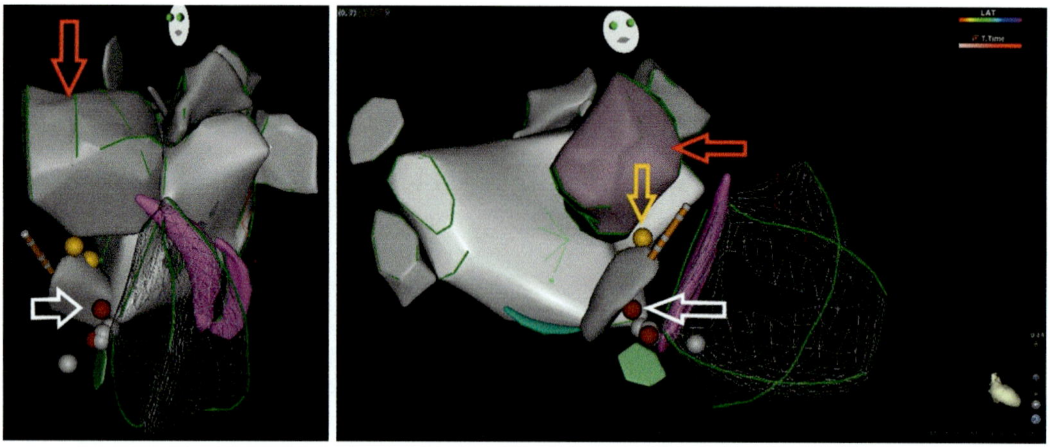

Fig. 8.4 Left (LAO view)/right (RAO view). Intracardiac echo-facilitated 3D anatomy of the left ventricle (mesh), mitral leaflets (purple); left atrium (grey); tendon of Todaro (dark grey); CS ostium (light green); fossa ovalis (turquoise); aortic root (red arrow); and His bundle (yellow arrow). The effective lesion site (white arrow) was located at the midseptum, within the triangle of Koch

be found in the aortic cusps, with no risk to damage the His in these locations), and using LAO and RAO views the ablation catheter is then prolapsed through the aortic valve, towards the left ventricle. The lack of visualization of the coronary arteries was pointed out as a limitation of non-fluoroscopic ablation using just an EAM; nevertheless if an angiography is not performed, this is also a limitation for fluoroscopy [46]. If the operator prefers, the ostium of the coronary arteries can be demarcated using the Carto-Sound module of the CARTO system, as intracardiac facilitated 3D EAM provides a noncontact tool for visualizing not just the ostium, if not the initial trajectory of these vessels, without the need of risk of performing an angiogram. This represents a clear advantage of advance EAM over fluoroscopy.

Mapping and Ablation

The identification of the earliest ventricular activation during anterograde AP conduction and earliest retrograde atria activation during ORT is the most common mapping approach [47–49].

Left FW APs: Mapping is facilitated by multielectrode recordings from the coronary sinus catheter. Although transseptal and transaortic approaches are complementary, the first may be preferred in the presence of peripheral vascular disease, aortic valve disease, or small ventricular chambers; however, as most of these patients are young, a retrograde approach has little risk for most of the patients; most of the APs are easily accessible through a retrograde access other than anterior or anterolateral APs that need longer sweep catheters when accessing from below. The transseptal approach provides better access to anterolateral or lateral AP locations. Transseptal access is directed at positions on or above the mitral annulus, with the electrodes parallel to the annulus. Although catheter mobility is greater, stability may be problematic. Catheter stability may be improved with the use of deflectable sheaths. For the transaortic approach, once the catheter is prolapsed it is curved through the aortic valve to prevent perforations of the coronary cusps or entry into the coronary arteries. The catheter is then directed (counterclockwise rotation) posterior at sites beneath the mitral annulus, the curve is loosened, and the catheter usually arrives at the AP ventricular insertion; retrograde ablation of AP is highly facilitated by multiplane simultaneous opposite incidences (Fig. 8.5a, b). Electrogram characteristics can predict successful ablation sites when mapping anterograde AP activation by the transaortic approach: (1)

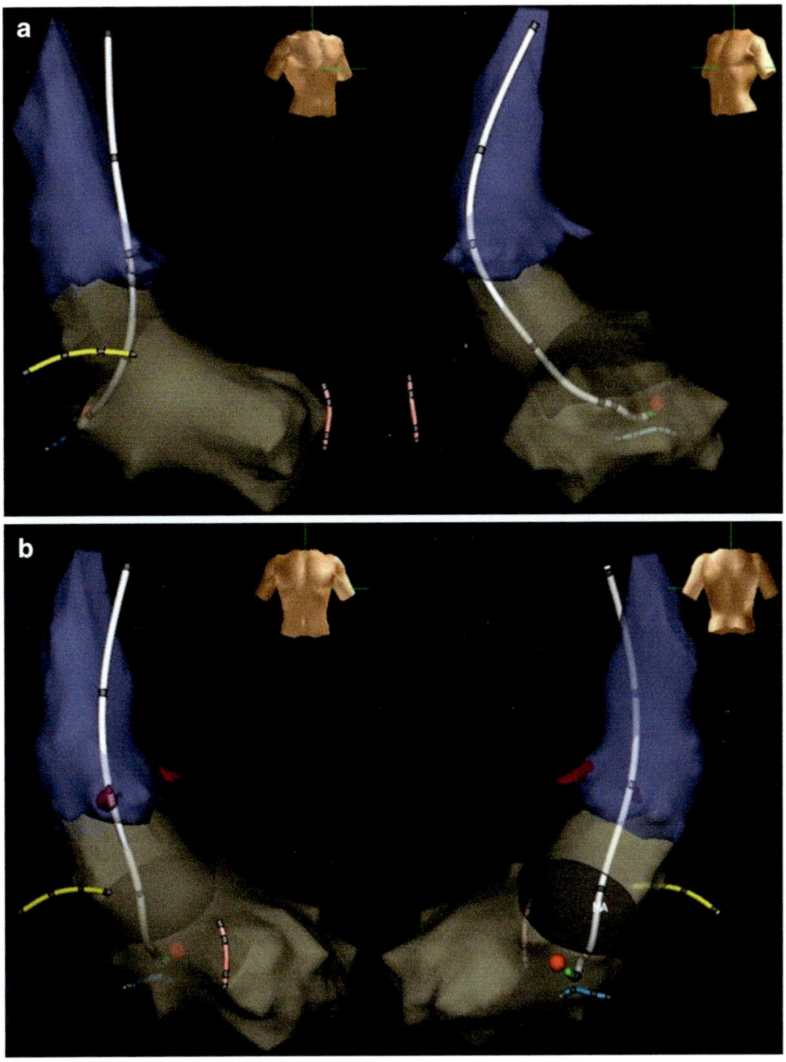

Fig. 8.5 (**a**) Standard RAO and LAO incidences, aiming to direct the catheter to the posterolateral area of the mitral annulus; aortic root and coronary arteries are depicted in blue. A customized multipole catheter was used, to be able to visualize most of the distal part of that catheter. (**b**) Posterior view (right) instead of anterior (left) incidence allows visualizing the precise location of the successful RF application (no fluoroscopy incidence can obtain this image); in case of catheter displacement, 3D mapping system features allow to regain the exact same location when needed

delta-to-ventricle interval; (2) atrial electrogram amplitude ($A > 1$ mV); (3) electrogram stability (10% change in EGM amplitude); (4) local AV electrogram interval (<40 ms); and (5) presence of a presumed AP potential [50]. The local VA electrogram interval during retrograde activation should be <30 ms [51]. Current and countercurrent pacing maneuvers are useful to discriminate between atrial and ventricular components of the electrogram, specially when the AP presents an oblique course across the AV annulus [52–54].

Right FW: Mapping and ablation of right free wall APs are difficult because of the absence of a venous structure around the tricuspid annulus and because of unstable contact. Mapping can be facilitated at these locations by employing a circular multielectrode halo catheter positioned near the annulus [55].

Posteroseptal APs: Features that suggest a successful ablation from the right endocardial approach include (1) negative delta wave in V1; (2) difference in VA time between the His recording and the earliest CS recording of less than 25 ms; (3) long RP tachycardias; (4) earliest VA less than 15 ms from the CS ostium; and (5) sharp/blunt CS EGM at earliest retrograde site. There are also features favoring the left endocardial approach: (1) R > S wave in V1; (2) difference in VA time between the His recording and the earliest CS recording of more than 25 ms; (3)

earliest retrograde atrial activation during ORT at middle CS; (4) earliest VA of more than 15 ms from the CS ostium; and (5) blunt/sharp CS EGM at earliest retrograde site [12]. In case of endocardial mapping failure, attention should turn to the coronary sinus system. Features that suggest an epicardial AP using the CS musculature include (1) the presence of a CS diverticulum; (2) a negative delta wave in lead II; (3) a steep positive delta wave in aVR; and (4) a deep S wave in V6. CS musculature connection can be present in up to 21% of PS APs, of which the most common occur in the middle cardiac vein (82%), followed by the posterior cardiac vein (11%), both veins (5%), and floor of the CS between these two veins (2%) [56, 57].

Anterior and midseptal APs: Superoparaseptal APs exhibit a predominantly positive delta wave in leads I, II, III, aVL, aVF, and V3–V6. Earliest anterograde activation occurs at or anterior to His recording locations, while the earliest retrograde activation occurs at the His bundle location (do not forget to map the aortic root as sometimes atrial earliest activation is found at this level). Midseptal AP ECG characteristics include delta waves which are predominantly positive in leads I, II, aVL, and V2–V6, with a negative complex in leads III and aVF, and negative or isoelectric in aVR and V1. The earliest anterograde ventricular and retrograde atrial activation occurs between the His bundle recording and the CS ostium [58–60].

Results of AP Non-fluoroscopic Catheter Ablation

The systematic use of a non-fluoroscopic approach is associated to procedural success rates of 99.1% [61]. Scaglione et al. reported a total of 44 consecutive pediatric patients treated with a non-fluoroscopic catheter-based ablation approach of APs [62]. Right chambers were accessed through a venous transfemoral approach while a retrograde transaortic approach was used to access the mitral annulus. Only three cases of left-sided APs were ablated through a patent foramen ovalis. In this experience, a total of 47 APs (left sided 45%) were ablated without the use of fluoroscopic guidance. Ablation without the use of fluoroscopy was successfully performed in every patient and no complication occurred. Recurrence rate was 14.8%.

A multicentre, randomized, controlled study on 262 pediatric patients undergoing electrophysiological study for SVT (72% AVRT) showed that procedures were performed without any use of fluoroscopy. Unfortunately, in this setting, left-sided APs requiring transseptal access were excluded [63].

Echocardiography is commonly used as an adjunct to fluoroscopy in the performance of transseptal puncture. Some authors state that echo guidance should be the standard of care for all transseptal procedures. Intracardiac localization of the sheath, dilator, and needle tip is better assessed by echo than by fluoroscopy [64].

The NO-PARTY trial has reported a potential 96% reduction in the estimated risks of cancer incidence and mortality and a significant reduction in estimated years of life lost and of life affected by a zero fluoroscopy approach compared with the conventional approach. A minimized fluoroscopy approach was associated with a significant reduction in patients' and operator radiation dose. The acute success (97%) and complication (1%) rates were not different between the minimized fluoroscopy and conventional approach. The reduction in patients' exposure shows a 96% reduction in the estimated risks of cancer incidence and mortality. Undergoing a conventional fluoroscopic EP procedure at 35 years of age results in almost 1 week of "life lost" and about 2 weeks of "life affected" per patient, in contrast with 5 h and half a day, respectively, with a minimal fluoroscopy approach.

Limitations

On the rare limitations of a total non-fluoroscopic approach we have issues with vascular access in the elderly population; the unexpected occurrence of an anatomical anomaly that might require fluoroscopic delineation (such as a CS aneurysm requiring CS angiography); and implanted pacemakers or implantable cardioverter-defibrillators, as they need fluoroscopic catheter guidance to prevent inadvertent permanent lead dislodgement or entrapment.

Conclusion

There is no major risk to try to reduce or to completely eliminate fluoroscopy in AP's ablation cases; most of the cases can be achieved with a simple three-catheter setting (ablation, coronary sinus, and right ventricular apex ones) approach; even for left-sided APs, if retrograde access is not effective or not preferred, PFO or transseptal access can be obtained with minimal or no fluoroscopy using ICE or TEE; and EAM features as marking target sites or catheter position help to gain efficiency and to make life at the EP lab easier and safer for patients and EP team.

References

1. Anderson R, Ho S. Anatomy of the atrioventricular junctions with regard to ventricular preexcitation. Pacing Clin Electrophysiol. 1997;20:2072–6.
2. Anselmino M, Sillano D, Casolati D, et al. A new electrophysiology era: zero fluoroscopy. J Cardiovasc Med (Hagerstown). 2013;14(3):221–7.
3. Gaita F, Guerra PG, Battaglia A, et al. The dream of near-zero X-rays ablation comes true. Eur Heart J. 2016;37(36):2749–55.
4. Casella M, Dello Russo A, Russo E, et al. X-ray exposure in cardiac electrophysiology: a retrospective analysis in 8150 patients over 7 years of activity in a modern, large-volume laboratory. J Am Heart Assoc. 2018;7(11):e008233.
5. Yang L, Sun G, Chen X, et al. Meta-analysis of zero or near-zero fluoroscopy use during ablation of cardiac arrhythmias. Am J Cardiol. 2016;118(10):1511–8.
6. Scaglione M, Ebrille E, Clemente FD, et al. Catheter ablation of atrial fibrillation without radiation exposure using a 3D mapping system. J Atr Fibrillation. 2015;7(5):1167. https://doi.org/10.4022/jafib.1167.
7. Reddy VY, Morales G, Ahmed H, et al. Catheter ablation of atrial fibrillation without the use of fluoroscopy. Heart Rhythm. 2010;7(11):1644–53.
8. Anderson RH, Brown NA. The anatomy of the heart revisited. Anat Rec. 1996;246:1–7.
9. Anderson RH, Brown NA, Webb S. Development and structure of the atrial septum. Heart. 2002;88:104–10.
10. Anderson RH, Webb S, Brown NA, et al. Development of the heart. 2. Septation of the atriums and ventricles. Heart. 2003;89:949–58.
11. Klein G, Hackel D, Gallagher J. Anatomic substrate of impaired conduction over an accessory atrioventricular pathway in the Wolff-Parkinson-White syndrome. Circulation. 1980;61:1249–56.
12. Chauvin M, Shah D, Haïssaguerre M, et al. The anatomic basis of connections between the coronary sinus musculature and the left atrium in humans. Circulation. 2000;101:647–52.
13. Arruda M, McClelland J, Beckman K, et al. Atrial appendage-ventricular connections: a new variant of preexcitation. Circulation. 1994;90:1–126.
14. De Chillou C, Rodriguez L, Schlapfer J, et al. Clinical characteristics and electrophysiologic properties of atrioventricular accessory pathways: importance of the accessory pathway location. J Am Coll Cardiol. 1992;20:666–71.
15. Jackman WM, Friday KJ, Fitzgerald DM, et al. Localization of left free-wall and posteroseptal accessory atrioventricular pathways by direct recordings of accessory pathway activation. Pacing Clin Electrophysiol. 1989;12:204–14.
16. Wang X, McCelland J, Beckman K, et al. Left free-wall accessory pathway ablation from the coronary sinus: unique coronary sinus electrogram pattern. Circulation. 1992;86:I–586.
17. Becker AE, Anderson RH. The Wolff-Parkinson-White syndrome and its anatomical substrates. Anat Rec. 1981;201:169–77.
18. Becker A, Anderson R, Durrer D, et al. The anatomical substrates of Wolff-Parkinson-White syndrome: a clinical correlation in seven patients. Circulation. 1978;57:870–9.
19. Shinbane J, Lesh M, Stevenson W, et al. Anatomic and electrophysiologic relation between the coronary sinus and mitral annulus: implications for ablation of left-sided accessory pathways. Am Heart J. 1998;135:93–8.
20. Sun Y, Arruda M, Otomo K, et al. Coronary sinus-ventricular accessory connections producing posteroseptal and left posterior accessory pathways: incidence and electrophysiological identification. Circulation. 2002;106:1362–7.
21. Casella M, Dello Russo A, Pelargonio G, et al. Near zerO fluoroscopic exPosure during catheter ablAtion of supRavenTricular arrhYthmias: the NO-PARTY multicentre randomized trial. Europace. 2016;18(10):1565–72.
22. Mahaim I, Winston MR. Recherches d'lanatomic comparee et du pathologic experimentale sur les connexions hautes du faisceau de His-Tawara. Cardiologia. 1941;5:189–260.
23. Haïssaguerre M, Gaita F, Fischer B, et al. Radiofrequency catheter ablation of left lateral accessory pathways via the coronary sinus. Circulation. 1992;86:1464–8.
24. Chen S, Tai C. Ablation of atrioventricular accessory pathways: current technique—state of the art. Pacing Clin Electrophysiol. 2001;24:1795–809.
25. Josephson M. Preexcitation syndromes. In: Josephson M, editor. Clinical cardiac electrophysiology: techniques

and interpretations. 3rd ed. Philadelphia, PA: Lippincott Williams & Wilkins; 2002. p. 322–424.
26. Haïssaguerre M, Gaita F, Marcus FI, et al. Radiofrequency catheter ablation of accessory pathways: a contemporary review. J Cardiovasc Electrophysiol. 1994;5:532–52.
27. Katsouras C, Greakas G, Goudevenos J, et al. Localization of accessory pathways by the electrocardiogram: which is the degree of accordance of three algorithms in use? Pacing Clin Electrophysiol. 2004;27:189–93.
28. Teo W, Klein G, Guiraudon G, et al. Predictive accuracy of electrophysiologic localization of accessory pathways. J Am Coll Cardiol. 1991;18:527–32.
29. Calkins H, Kim Y-N, Schmaltz S, et al. Electrogram criteria for identification of appropriate target sites for radiofrequency catheter ablation of accessory atrioventricular connections. Circulation. 1992;85:565–73.
30. Hirao K, Otomo K, Wang X, et al. Para-Hisian pacing: a new method for differentiating retrograde conduction over an accessory AV pathway from conduction over the AV node. Circulation. 1996;94:1027–35.
31. Miles WM, Yee R, Klein GJ, et al. The preexcitation index: an aid in determining the mechanism of supraventricular tachycardia and localizing accessory pathways. Circulation. 1986;74:493–500.
32. Yang Y, Cheng J, Glatter K, et al. Quantitative effects of functional bundle branch block in patients with atrioventricular reentrant tachycardia. Am J Cardiol. 2000;85:826–31.
33. Mahaim I, Benatt A. Nouvelles recherches sur les connexions superieures de la branch gauche du faisceau de His-Tawara avec cloison interventriculaire. Cardiologia. 1938;1:61–76.
34. Ellenbogen KA, O'Callaghan WG, Colavita PG, et al. Catheter atrioventricular junction ablation for recurrent supraventricular tachycardia with nodoventricular fibers. Am J Cardiol. 1985;55:1227–9.
35. Tchou P, Lehmann MH, Jazayeri M, Akhtar M. Atriofascicular connection or a nodoventricular Mahaim fiber? Electrophysiologic elucidation of the pathway and associated reentrant circuit. Circulation. 1988;77:837–48.
36. Gillette PC, Garson A Jr, Cooey DA, et al. Prolonged and decremental antegrade conduction properties in right anterior atrioventricular connections: wide QRS antidromic tachycardia of left bundle block pattern without Wolff- Parkinson-White configuration in sinus rhythm. Am Heart J. 1982;103:66.
37. Knight BP, Zivin A, Souza J, et al. A technique for the rapid diagnosis of atrial tachycardia in the electrophysiology laboratory. J Am Coll Cardiol. 1999;33:775–81.
38. Grogin HR, Lee RJ, Kwasman M, et al. Radiofrequency catheter ablation of atriofascicular and nodoventricular Mahaim tracts. Circulation. 1994;90:272–81.
39. Klein GJ, Guiraudon GM, Kerr CR, et al. "Nodoventricular" accessory pathway: evidence for a distinct accessory atrioventricular pathway with atrioventricular node-like properties. J Am Coll Cardiol. 1988;11:1035.
40. Kerst G, Weig HJ, Weretka S, et al. Contact force-controlled zero-fluoroscopy catheter ablation of right-sided and left atrial arrhythmia substrates. Heart Rhythm. 2012;9(5):709–14.
41. Mah DY, Miyake CY, Sherwin ED, et al. The use of an integrated electroanatomic mapping system and intracardiac echocardiography to reduce radiation exposure in children and young adults undergoing ablation of supraventricular tachycardia. Europace. 2014;16(2):277–83.
42. Razminia M, Manankil MF, Eryazici PL, et al. Nonfluoroscopic catheter ablation of cardiac arrhythmias in adults: feasibility, safety, and efficacy. J Cardiovasc Electrophysiol. 2012;23(10):1078–86.
43. Kerst G, Parade U, Weig HJ, et al. A novel technique for zero-fluoroscopy catheter ablation used to manage Wolff-Parkinson-White syndrome with a left-sided accessory pathway. Pediatr Cardiol. 2012;33(5):820–3.
44. Ferguson JD, Helms A, Mangrum JM, et al. Catheter ablation of atrial fibrillation without fluoroscopy using intracardiac echocardiography and electroanatomic mapping. Circ Arrhythm Electrophysiol. 2009;2(6):611–9.
45. Brooks AG, Wilson L, Chia NH, et al. Accuracy and clinical outcomes of CT image integration with CartoSound compared to electro-anatomical mapping for atrial fibrillation ablation: a randomized controlled study. Int J Cardiol. 2013;168(3):2774–82.
46. Merino JL. Tools or toys? The 20-year anniversary of the nonfluoroscopic mapping system dilemma. Rev Esp Cardiol. 2017;70(9):690–3.
47. Gallagher JJ, Smith WM, Kasell JH, et al. Role of Mahaim fibers in cardiac arrhythmias in man. Circulation. 1981;64:176–89.
48. Kuck K-H, Schluter M. Single-catheter approach to radiofrequency current ablation of left-sided accessory pathways in patients with Wolff-Parkinson-White syndrome. Circulation. 1991;84:2366–75.
49. Swartz F, Tracy CM, Fletcher RD. Radiofrequency endocardial catheter ablation of accessory atrioventricular pathway atrial insertion sites. Circulation. 1993;87:487–99.
50. Chen X, Borggrefe M, Shenasa M, et al. Characteristics of local electrogram predicting successful transcatheter radiofrequency ablation of left-sided accessory pathways. J Am Coll Cardiol. 1992;20:656–65.
51. Hindricks G, Kottkamp H, Chen X, et al. Localization and radiofrequency catheter ablation of left-sided accessory pathways during atrial fibrillation. J Am Coll Cardiol. 1995;25:444–51.
52. Bashir Y, Heald SC, Katritsis D, et al. Radiofrequency ablation of accessory atrioventricular pathways: predictive value of local electrogram characteristics for the identification of successful target sites. Br Heart J. 1993;69:315–21.

53. Cappato R, Schlüter M, Mont L, Kuck K-H. Anatomic, electrical and mechanical factors affecting bipolar endocardial electrogram: impact on catheter ablation of manifest left free-wall accessory pathways. Circulation. 1994;90:884–94.
54. Takahashi A, Shah D, Jais P, et al. Specific electrocardiographic features of manifest coronary vein posteroseptal accessory pathways. J Cardiovasc Electrophysiol. 1998;9:1015–25.
55. Michaud GF, Tada H, Chough S, et al. Differentiation of atypical atrioventricular node re-entrant tachycardia from orthodromic reciprocating tachycardia using a septal accessory pathway by the response to ventricular pacing. J Am Coll Cardiol. 2001;38:1163–7.
56. Jackman WM, Wang X, Friday KJ, et al. Catheter ablation of accessory atrioventricular pathways (Wolff-Parkinson-White syndrome) by radiofrequency current. N Engl J Med. 1991;324:1605–11.
57. Calkins H, Yong P, Miller J, et al. Catheter ablation of accessory pathways, atrioventricular nodal reentrant tachycardia, and the atrioventricular junction: final results of a prospective, multicenter clinical trial. Circulation. 1999;99:262–70.
58. Xie B, Heald SC, Camm AJ, et al. Successful radiofrequency ablation of accessory pathways with the first energy delivery: the anatomic and electrical characteristics. Eur Heart J. 1996;17:1072–9.
59. Langberg JJ, Calkins H, Kim Y-N, et al. Recurrence of conduction in accessory atrioventricular connections after initially successful radiofrequency catheter ablation. J Am Coll Cardiol. 1992;19:1588–92.
60. Coppess MA, Altemose GT, Jayachandran JV, et al. Unusual features of intermediate septal bypass tracts. J Cardiovasc Electrophysiol. 2000;11:730–5.
61. Álvarez M, Bertomeu-González V, Arcocha MF, et al. Nonfluoroscopic catheter ablation. Results from a prospective multicenter registry. Rev Esp Cardiol (Engl Ed). 2017;70(9):699–705.
62. Scaglione M, Ebrille E, Caponi D, et al. Zero-fluoroscopy ablation of accessory pathways in children and adolescents: CARTO3 electroanatomic mapping combined with RF and cryoenergy. Pacing Clin Electrophysiol. 2015;38(6):675–81.
63. Clark J, Bockoven JR, Lane J, et al. Use of three-dimensional catheter guidance and trans-esophageal echocardiography to eliminate fluoroscopy in catheter ablation of left-sided accessory pathways. Pacing Clin Electrophysiol. 2008;31(3):283–9.
64. Huo Y, Christoph M, Forkmann M, et al. Reduction of radiation exposure during atrial fibrillation ablation using a novel fluoroscopy image integrated 3-dimensional electroanatomic mapping system: a prospective, randomized, single-blind, and controlled study. Heart Rhythm. 2015;12(9):1945–55.

Focal Atrial Tachycardia

9

Charles Dussault and Jean-Francois Roux

Focal atrial tachycardias, defined as a regular atrial arrhythmia not requiring the AV node or the ventricles, represent 5–15% of supraventricular tachycardia (SVT) cases. They therefore represent a relatively rare form of arrhythmia compared to reentrant SVTs. In the vast majority of cases, they arise in patients with structurally normal hearts. While evenly distributed between genders, younger patients are more commonly affected with these arrhythmias, increasing the interest in fluoro-reduction strategies. The potential sites of origin for these arrhythmias are diverse. Recognized mechanisms for focal atrial tachycardia include triggered activity, abnormal automaticity, and microreentry.

Hazards of radiation exposure have been specifically documented for patients undergoing RF ablation for supraventricular tachycardias, with an increased incidence of fatal malignancies most notably affecting the lungs. This particular risk appears to be increased in obese subjects [1].

To further describe the mechanism of a focal AT, response to various pacing and pharmacological maneuvers can be assessed (Table 9.1). Activation mapping is the cornerstone of focal atrial tachycardia localization. Technological advancements in the field of electroanatomical mapping now allow the localization of non-sustained atrial arrhythmia foci that would otherwise be impossible to map and successfully ablate. High-density mapping has also made possible the identification as well as definition of microreentrant arrhythmias. The three-dimensional display of the atria is of paramount importance in eliminating fluoroscopy. Electroanatomical mapping systems use a color-coded display showing the earliest site of activation as the red region with activation spreading in a radial (centrifugal) direction.

ECG Localization of Atrial Tachycardia

When a fluoroless approach is contemplated, surface ECG localization of the arrhythmia focus ahead of it is critically important. Although significant overlap exists, available algorithms are helpful in identifying the most likely site of origin of the arrhythmia. In order to fully delineate the potential risks of the procedure, it is particularly important to identify arrhythmias likely to originate from the left atrium or the parahisian region. Of note, an isoelectric p-wave in lead V1 suggests a focus near the AV node, while a positive p-wave in leads V1 to V5 is more suggestive of a left atrial origin [2].

Our standard approach consists of using the patches needed for a 3D mapping system on all

C. Dussault (✉) · J.-F. Roux
Cardiology Division, Department of Medicine, Université de Sherbrooke, Sherbrooke, QC, Canada
e-mail: Charles.dussault@usherbrooke.ca; Jean-Francois.Roux@usherbrooke.ca

R. Proietti et al. (eds.), *Cardiac Electrophysiology Without Fluoroscopy*, https://doi.org/10.1007/978-3-030-16992-3_9

Table 9.1 Atrial tachycardia mechanisms

	Initiation	Response to entrainment/overdrive	Other
Triggered	Rapid atrial pacing/ PES	Transient suppression or termination	Adenosine response
Increased automaticity	Isoproterenol	Transient suppression	Warm-up/cool-down
Microreentrant	Rapid atrial pacing/ PES	Entrainment possible	Adenosine response possible

suspected cases, as if an atrial tachycardia arises, all is already in place to perform a 3D mapping cartography, navigation, and ablation, thus reducing or eliminating the need of fluoroscopy.

Evidence Supporting Fluoroless Ablation of Focal Atrial Tachycardia

Razminia et al. [3] published their 5-year experience with fluoroless catheter ablation for various cardiac arrhythmias including ATs, demonstrating both the efficacy and the safety of this approach. One hundred and eleven patients underwent focal AT ablation with an acute success rate of 100%. They used either Carto 3 (Biosense Webster) or EnSite (Abbott) as their EA mapping system and used an intracardiac ultrasound probe for left side. Ablation catheters were either conventional or irrigated RF and contact force was not mandatory. The sites of origin of these arrhythmias were highly variable, with 39 coming from the right atrium, 42 from the left atrium, 4 from the noncoronary sinus, and 26 from within the coronary sinus. The median procedure duration was 146 min (range 54–371 min). Of note, procedure duration was shown to be highly operator dependent and significantly decreased over time, decreasing from a mean of 209.6 min during the first year of the study to 105.3 min 5 years later.

After an average follow-up of 18.4 months, the recurrence rate was 5.4%, which is comparable to what is expected following fluoroscopy-guided ablation procedures. As for safety, only one major complication occurred among the 60 patients who underwent ablation of a focal AT as the primary arrhythmia (tamponade requiring pericardiocentesis during left-sided AT ablation). This reported 1.7% complication rate compared to accepted complication rates for this type of procedure [4].

Technical Considerations

As for other EP procedures using 3D mapping, the diagnostic study for focal AT requires the use of a coronary sinus catheter that will serve as reference for the EA mapping system. In order to position the remaining diagnostic catheters, the ablation catheter is advanced in the right atrium and a geometry of the right atrium is created with precise delineation of the tricuspid annulus. A particular attention is devoted to mapping of the His region, where tags will be highlighted at sites demonstrating His bundle potentials. The remaining diagnostic catheters can then be safely positioned as required at the right ventricular apex, His bundle region, and high right atrium. Using this technique, successful catheter positioning without fluoroscopy has been reported to approach 100% (please refer to the chapter on catheter positioning for details on any of the available 3D mapping system utilization).

A standard EP study can then be performed to induce the clinical arrhythmia and diagnose the atrial tachycardia. Once the diagnosis is confirmed, activation sequences in the atrium based on diagnostic catheters should suggest a likely region of origin for the arrhythmia. The ablation catheter will then be used to delineate the exact focus of the arrhythmia by identifying the earliest activation point.

If the foci are localized in the right atrium, the only consideration before ablation is the distance to the His bundle; as all available His potentials are recorded in the 3D mapping system, it is easy to safety ablate while visualizing at all times the catheter ablation in he 3D mapping system, with multiangled views as needed. We suggest a 1 cm distance from any His recorded in the atrial anatomy as a safety margin to ablate with radiofrequency; closer foci can be approached safely with cryoablation.

If the foci are localized in the left side, the complete elimination of fluoroscopy needs either a patent foramen ovale (present in as high as 20% of patients) or an intracardiac ultrasound (ICE) to perform a transseptal puncture; otherwise, minimal fluoroscopy can be used to achieve left access and the case can be continued without X-rays as in any right-sided approach (please refer to the atrial fibrillation ablation chapter for details on transseptal access).

In our series, with 37 atrial tachycardias approached initially without fluoroscopy, we were able to achieve (without ICE) a 83.8% success in eliminating completely the need of fluoroscopy (left-sided access requires fluoroscopy for the transseptal puncture and ablation proceeded then without X-rays even if these cases were counted as a "failure" to perform a 100% fluoroscopy-free procedure) [5].

Finally, we suggest also (unless the activation sequence shows a pulmonary vein foci as the clear origin of the arrhythmia) to map the coronary cusps as between 10 and 15% of septal localizations can be approached from the aortic cusps. Finally care on energy titration or source of energy is required for locations near the septal tricuspid annulus, as ablating form this region could occlude the right coronary artery or the AV node artery, ending in complete AV block in a region far from the His or the AV node [6].

Conclusion

Atrial tachycardia ablation either in the right of the left side is feasible and safe with a minimal or complete elimination of fluoroscopy, as all of these substrates need a 3D mapping system to perform the procedure. Left atrial access is also feasible without fluoroscopy using ICE, but minimal fluoroscopy can be used for transseptal puncture and then continuing without fluoroscopy for the rest of the procedure.

References

1. Kovoor P, et al. Risk to patients from radiation associated with radiofrequency ablation for supraventricular tachycardia. Circulation. 1998;98:1534–40.
2. Zipes D, Jalife J. Cardiac electrophysiology: from cell to bedside. 6th ed. Philadelphia: Saunders; 2013.
3. Razminia M, et al. Fluoroless catheter ablation of cardiac arrhythmias: a 5 year experience. PACE. 2017;40:425–33.
4. Bohnen M, et al. Incidence and predictors of major complications from contemporary catheter ablation to treat cardiac arrhythmias. Heart Rhythm. 2011;8:1661–6.
5. Ayala Valani L, et al. Real life EP lab without fluoroscopy. Eur Heart J. 2018;39(Issue Suppl. 1):P6646.
6. Mykytsey A, et al. Right coronary artery occlusion during RF ablation of typical atrial flutter. J Cardiovasc Electrophysiol. 2010;21(7):818–21.

10 Ablation of Atrial Flutter with Zero Fluoroscopy Approach

Vincenzo Russo, Roberta Bottino, Anna Rago, Riccardo Proietti, Antonio Cassese, Carmine Ciardiello, and Gerardo Nigro

Introduction

Over the last 20 years, interventional electrophysiology (EP) has expanded significantly in the field of diagnostic studies, ablations, and device implantation. During any intracardiac procedure, real-time visualization of catheters is critical. In the field of catheter ablation of cardiac arrhythmias, the procedure is traditionally performed using fluoroscopic guidance for catheter placement. During interventional studies, fluoroscopy involves 95% of the total X-ray operation time in EP, causing roughly 40% of the total radiation exposure to the staff and the patients [1]. The resulting exposure of both patients and medical staff to ionizing radiations could induce biological effects in a stochastic (carcinogenic and genetic effects) or in a deterministic (also called tissue reactions) way [2]. It has been well established that radiation exposure increases the lifetime risk of deterministic effects such as skin injuries and cataracts [3–6]. For those effects, there is a threshold of dose (below this threshold, the effect is not produced) and the severity increases with the dose [2]. Also, radiation exposure increases the lifetime risk of stochastic effects such as damage to cells and their Deoxyribonucleic acid (DNA) with higher incidence of genetic defects and cancers [4, 7, 8]. For stochastic effects the most widely accepted model is the "Linear Non-Threshold" model: any small amount of radiation involves an increase in cancer risk without any threshold, and the probability increases linearly with increasing radiation dose [2]. Radiofrequency (RF) ablation can be of long duration, with an average effective radiation dose of 15 mSv, the equivalent of 150 chest X-rays, being remarkably higher even than that of common CT, and is considered to increase the occurrence of malignant tumors [7, 9]. Studies have shown that the radiation exposure received from 53 to 60 min of fluoroscopy during ablation procedures might result in 0.7–1.4 fatal malignancies per 1000 women and 1.0–2.6 per 1000 men [10, 11]. In addition, orthopedic diseases attributed to the use of heavy protective lead apparel have been documented [12]. Radiation exposure presents even more risk for individuals with certain conditions such as pregnant women, patients with immune system dysfunction, and pediatric population [9]. In the following paragraphs we will show the available data on fluoroless catheter ablation of atrial flutter.

Vincenzo Russo and Roberta Bottino contributed equally to this work.

V. Russo (✉) · R. Bottino · A. Rago · A. Cassese
G. Nigro
Department of Cardiology, University of Campania "Luigi Vanvitelli", Monaldi Hospital, Naples, Italy
e-mail: v.p.russo@libero.it; gerardo.nigro@unincampania.it

R. Proietti
Department of Cardiology, University of Padua, Pauda, Italy

C. Ciardiello
HT Med, Pozzuoli (Naples), Italy

R. Proietti et al. (eds.), *Cardiac Electrophysiology Without Fluoroscopy*,
https://doi.org/10.1007/978-3-030-16992-3_10

Typical Atrial Flutter and Main Atypical Atrial Flutter Forms

Atrial flutter (AFL) refers to a heterogeneous group of atrial arrhythmias defined mechanistically by a macroreentrant circuit around fixed anatomical barriers or functional conduction blocks [13, 14].

Typical AFL is a regular, organized atrial tachycardia confined to the right atrium, with the wave front traveling around the tricuspid annulus, with a ventricular rate response limited by the atrioventricular (AV) node conductions, usually presenting a 2:1 or 3:1 response [15]. It originates in a well-known right atrial macroreentrant circuit bounded by the tricuspid annulus anteriorly, limited by anatomical barriers posteriorly such as both the superior and inferior cava veins and the coronary sinus [15]. The circuit involves the cavotricuspid isthmus (CTI) as the critical zone of slow conduction enabling reentry to be sustained [16–19]. The CTI is situated between the inferior aspect of the tricuspid annulus and the ostium of the inferior vena cava. The most common direction of activation of the typical AFL circuit is counter clockwise when viewed from a left anterior oblique (LAO) fluoroscopic perspective: the wave front proceeds in a lateral to septal direction along the isthmus between the inferior vena cava (IVC) and the tricuspid valve (TV) and then proceeds along the septum in a caudocranial direction [20]. When the wavefront from a LAO perspective proceeds in the opposite direction, the activation will be clockwise (reverse typical atrial flutter −10% of clinical cases) [20].

Atypical AFL includes macroreentrant tachycardias in which the wave front does not travel around the tricuspid annulus but around various anatomical boundaries resulting from atrial remodelling (fibrous scarring) due to severe structural heart disease or scarring after previous cardiac surgery and atrial fibrillation ablation [14]. Atypical right atrial flutter includes the following: lower loop reentry, fosa ovalis flutter, superior vena cava flutter, and upper loop reentry [21–24].

Lower loop reentry atrial flutter (LLR) uses a circuit that includes the CTI, as common atrial flutter, but it shortens the circuit through a gap in the crista terminalis [14].

Upper loop reentry was also described using a circuit through a gap in the crista terminalis and then in the posterior right atrium wall. The electrocardiogram pattern mimics a clockwise typical flutter but the cycle length is usually shorter, as in lower loop reentry [21, 22].

An infrequent form of right atrial atypical flutter is confined within the superior vena cava and from it the atria are passively activated [23].

In the group of atrial flutters called "incisional flutters" the circuit uses previous surgery-related scars. This kind of flutter is mostly seen in patients with history of surgical correction of congenital heart diseases [24, 25].

Finally, atypical AFL may originate in the left atrium, in which the leading wave front is confined. It occurs mainly in patients with underlying structural heart disease accounting for 10% of AFLs [26]. The most frequent left AFLs are perimitral, with the arrhythmia rotating in a zone of conduction block including the pulmonary veins, or an electrically silent area [26, 27]. In some patients, the circuits are more complex, with two or three loops rotating concomitantly (peripulmonary veins, septal, roof, and posterior wall macroreentrys) [26].

Atrial Flutter Ablation: Conventional and Fluoroless Techniques

The incidence of AFL increases with age from 0.05% in patients <50 years to 5.87% in those ≥80 years with an overall incidence in the general population of 0.88% [28]. AFL is frequently associated with other cardiovascular conditions such as hypertension, coronary artery disease, chronic pulmonary disease, and sick sinus syndrome [25]. Regarding treatment, the superiority of catheter ablation over use of antiarrhythmic drugs with respect to freedom from AFL recurrences during long-term follow-up has been demonstrated in randomized clinical trials [29, 30]. According to the 2016 ESC Guidelines, management of typical AFL with ablation of the CTI is recommended for patients failing antiarrhythmic drug therapy or as first-line treatment considering patient preference [31]. During an AFL ablation procedure, a contiguous linear lesion across the CTI is created, deploying continuous RF lesions in order to interrupt the macroreentrant circuit by connecting the non-excitable tissue of the tricuspid annulus and the IVC. Bidirectional conduction block across the CTI is a generally accepted procedural end point to prove the electrophysiological interruption of the circuit and can be achieved in approximately 95% of patients [14, 32, 33].

Traditionally AFL ablation is performed using fluoroscopic guidance for catheter placement. The conventional fluoroscopy AFL ablation provides instantaneous localization of intracardiac tools and shows real-time relationship of these tools to moving cardiac structures, but has some important limitations such as radiation exposure to patients and healthcare personnel [7, 34, 35] and the solely 2D orientation. During AFL ablation fluoroscopy time usually exceeds 15 min [32, 33, 36, 37] with longer fluoroscopy times in case of complex anatomy of the CTI [38]. The capability of 2-D orientation only may result in an arduous catheter navigation and inappropriate catheter tip–tissue contact. To overcome these problems, various measures including the use of new three-dimensional electroanatomical mapping (3D-EAM) software, intracardiac echocardiography (ICE), transesophageal echocardiography (TEE), and contact-force sensing catheters have led to a significant reduction or complete elimination of fluoroscopy in most patients [39]. Intracardiac echocardiogram (ICE) uses high-frequency ultrasound and allows identification of anatomic structures and provides accurate catheter location in the form of real-time images [40]. ICE has proven to be an invaluable tool for guiding transseptal puncture and catheter manipulation especially in left atrial and ventricular ablation procedures. 3D-EAM different systems are employed to facilitate mapping and ablation. These mapping systems can also merge cardiac chamber anatomy acquired with a mapping catheter with a pre-acquired anatomical image, such as a fluoroscopic, magnetic resonance imaging (MRI), or CT image. These computerized systems enable the creation of a 3D geometry of cardiac structures allowing physicians to navigate catheters within an accurate shell of patient's anatomy and zero or near zero fluoroscopy catheter guidance.

Each EAM system has its strengths and weaknesses, and the system chosen must depend upon what data is required for procedural success (activation mapping, substrate mapping, cardiac geometry), the anticipated arrhythmia, the compatibility of the system with adjunctive tools (i.e., diagnostic and ablation catheters), and the operator's familiarity with the selected system.

Current 3D-EAM used for electrophysiology catheter visualization include the following: CARTO (Biosense Webster Inc., Diamond Bar, CA), EnSiteNavX and Mediguide technologies (Abbott, Abbott Park, IL), and Rhythmia (Boston Scientific, San Jose, CA).

The Carto system, in its present third generation (Carto 3), is based on six skin patches positioned on patient's chest and back that create an electrical-based location field. These patches, by a location pad technology (with nine coils), also create a magnetic field. Therefore, the combination consists in an electromagnetic field in which catheter movements can be detected. As the catheter moves around the chamber, a multitude of such associated locations are created and stored by the system. Also with this system, activation mapping information, during arrhythmias or sinus rhythm, may be projected to the map with a color-coded mode useful for guiding the ablation to the origin of the arrhythmia [41].

The EnSiteNavX (Fig. 10.1a, b) relies on three pairs of nominally orthogonal skin patches in *x*–*y* and *z*-axis positioned on the patient's chest. These patches create an electrical location field on the patient's thorax. An additional patch positioned on the abdomen serves as a reference during advancement of the catheters in the iliofemoral venous axis. The system collects electrical data from standard electrophysiology catheters and uses this information to track or navigate their movement, construct 3D models of the chamber, and create activation and voltage

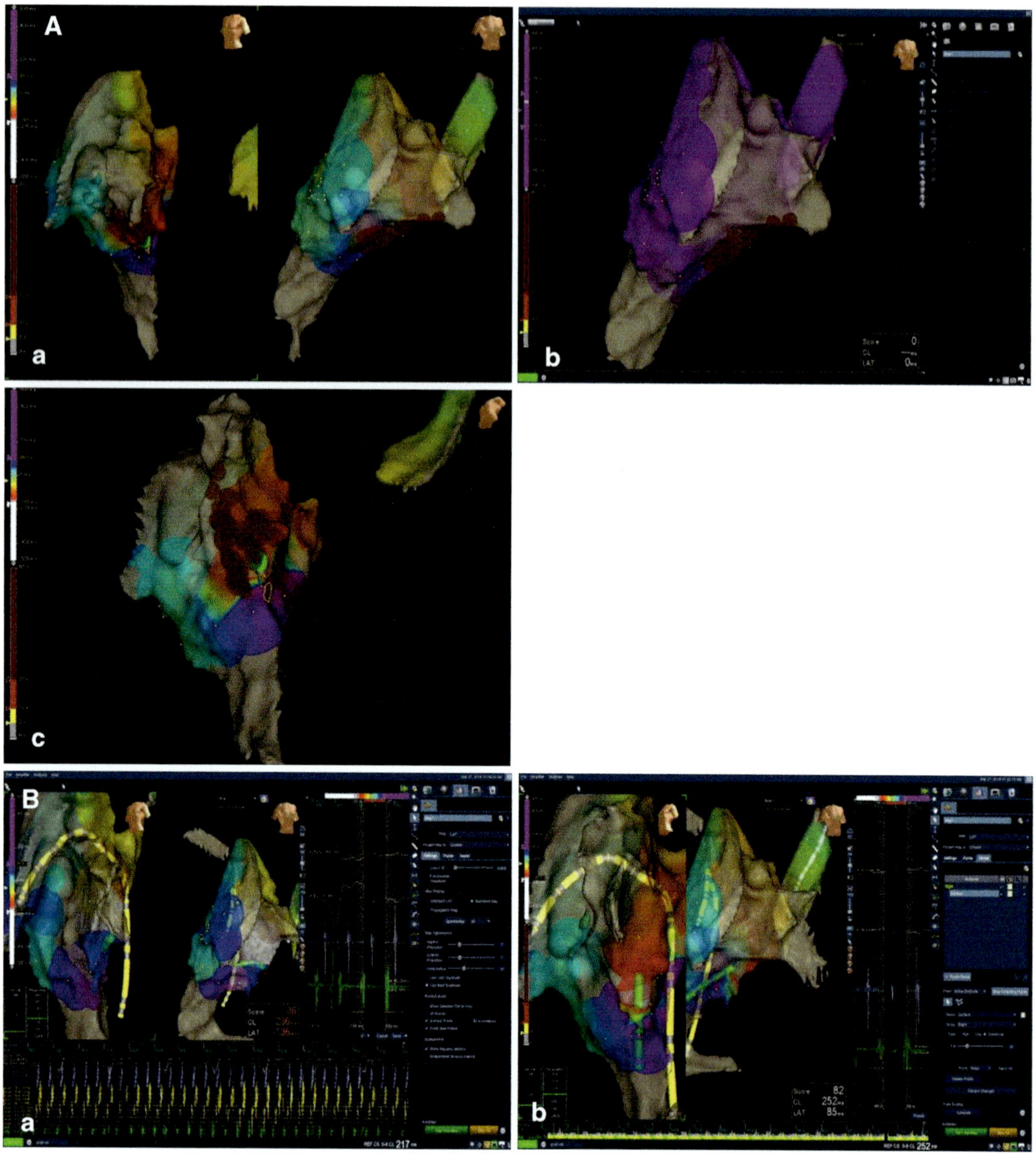

Fig. 10.1 (**A**) Common typical atrial flutter ablation, guided by EnSite Precision Cardiac Mapping System. (**a**) Right atrium electrical activation map in left anterior oblique (LAO) and in right anterior oblique (RAO) projections. (**b**) Propagation map of the right atrium in RAO projection. (**c**) Lesion line after cavotricuspid isthmus (CTI) ablation in left cranial oblique projection. The earliest activation (**light red**) is located on the right side of the lesion line, near the lower zone of interatrial septum; the latest activation (**purple**) is located on the left side of the lesion line (in the lower zone of the lateral wall). (**B**) (**a**) Proximal-to-distal coronary sinus activation sequence confirming the counterclockwise circuit of common typical flutter. The ablation target is the cavotricuspid isthmus. (**b**) The window of interest shows the mesodiastolic potential on the ablation catheter corresponding to the atrial signal

maps. Catheter positioning system is based on a dynamic electromagnetic field integrated with a miniaturized single coil sensor mounted on dedicated electrophysiology catheters and a reference sensor attached to the patient's chest [41].

The MediGuideT technology (no longer commercialized) consists of three components: a transmitter unit generating a low-intensity dynamic 3D electromagnetic field; miniaturized passive single coil sensors (<1 mm^3) embedded in intracardiac devices such as conventional electrode or ablation catheters; and an electromagnetic field reference sensor affixed to the patient's chest at the level of the sternum similar to an ECG electrode in size. The electromagnetic fields induce voltages on the passive device sensors. According to these voltages, the system computes position and orientation of each sensor within the 3D tracking volume with respect to the transmitter assembly with a time latency of 1 ms. The electromagnetic field transmitters are mounted on the fluoroscopy detector of a conventional X-ray imaging system aligning the fluoroscopy space with the 3D electromagnetic sensor field. As a result, the sensor-equipped EP catheter can either be seen on fluoroscopy or tracked nonfluoroscopically at the identical position by the 3D electromagnetic sensor field. With the use of prerecorded fluoroscopy cine loops, real-time catheter location data obtained from the electromagnetic sensor field are visualized nonfluoroscopically within the X-ray environment [41] to navigate in more familiar (X-ray) environment, with real-time catheter tracking, but with saved (not real time) fluoroscopic shadows.

Rhythmia™ is a novel, high-density automated electroanatomic contact mapping system. The system utilizes a 64-pole steerable basket catheter (magnetically located) that is used to create a shell of the chamber of interest and simultaneously collect very high-density, low-noise electrogram information. Electrogram collection is automated, so activation patterns and scar maps containing several thousand points are acquired routinely. Location of any ablation catheter is currently impedance based and requires an intracardiac catheter as a positional reference (e.g., a coronary sinus catheter), although there are also magnetic-guided proprietary catheters (Intella Tip and Intella MiFi Tip) available. While it is possible to use any ablation catheter, activation and substrate mapping can be performed only with a dedicated catheter (Intella-Map OrionTM), an high resolution mapping basket catheter with 64 low-noise electrodes and 2.5 mm inter-electrodes pacing. Thanks to the latter and an advanced point acquisition software and process, this system is able to generate, by automated and continuous mapping, a very high resolution 3D electroanatomical maps [41].

However, some limitations of 3D mapping systems should be mentioned: these systems work as independent tools unrelated to the standard working environment of live fluoroscopy; it only provides static models and maps while intracardiac locations are affected by multiple components of organ motion (e.g., cardiac cycle, respiration). Even in Mediguide system and in Carto-UniVu system pre-acquired fluoroscopy loops only provide an illusion of real-time imaging, and acute clinical variations, such as a pericardial tamponade or a pneumothorax, will not be real-time depicted. Additionally, 3D mapping systems increases procedural costs being associated with a more complex workflow, especially in the setting of simple EP studies such as AFL ablation [32].

Another way to reduce radiation exposure to the operator is the use of remote navigation systems; with these systems, the interventional electrophysiologist is sitting in a control room remote from X-ray exposure while catheter navigation is allowed by magnetic or robotic navigation (manipulation of steerable sheaths via a robotic arm) [42]. The prolonged procedure duration, the requirement for additional technical equipment, and the lower success rate are major limitations of remote navigation technologies [43].

Fluoroless or near Zero-Ray Ablation: Hands on

The first challenge is catheter positioning, please refer to the chapter on catheter placement for further details; briefly, and no matter the system used, the first catheter is advanced gently from the groin through the inferior vena cava (IVC) until atrial EGMs are detected; if advanced too fast, the catheter would pass to the superior vena cava (SVC); at the beginning of the experience, to measure the distance from the groin to the chest with the catheter on the outside could help to give an idea on how much the catheter needs to be advanced until the atrium is reached (in Carto or Rhythmia a mark of the catheter placed at the lower sternum, outside the chest, could give also an idea on how far the catheter needs to be advanced in the inferior vena cava); if IVC valves prevent atrial access, a softer and smaller quadripolar catheter could be used, advanced until atrial signals are seen, then stiffer catheters advance become easier as valves are now open; in the very beginning, we can leave some "marks" while the first catheter advances, to show the road through the atrium. Once the roving catheter is on the atrium, the virtual anatomy can be created: IVC and SVC are "drawn" rotating the catheter with a gentle curve, followed by the right atrium; since the beginning, simultaneous RAO and LAO views help to orientate the movement of the roving catheter. Tricuspid valve is easily depicted once annotated on places where there are simultaneous atrial and ventricular signals. His bundle is located and marked at his usual position, also guided by EGMs; the catheter is then flexed posteriorly or down, and advanced anteriorly to obtain big ventricular signals; then a gentle retraction, clockwise torque, and freeing simultaneously the curve allows the access to the coronary sinus, the catheter is then advanced to create CS virtual anatomy as far as possible. The other catheters needed are advanced in the same way as described before; depending on the system used, the reference catheter can be switched to the decapolar catheter placed in the CS, if needed. We are ready to start the EP study to prove the origin of the flutter (if the patient is in flutter), and the absence of other mechanisms or substrates (if the patient is in sinus rhythm).

To reduce the cost associated to 3-D mapping systems use for every flutter ablation, a two catheter only approach could be implemented for flutter ablation (for Carto, NavX, and Rhythmia using Intella Tip catheters; Rhythmia Orion basket catheter is currently used in some EP labs to approach patients with recurrences only). A multipolar catheter is placed in the coronary sinus either at the beginning or once the atrial anatomy is already constructed, with detail in the cavotricuspid isthmus, to well depict its length, characteristics (concave, convex, pouches inside, etc.).

If the patient is in flutter, and the coronary sinus catheter in place, two approaches can be used: slightly faster than the flutter cycle length stimulation is applied to measure the post pacing intervals (PPI) in the distal coronary sinus, the proximal coronary sinus and in any place of the putative circuit around the tricuspid annulus, it can easily prove the circuit confined to the right atrium; alternatively, an activation map of the right atrium can be constructed dragging the ablation catheter in different right atrial locations and acquiring EGMs either manually or with the software of different 3-D mapping systems; if the Rhythmia Orion is used, a very detailed activation map can be created to depict the flutter circuit in the right atrium. Once the circuit is confirmed as typical, the RAO view is used to depict catheter position in the anterior (ventricular) posterior (inferior vena cava) axis; the LAO view is also useful (with some caudal tilt to better observe the isthmus from "below") to maintain the isthmus line as straight as possible. The catheter is pulled back while ablating, since ventricular aspect appears in the EGMs (big V and almost no A), until it drops into the inferior vena cava. The flutter usually stops during the construction of the line. If the patient is in sinus rhythm (or once the flutter is stopped while burning), with the two catheter approach, the coronary sinus is used to pace at the slowest cycle length possible; the ablation catheter is used to apply RF until local EGM amplitude reduction, and specially until widely separated double potentials, or local EGM displacement from close to the pacing artifact, to a distant from the pacing artifact, once the isthmus is blocked and the activation must proceed giving a complete turn around the valve. Alternatively, differential pacing from either site of the line or new activations maps can be created while stimulating from the coronary sinus, to confirm the complete block at the isthmus level. Using the fluoro free two catheters approach, the total duration (patient in and patient out, 184 patients) of a flutter ablation had a median time of 105 min (range 35–210 min), not different of our historical control (with fluoroscopy before 2008) of 101 min; we could eliminate fluoroscopy in 95% of patients.

Fluoroless or near Zero-Ray Ablation: Current Major Results

Fluoroscopy Plus 3D Guided Procedures

Several studies have demonstrated the feasibility, safety, and efficacy of 3D guided procedure catheter ablation in AFL (Table 10.1).

In this regard in 2013 Shurrab et al. [44] conducted a metanalysis in order to compare success, procedure time, and complications of fluoroscopy plus 3D guided to fluoroscopically-only guided supraventricular arrhythmias ablation procedures. Studies from 1990 to 2010 were identified, 10 eligible studies comparing fluoroscopy-only and 3D-guided ablation in AFL were found. Of the 561 AFL, 292 underwent a 3D guided procedure (CARTO: 194, NavX/EnsiteNavX:72, Localisa:26). The acute success rate was 97% vs. 93% (fluoroscopy+3D-guided ablation vs. fluoroscopically-only guided; $p = 0.57$); the long-term success rate was not statistically different (93% vs. 96%, fluoroscopy- and 3D-guided ablation vs. fluoroscopically-only guided, $p = 0.90$, follow-up between 1.5 and 16 months). Fluoroscopic time and radiation exposure were significantly reduced for ablation of AFL with 3D systems ($p < 0.001$ and $p = 0.002$, respectively) while ablation and procedure time were not statistically different between 3D and conventional system (ablation time: 56 vs. 55 min, $p = 0.43$; average procedure time: 117 min vs. 115 min, $p = 0.75$). Only one major complication was reported in the AFL 3D group showing no significant difference between the two groups. Globally the study demonstrated that success, procedure time, and complications are similar between fluoroscopy only and 3D-guided plus fluoroscopy ablations, while fluoroscopic time and radiation exposure are significantly reduced for ablation of AFL with 3D systems. Similar results were obtained in a recent study conducted by Brunelli and colleagues [45].

Near Zero and Zero-Fluoroscopy Procedures

Supraventricular Arrhythmias

Regarding zero-fluoroscopic techniques, results of recent studies show feasibility, safety, and efficacy of non-fluoro supraventricular arrhythmias ablation [39, 46–54]. Yang et al. [55] conducted in 2016 a meta-analysis in order to compare fluoroscopic time, ablation time, procedure duration, immediate success, long-term success, complications, and recurrence rate in the treatment of cardiac arrhythmias between procedures using zero or near-zero fluoroscopy and conventional ablation. Studies were retrieved between 1974 and 2016. Zero fluoroscopy was defined as the achievement of ablation entirely without use of any fluoroscopy. Near-zero fluoroscopy was interpreted as planning for a procedure with no fluoroscopy, but very limited radiation use if considered necessary by the operator. Ten eligible studies were found. Seven out of ten studies [39, 46, 47, 49–52] took into account AFL ablation procedures and three out of seven were randomized prospective trials [46, 47, 49]. Overall, fluoroscopic time was reduced in zero or near-zero fluoroscopy ablation by a standard mean difference (SMD) of −1.62. Radiation dose was dramatically lower in the zero or near-zero fluoroscopy ablation group than that in the conventional group. Procedure duration was not significantly different. Ablation time was reduced in non-randomized trials but not in randomized trials. Acute success, complication, and recurrence rates did not show significant differences between the two groups regardless of the arrhythmia considered. Similar results were obtained from more recent studies [56–59].

Atrial Flutter

As regard directly AFL ablation several recent studies compared results of different non-fluoro 3D EAM systems. Macıas et al. [60] evaluate the feasibility and safety of a zero-fluoroscopy approach to CTI catheter ablation using the Carto 3 system compared to the Ensite-NavXTM system. The study

Table 10.1 Characteristics of the studies

Author/reference	Year of publication	Study design	Arrhythmias studied (%)	Fluoroless system used (n)	Population features	Fluoroscopy time (min)	Procedure duration (min)	Main efficacy results	Main safety results (major complications)	Follow-up
Bastian et al. [61]	2017	Prospective study	AFL (100%)	**EAM:** **Carto 3** (267) **EnSite NavX** (88)	$N = 355$ **Carto 3** Mean age: 65.1 ± 12.5 **EnSite NavX** Mean age: 67 ± 14.4	**Carto** 7.1 ± 6.6 **EnSite NavX** 0.8 ± 1.9	**Carto** 95.3 ± 48.3 **EnSite NavX** 93.4 ± 42.5	"Zero-fluoroscopy" approach higher in the **Ensite NavX** group ($p < 0.001$)	0	*Data not shown*
Stec et al. [56]	2017	Prospective study	**Ensite NavX** AFL (23%) AVNRT (52%) AP (21%) AT (4%) **X-ray procedures** AFL (31%) AVNRT (42%) AP (21%) AT (6%)	**EAM:** **Ensite NavX** (1512)	$N = 2242$ **Ensite NavX** Mean age: 47 ± 20 **X-ray procedures** Mean age: 52 ± 18	**Ensite NaveX** 0.5 ± 2.5 min **X-ray procedures** 8.1 ± 8.3	**Ensite NaveX** 51.3 ± 27.2 **X-ray procedures** 63.2 ± 38.7 ($p < 0.001$)	Acute success: **Ensite NaveX** 97.3% **X-ray procedures** 98.3%	0	*Data not shown*
Deutsch et al. [63]	2017	Prospective study	AFL (100%)	**EAM:** **Ensite Velocity NavX** (219)	$N = 460$ **Ensite NavX + MVG** $n = 164$; mean age: 63.7 ± 9.5; 30% female **Ensite NavX + PBT** $n = 55$; mean age: 63.9 ± 10.7; 39% female **ALARA + MVG** $n = 36$; mean age: 64.2 ± 9.6; 39% female **ALARA + PBT** $n = 205$; mean age: 64.7 ± 9.1; 30% female	**NXR + MVG** 0.3 ± 1.6 **NXR + PBT** 0.2 ± 1.1 **ALARA + MVG** 7.7 ± 6.0 **ALARA + PBT** 9.1 ± 7.2	**NXR + MVG** 45 ± 17.6 **NXR + PBT** 47.2 ± 15.7 **ALARA + MVG** 52.6 ± 23.7 **ALARA + PBT** 59.8 ± 24.0	Acute success: 99% in all groups	0	*Data not shown*

Brunelli et al. [45]	2017	Prospective study	AFL (66%) AVNRT (32%) AP (2%) (data available only as rate of total pts)	**EAM:** **Ensite NavX** (97)	*N* = 137 Mean age: 66 ± 15 41% female	**Ensite NavX** 0 **X-ray procedures** 11	**Ensite NavX** 90 (60–120) **X-ray procedures** 68 (50–93)	Acute success: 99.27% in both group **EnSite NavX** Zero fluoroscopy achieved in 52%	0	*Data not shown*
Seizer et al. [52]	2016	Retrospective study	**EnSite NavX** AFL (12.08%) AVNRT (52.75%) WPW (23.08%) AT (8.79%) **X-ray procedures** AFL (15.03%) AVNRT (48.39%) WPW (33.33%) AT (8.79%)	**EAM:** **EnSite NavX** (91)	*N* = 184 **Ensite NavX** Mean age: 36.0 ± 22.1 50.7% female **X-ray procedures** Mean age: 52.1 ± 19.1 50.7% female	**EnSite NavX** 0 **X-ray procedures** 13.3 ± 12.2	**EnSite NavX** 102.6 ± 35.5 **X-ray procedures** 128.3 ± 90.3	Acute success rate: **EnSite NavX** 100%	0	389 ± 217 days
Giaccardi et al. [51]	2016	Prospective study	**EnSite Velocity NavX** AFL (45.12%) AVNRT (34%) AP (8.75%) AT (4.38%) Others (7.75%) **X-ray procedures** AFL (23.45%) AVNRT (60.69%) AP (15.17%) AT (0%) Others (0.69%)	**EAM:** **EnSite Velocity NavX** (297)	*N* = 442 Mean age: 58 ± 19	**EnSite Velocity NavX** 14 ± 6 (s) **X-ray procedures** 19.32 ± 13.88 ($P < 0.0001$)	**EnSite Velocity NavX** 91 ± 52 min **X-ray procedures** 87 ± 57 min ($P = 0.41$)	Acute success rate: **EnSite Velocity NavX** 97% **X-ray procedures** 96% ($p = 0.46$)	13 (not specifically related to X-ray procedure)	*Data not shown*

(continued)

Table 10.1 (continued)

Author/reference	Year of publication	Study design	Arrhythmias studied (%)	Fluoroless system used (*n*)	Population features	Fluoroscopy time (min)	Procedure duration (min)	Main efficacy results	Main safety results (major complications)	Follow-up
Casella et al. [46]	2016	Prospective RCT	**EnSite NavX** AFL (8%) AVNRT (63%) AP (16%) AT (2%) **X-ray procedures** AFL (5%) AVNRT (62%) AP (20%) AT (2%)	**EAM:** **EnSite NavX** (134)	$N = 262$ **Ensite NavX** Mean age: 36.3 + 10.4 59% female **X-ray procedures** Mean age: 35.4 + 10.4 57% female	**Ensite NavX** 0 **X-ray procedures** 14.32 (9.08–22.43)	*Data not shown*	Acute success: 99% in both groups	0	From 1 to 6 months
Schoene et al. [62]	2015	Prospective study	AFL (100%)	**EAM** **MediGuide** (20)	$N = 40$ **MediGuide** Mean age: 62.7 ± 12 Male 17 **X-ray procedures** Mean age: 67.7 ± 12 Male 17	**MediGuide** 0.3 **X-ray procedures** 5.7 ($P < 0.001$)	**MediGuide** 49.5 min **X-ray procedures** 33.5 min ($P < 0.001$)	Acute success rate: 100% in both groups 6 months: **MediGuide** 95% **X-ray procedures** 90%	0	6 months
Macias et al. [60]	2014	Prospective study	AFL (100%)	**EAM:** **Carto3** (20) **EnSite NavX** (40)	$N = 60$ **Carto 3** Mean age: 60.2 ± 9.9 20% female **Initial Ensite NaveX** Mean age: 61.9 ± 9.6 20% female **Late Ensite NaveX** Mean age: 61.9 ± 9.6 20% female	**Carto 3** 0.33 ± 1.3 min **Initial Ensite NavX** 4.1 ± 12.5 min **Late Ensite NavX** 0.08 ± 0.35 min	**Carto 3** 158 ± 54 min **Initial Ensite NavX** 147 ± 46 min **Late Ensite NavX** 123 ± 37 min	Acute success: **Carto 3** 95% **EnSite NavX** 100% Recurrences: **Carto 3** 5.2% **EnSite NavX** 5% Not statistical difference in achieving zero fluoroscopy rate between groups	**Carto 3** 0% **Initial Ensite** 5% **Late Ensite** 0%	6 months

Stec et al. [50]	2014	Prospective study	**Ensite Velocity NavX** AFL (12.7%) AVNRT (61.17%) WPW (27.13%) AT (5.85%) Others (6.91%) **X-ray procedures** AFL (27.87%) AVNRT (49.3%) AP (22.69%) AT (3.36%) Others (3.5%)	**EAM:** **Ensite Velocity NavX** (188)	$N = 902$ **Ensite Velocity NavX** Mean age: 45 ± 21 54.8% female **X-ray procedures** Mean age: 52 ± 18 54.1% female	**Ensite Velocity NavX** 0.2 ± 0.9 min **X-ray procedures** 8.1 ± 7.4 X-ray group	**Ensite Velocity NavX** 36.9 ± 23.4 **X-ray procedures** 63.1 ± 29.2	Acute success rate: 98% In both groups Long-term success rate: **Ensite Velocity NavX** 93.6% **X-ray procedures** 94%	0	Mean follow-up (months): **Ensite Velocity NavX** 8.0 ± 5.2 **X-ray procedures** 11.0 ± 5.7
Shurrab et al. [44]	2013	Meta-analysis	AFL AF AVNRT AVRT WPW Others (overall rates are not available for each arrhythmia)	**EAM:** **Carto** (472) **EnSite NavX:** (168) **Localisa** (26)	$N = 1292$ Mean age Not available	**EAM:** 8 **X-ray procedures:** 20 **EAM vs. X-ray procedures:** **AFL** ($p < 0.001$) **AVNRT** ($p < 0.02$) **WPW** ($p < 0.001$)	**EAM:** **AFL:** 117 **AF** 149 **AVNRT:** 98 **AVRT:** 112 **X-ray procedures:** **AFL** 122 **AF** 30 **AVNRT** 97 **AVRT** 101	Acute success: **EAM** **AFL** 97% **AF** **100%** **X-ray procedures:** **AFL** 93% **AF** 100% Chronic success: **EAM** **AFL** 93% **AF** 84% **X-ray procedures:** **AFL** 96% **AF** 76%	**EAM** 5 **X-ray procedures:** 2 ($p < 0.29$)	Between 1.5 and 16 months

(continued)

Table 10.1 (continued)

Author/ reference	Year of publication	Study design	Arrhythmias studied (%)	Fluoroless system used (*n*)	Population features	Fluoroscopy time (min)	Procedure duration (min)	Main efficacy results	Main safety results (major complications)	Follow-up
Razminia et al. [39]	2012	Retrospective study	**NXR procedures** AFL (16.67%) AVNRT (16.67%) AVRT (10%) AF (36.67%) AT (15%) **X-ray procedures** AFL (16.67%) AVNRT (16.67%) AVRT (10%) AF (36.67%) AT (15%)	**EAM:** **EnSite NavX** **ICE:** **AcuNav** **IE:** **EP-WorkMate** (60)	$N = 120$ **EnSite NavX/ AcuNav** Age 55 ± 15 years 47% female **X-ray procedures** Age 56 ± 15 37% female	**EnSite NavX** 0 min **AcuNav** 17 ± 15 min	Data not detailed (show in plot) No difference between two groups	Acute success rate: **EnSite NavX** 98% **X-ray procedures** 100%	**EnSite NavX** 1 **X-ray procedures** 2	*Data not shown*
Vollmann et al. [43]	2009	Prospective study	AFL (100%)	**RMN** (45)	$N = 90$ **RMN** Mean age: 68 ± 8 20% female **X-ray procedures** Mean age: 68 ± 9 27% female	**RMN** 7.6–19.9 **X-ray procedures** 11.5–23.1	**RMN** 113.5 ± 34.8 **X-ray procedures** 77.2 ± 24.1 ($P < 0.0001$)	Acute success: **RMN** 84% **X-ray procedures** 91% Long-term success: **RMN** 73% **X-ray procedures** 89%	**RMN** 0 **X-ray procedures** 1	At 1 day + 91 ± 19 days + 189 ± 35 days

Hindricks et al. [32]	2009	Prospective study	AFL (100%)	**EAM:** **Carto** (105)	$N = 210$ **Carto** Mean age: 62 ± 10 10% female **X-ray procedures** Mean age: 62 ± 10 21% female	**Carto** 7.7 ± 7.3 min X-ray **procedures** 14.8 ± 11.9	**Carto** 99 ± 57 min **X-ray procedures** 88 ± 54	Acute success: **Carto** 94% **X-ray procedures** 97% ($p > 0.05$) Long-term success **Carto** 6.6% **X-ray procedures** 5.7% ($p > 0.05$)	0	6 months

Studies are reported by year of publication. *EAM* electroanatomic mapping, *AFL* atrial flutter, *AF* atrial fibrillation, *AVNRT* atrioventricular nodal reentry tachycardia, *AVRT* atrioventricular reentry tachycardia, *WPW* Wolff-Parkinson-White, *AP* accessory pathways, *AT* atrial tachycardia, *ALARA* as reasonable achievable fluoroscopic approach, *MVG* multi-voltage gradient, *PBT* pull-back technique, *NXR* non-X-Ray, *RMN* remote magnetic catheter navigation, *pts* patients compared results of three different groups: Group A consisted of 20 consecutive procedures guided by CartoR 3 system, compared with two case-control groups matched from 146 procedures guided with the Ensite-NavXTM system. Group B consisted of 20 matched procedures from the first 50 procedures performed in the electrophysiology unit, and Group C consisted of 20 matched procedures from the last 50 procedures. Outcomes analyzed were acute success immediately after ablation (bidirectional block) and at 24 h, and procedure times, complications, and recurrence rate at 6 month. A zero fluoroscopy approach was attempted in over 60 consecutive typical atrial flutter ablations cases. In this series, no fluoroscopy was achieved in 90% of cases, used only in case of challenging catheter positioning. Acute success rate was 95% for group A, 100% for group B, 100% for group C, showing no significant differences between groups ($p = 0.36$). Only one complication was seen in the group B. Also, recurrence rate was similar between all groups with no significant differences demonstrated (5.2% group A, 0% group B, 5% group C, $p = 0.57$). The study concluded that a zero-fluoroscopy approach to CTI catheter ablation using the Carto 3 system is feasible in most procedures with similar results to the zero-fluoroscopy approach using the Ensite-NavXTM system.

Even more recently, Bastian et al. [61] conducted a study in order to evaluate the effects of the use of different 3D-EAM systems on procedure duration and radiation exposure in typical atrial flutter ablation. There was no intended complete suppression of fluoroscopy. The study was conducted on 355 consecutive patients undergoing typical atrial flutter ablation. Of these 355 patients, 267 patients using Carto_3 (Biosense Webster, Diamond Bar, CA) were compared to 88 patients using EnsiteNavX/Precision (Abbott, SJM, St Paul, MN). The success in obtaining total elimination of fluoroscopy approach was significantly higher in the Ensite group (17.2% vs. 65.1%, $p < 0.001$), while procedure time shows no significant differences between groups ($p = 0.75$). The authors acknowledge the fact of catheter visualization since the groin level with NavX could have influenced the higher rate of complete X-ray elimination.

The 6 months prospective randomized study by Schoene et al. [62] compared the effects of using Mediguide technology versus standard fluoroscopy on procedural parameters in 40 patients undergoing radiofrequency ablation of typical atrial flutter. The primary endpoints were defined as radiation dose and fluoroscopy time. The secondary endpoints included procedure duration. Safety outcomes involved death, pericardial effusion, minor or major strokes, and/or bleeding within 24 h after the ablation procedure. Results show a significant reduction in radiation exposure and fluoroscopic time duration ($P < 0.001$). The median procedure duration in all patients was 45 min, no significant differences were observed between groups (49.5 vs. 33.5, $p = 0.053$). During the 24 h post ablation, no major complications including death, pericardial effusions, bleedings, or strokes occurred in either group. Recurrences at 6 months follow-up, were 95% in the Mediguide group and 90% in the control group, showing no significant differences between the two. Overall, data shows that Mediguide system is as effective as conventional AFL ablation procedure, reducing both fluoroscopy time and X-ray dose without lengthening the procedure time.

Searching the best ablation technique to achieve the lower exposure to radiation with the highest success rate, the prospective observational study by Deutsch et al. [63] demonstrated that the most optimal ablation method for CTI-dependent AFL seems to be the maximum voltage gradient technique (MVG). The result was obtained assessing two different navigation methods: No-X-Ray [NXR] and fluoroscopy based as low as reasonable achievable [ALARA] and two different mapping and ablation systems (multi-voltage guided [MVG] and pull-back technique [PBT]. Four different groups (NXR + PBT, NXR + MVG, ALARA + PBT, ALARA + PBT) were created to evaluate the feasibility and effectiveness of CTI ablation during implementation of the NXR approach and the maximum voltage-guided technique for ablation of AFL. Compared with ALARA, the procedure time decreased in NXR groups

(45.4 ± 17.6 and 47.2 ± 15.7 min vs. 52.6 ± 23.7 and 59.8 ± 24.0 min, $P < .01$). In addition, in NXR groups there were a significant reduction in fluoroscopy exposure (from 0.2 ± 1.1 [NXR + PBT] and 0.3 ± 1.6 [NXR + MVG] to 7.7 ± 6.0 min [ALARA + MVG] and 9.1 ± 7.2 min [ALARA + PBT], $P < .001$), most of all in the MVG technique subgroup. However these results need a better evaluation.

Some studies reported higher cost for zero or near-zero fluoroscopy technique [32, 52]. In the prospective, multicenter, randomized controlled trial by Casella et al. [46], the risks of cancer incidence and mortality from a minimally fluoroscopic approach procedure appeared reduced by 96% compared with conventional procedure. Also, a dramatic reduction has been calculated in years of life lost (YLL) and years of life affected (YLA) in minimally fluoroscopic approach group in comparison with conventional group. Because of these considerations the use of minimally fluoroscopic approach could also be seen as an increase in life expectancy and in the period of life without cancer; for these reasons cost-effectiveness analysis shows that the benefits of minimally fluoroscopic approach for patients and professionals are likely to justify its additional costs.

As previously described, other systems are today available for lowering radiation exposure to healthcare staff as remote navigation systems. Vollmann et al. [43] evaluated the efficacy of remote magnetic catheter navigation (RMN) for CTI ablation versus conventional system in a randomized clinical trial. The RMN-guided ablation was associated with reduced radiation exposure (median, 10.6 min; interquartile range [IQR], 7.6–19.9, vs. 15.0 min; IQR, 11.5–23.1; $P = 0.043$) but prolonged ablation (55 min; IQR, 28–76, vs. 17 min; IQR, 7–31; $P < 0.0001$) and procedure duration (114 ± 35 vs. 77 ± 24 min, $P < 0.0001$) and similar procedure times as compared with conventional catheter navigation. Additionally, long-term success (at 6 months) was lower in the RMN group (73% vs. 89%, $P = 0.063$) appearing less effective irrespective of CTI anatomy than conventional technique.

Conclusion

Catheter ablation is the treatment of choice in the vast majority of patients with typical or reverse typical AFL. Radiation exposure to patients and medical staff during an ablation procedure remains a major concern especially in pregnant women, children, and immunosuppressed patients. Remote catheter navigation and 3D mapping systems have the potential to significantly reduce X-ray exposure and has been demonstrated to be as feasible, safe, and effective as conventional fluoroscopic approach. In the setting of an AFL ablation procedure these technologies could be limited by a more complex workflow and increased procedural costs. High volume of a single vendor and a two catheter approach can reduce costs, and everyday use of the 3-D systems can speed also the workflow in flutter ablation.

References

1. Heidbuchel H, Wittkampf FH, Vano E, Ernst S, Schilling R, Picano E, et al. Practical ways to reduce radiation dose for patients and staff during device implantations and electrophysiological procedures. Europace. 2014;16:946–64. https://doi.org/10.1093/europace/eut409.
2. The 2007 Recommendations of the International Commission on Radiological Protection. ICRP publication 103. Ann ICRP 2007;37:1–332.
3. Vano E, Arranz L, Sastre JM, Moro C, Ledo A, Garate MT, et al. Dosimetric and radiation protection considerations based on some cases of patient skin injuries in interventional cardiology. Br J Radiol. 1998;71:510–6.
4. Rehani MM, Ortiz-Lopez P. Radiation effects in fluoroscopically guided cardiac interventions: keeping them under control. Int J Cardiol. 2006;109:147–51.
5. Park TH, Eichling JO, Schechtman KB, Bromberg BI, Smith JM, Lindsay BD. Risk of radiation induced skin injuries from arrhythmia ablation procedures. Pacing Clin Electrophysiol. 1996;19(9):1363.
6. McFadden SL, Mooney RB, Shepherd PH. X-ray dose and associated risks from radiofrequency catheter ablation procedures. Br J Radiol. 2002;75:253–65.
7. Kovoor P, Ricciardello M, Collins L, Uther JB, Ross DL. Risk to patients from radiation associated with radiofrequency ablation for supraventricular tachycardia. Circulation. 1998;98:1534–40.
8. Calkins H, Niklason L, Sousa J, el-Atassi R, Langberg J, Morady F. Radiation exposure during radiofrequency catheter ablation of accessory atrioventricular connections. Circulation. 1991;84:2376–82.

9. Picano E, Vañó E, Rehani MM, Cuocolo A, Mont L, Bodi V, et al. The appropriate and justified use of medical radiation in cardiovascular imaging. A position document of the ESC associations of cardiovascular imaging, percutaneous cardiovascular interventions and electrophysiology. Eur Heart J. 2014;35:665–72.
10. Lickfett L, Mahesh M, Vasamreddy C, Bradley D, Jayam V, Eldadah Z, et al. Radiation exposure during catheter ablation of atrial fibrillation. Circulation. 2004;110:3003–10.
11. Rosenthal LS, Mahesh M, Beck TJ, Saul JP, Miller JM, Kay N, et al. Predictors of fluoroscopy time and estimated radiation exposure during radiofrequency catheter ablation procedures. Am J Cardiol. 1998;82:451–8.
12. Klein LW, Miller DL, Balter S, Laskey W, Haines D, Norbash A, et al. Occupational health hazards in the interventional laboratory: time for a safer environment. Radiology. 2009;250:538–44.
13. Kottkamp H, Hindricks G. Catheter ablation of atrial flutter. Thorac Cardiovasc Surg. 1999;47(3):357–61.
14. Lee G, Sanders P, Kalman JM. Catheter ablation of atrial arrhythmias: state of the art. Lancet. 2012;380(9852):1509–19.
15. Saoudi N, Cosio F, Waldo A, Chen SA, Lesaka Y, Lesh M, et al. Classification of atrial flutter and regular atrial tachycardia according to electrophysiologic mechanism and anatomic bases: a statement from a joint expert group from the Working Group of Arrhythmias of the European Society of Cardiology and the North American Society of Pacing and Electrophysiology. J Cardiovasc Electrophysiol. 2001;12:852–66.
16. Olgin JE, Kalman JM, Saxon LA, Lee RJ, Lesh MD. Mechanism of initiation of atrial flutter in humans: site of unidirectional block and direction of rotation. J Am Coll Cardiol. 1997;29(2):376–84.
17. Cosio FG, Arribas F, Barbero JM, Kallmeyer C, Goicolea A. Validation of double-spike electrograms as markers of conduction delay or block in atrial flutter. Am J Cardiol. 1988;61(10):775–80.
18. Kalman JM, Olgin JE, Saxon LA, Fisher WG, Lee RJ, Lesh MD. Activation and entrainment mapping defines the tricuspid annulus as the anterior barrier in typical atrial flutter. Circulation. 1996;94(3):398–406.
19. Olshansky B, Okumura K, Hess PG, Waldo AL. Demonstration of an area of slow conduction in human atrial flutter. J Am Coll Cardiol. 1990;16(7):1639–48.
20. Földesi C, Pandozi C, Peichl P. Atrial flutter: arrhythmia circuit and basis for radiofrequency catheter ablation. Ital Heart J. 2003;4:395–403.
21. Yang Y, Cheng J, Bochoeyer A, Hamdan MH, Kowal RC, Page R, et al. Atypical right atrial flutter patterns. Circulation. 2001;103(25):3092–8.
22. Bochoeyer A, Yang Y, Cheng J, Lee RJ, Keung EC, Marrouche NF, et al. Surface and electrocardiographic characteristics of right and left atrial flutter. Circulation. 2003;108(1):60–6.
23. Merino JL, Peinado R, Abello M, Gnoatto M, Vasserot MG, Sobrino JA. Superior vena cava flutter: electrophysiology and ablation. J Cardiovasc Electrophysiol. 2005;16(6):568–75.
24. Kall JG, Rubenstein DS, Kopp DE, Burke MC, Verdino RJ, Lin AC, et al. Atypical atrial flutter originating in the right atrial free wall. Circulation. 2000;101(3):270–9.
25. Wellens HJ. Contemporary management of atrial flutter. Circulation. 2002;106:649–52.
26. Jaïs P, Shah DC, Haïssaguerre M, Hocini M, Peng JT, Takahashi A, et al. Mapping and ablation of left atrial flutters. Circulation. 2000;101(25):2928–34.
27. Ohtani K, Yutani C, Nagata S, Koretsune Y, Hori M, Kamada T. High prevalence of atrial fibrosis in patients with dilated cardiomyopathy. J Am Coll Cardiol. 1995;25:1162–9.
28. Granada J, Uribe W, Chyou PH, Maassen K, Vierkant R, Smith PN, et al. Incidence and predictors of atrial flutter in the general population. J Am Coll Cardiol. 2000;36(7):2242–6.
29. Natale A, Newby KH, Pisanó E, Leonelli F, Fanelli R, Potenza D, et al. Prospective randomized comparison of antiarrhythmic therapy versus first-line radiofrequency ablation in patients with atrial flutter. J Am Coll Cardiol. 2000;35(7):1898–904.
30. Da Costa A, Thévenin J, Roche F, Romeyer-Bouchard C, Abdellaoui L, Messier M, et al. Results from the Loire-Ardèche-Drôme-Isère-Puy-de-Dôme (LADIP) trial on atrial flutter, a multicentric prospective randomized study comparing amiodarone and radiofrequency ablation after the first episode of symptomatic atrial flutter. Circulation. 2006;114(16):1676–81.
31. Kirchhof P, Benussi S, Kotecha D, Ahlsson A, Atar D, Casadei B, et al. 2016 ESC Gguidelines for the management of atrial fibrillation developed in collaboration with EACTS. Eur Heart J. 2016;37:2893–962. https://doi.org/10.1093/eurheartj/ehw210.
32. Hindricks G, Willems S, Kautzner J, De Chillou C, Wiedemann M, Schepel S, et al. Effect of electroanatomically guided versus conventional catheter ablation of typical atrial flutter on the fluoroscopy time and resource use: a prospective randomized multicenter study. J Cardiovasc Electrophysiol. 2009;20(7):734–40. https://doi.org/10.1111/j.1540-8167.2009.01439.x.
33. Willems S, Weiss C, Ventura R, Rüppel R, Risius T, Hoffmann M, et al. Catheter ablation of atrial flutter guided by electroanatomic mapping (CARTO): a randomized comparison to the conventional approach. J Cardiovasc Electrophysiol. 2000;11(11):1223–30.
34. Wagner LK, Eifel PJ, Geise RA. Potential biological effects following high X-ray dose interventional procedures. J Vasc Interv Radiol. 1994;5(1):71–84.
35. Lindsay BD, Eichling JO, Ambos HD, Cain ME. Radiation exposure to patients and medical personnel during radiofrequency catheter ablation for supraventricular tachycardia. Am J Cardiol. 1992;70(2):218–23.
36. Anselme F, Savouré A, Cribier A, Saoudi N. Catheter ablation of typical atrial flutter: a randomized comparison of 2 methods for determining com-

plete bidirectional isthmus block. Circulation. 2001;103(10):1434–9.
37. Kottkamp H, Hügl B, Krauss B, Wetzel U, Fleck A, Schuler G, et al. Electromagnetic versus fluoroscopic mapping of the inferior isthmus for ablation of typical atrial flutter: a prospective randomized study. Circulation. 2000;102(17):2082–6.
38. Da Costa A, Faure E, Thévenin J, Messier M, Bernard S, Abdel K, et al. Effect of isthmus anatomy and ablation catheter on radiofrequency catheter ablation of the cavotricuspid isthmus. Circulation. 2004;110(9):1030–5.
39. Razminia M, Manankil MF, Eryazici PL, Arrieta-Garcia C, Wang T, D'Silva OJ, et al. Nonfluoroscopic catheter ablation of cardiac arrhythmias in adults: feasibility, safety, and efficacy. J Cardiovasc Electrophysiol. 2012;23:1078–86.
40. Saliba W, Thomas J. Intracardiac echocardiography during catheter ablation of atrial fibrillation. Europace. 2008;10(Suppl 3):42–7.
41. Gaita F, Guerra PG, Battaglia A, Anselmino M. The dream of near-zero X-rays ablation comes true. Eur Heart J. 2016;37(36):2749–55.
42. Schmidt B, Chun KR, Tilz RR, Koektuerk B, Ouyang F, Kuck KH. Remote navigation systems in electrophysiology. Europace. 2008;10(Suppl 3):iii57–61. https://doi.org/10.1093/europace/eun234.
43. Vollmann D, Lüthje L, Seegers J, Hasenfuss G, Zabel M. Remote magnetic catheter navigation for cavotricuspid isthmus ablation in patients with common-type atrial flutter. Circ Arrhythm Electrophysiol. 2009;2(6):603–10. https://doi.org/10.1161/CIRCEP.109.884411.
44. Shurrab M, Laish-Farkash A, Lashevsky I, Morriello F, Singh SM, Schilling RJ, et al. Three-dimensional localization versus fluoroscopically only guided ablations: a meta-analysis. Scand Cardiovasc J. 2013;47(4):200–9. https://doi.org/10.3109/14017431.2013.797099.
45. Brunelli M, Doroshenko Y, Baldauf T, Ngoli S, Bastian D, Walaschek J, et al. Zero or near zero fluoroscopy for catheter ablation of supraventricular right atrial tachycardia can be achieved with the use of a three-dimensional mapping system. Europace. 2017;19(Suppl_3):iii191.
46. Casella M, Dello Russo A, Pelargonio G, Del Greco M, Zingarini G, Piacenti M, et al. Near zerO fluoroscopic exPosure during catheter ablAtion of supraventricular arrhYthmias: the NO-PARTY multicentre randomized trial. Europace. 2016;18(10):1565–72.
47. Earley MJ, Showkathali R, Alzetani M, Kistler PM, Gupta D, Abrams DJ, et al. Radiofrequency ablation of arrhythmias guided by nonfluoroscopic catheter location: a prospective randomized trial. Eur Heart J. 2006;27:1223–122.
48. Bulava A, Hanis J, Eisenberger M. Catheter ablation of atrial fibrillation using zero-fluoroscopy technique: a randomized trial. Pacing Clin Electrophysiol. 2015;38:797–806.
49. Sun X, Xu J, Su H, Fan X, Liu F, An C, et al. Near-zero exposure radiofrequency ablation of paroxysmal supraventricular tachycardia guided by EnSiteNavX mapping. Sci Res Essays. 2011;6:5253–60.
50. Stec S, Sledz J, Mazij M, Ras M, Ludwik B, Chrabaszcz M, et al. Feasibility of implementation of a "simplified, No-X-Ray, no-lead apron, two-catheter approach" for ablation of supraventricular arrhythmias in children and adults. J Cardiovasc Electrophysiol. 2014;25:866–74.
51. Giaccardi M, Del Rosso A, Guarnaccia V, Ballo P, Mascia G, Chiodi L, et al. Near-zero xray in arrhythmia ablation using a 3-dimensional electroanatomic mapping system: a multicenter experience. Heart Rhythm. 2016;13:150–6.
52. Seizer P, Bucher V, Frische C, Heinzmann D, Gramlich M, Muller I, et al. Efficacy and safety of zero-fluoroscopy ablation for supraventricular tachycardias: use of optional contact force measurement for zero fluoroscopy ablation in a clinical routine setting. Herz. 2016;41(3):241–5. https://doi.org/10.1007/s00059-015-4358-4.
53. Smith G, Clark JM. Elimination of fluoroscopy use in a pediatric electrophysiology laboratory utilizing three-dimensional mapping. Pacing Clin Electrophysiol. 2007;30:510–8.
54. Alvarez M, Tercedor L, Almansa I, Ros N, Galdeano RS, Burillo F, et al. Safety and feasibility of catheter ablation for atrioventricular nodal re-entrant tachycardia without fluoroscopic guidance. Heart Rhythm. 2009;6:1714–20.
55. Yang L, Sun G, Chen X, Chen G, Yang S, Guo P, et al. Meta-analysis of zero or near-zero fluoroscopy use during ablation of cardiac arrhythmias. Am J Cardiol. 2016;118:1511–8. https://doi.org/10.1016/j.amjcard.2016.08.014.
56. Stec S, Deutsch KJ, Karbarz D, Klank-Szafran M, Sledz J, Mazij M, et al. Zero-fluoroscopy approaches the gold standard for catheter ablation of regular supraventricular tachycardias—experience beyond 1500 procedures. Eur Heart J. 2017;38(Supplement):179.
57. Bigelow AM, Smith PC, Timberlake DT, McNinch NL, Smith GL, Lane JR, et al. Procedural outcomes of fluoroless catheter ablation outside the traditional catheterization lab. Europace. 2017;19(8):1378–84. https://doi.org/10.1093/europace/euw207.
58. Walsh KA, Galvin J, Keaney J, Keelan E, Szeplaki G. Single Centre experience with a zero-fluoroscopic ablation strategy using a novel magnetic field and impedance-based 3D mapping system for supraventricular tachycardia. Europace. 2017;319:295–6.
59. Razminia M, Willoughby MC, Demo H, Keshmiri H, Wang T, D'Silva OJ, et al. Fluoroless catheter ablation of cardiac arrhythmias: a 5-year experience. Pacing Clin Electrophysiol. 2017;40(4):425–33. https://doi.org/10.1111/pace.13038.
60. Macías R, Uribe I, Tercedor L, Jiménez-Jáimez J, Barrio T, Álvarez M. A zero-fluoroscopy approach to cavotricuspid isthmus catheter ablation: comparative analysis of two electroanatomical mapping systems. Pacing Clin Electrophysiol. 2014;37(8):1029–37. https://doi.org/10.1111/pace.12376.

61. Bastian D, Vitali-Serdoz L, Poli S, Walascheck J, Brunelli M, Richter P, et al. Effects of different 3D electro-anatomic mapping systems on fluoroscopy exposure and procedural duration in typical atrial flutter ablation. JACC Clin Electrophysiol. 2017;3(10 Suppl):S3–4.
62. Schoene K, Rolf S, Schloma D, John S, Arya A, Dinov B, Richter S, Bollmann A, Hindricks G, Sommer P. Ablation of typical atrial flutter using a non-fluoroscopic catheter tracking system vs. conventional fluoroscopy—results from a prospective randomized study. Europace. 2015;17(7):1117–21. https://doi.org/10.1093/europace/euu398.. Epub 2015 Mar 3
63. Deutsch K, Śledź J, Mazij M, Ludwik B, Labus M, Karbarz D, et al. Maximum voltage gradient technique for optimization of ablation for typical atrial flutter with zero-fluoroscopy approach. Medicine (Baltimore). 2017;96(25):e6939. https://doi.org/10.1097/MD.0000000000006939.

11 Non-fluoroscopic Catheter Ablation of Atrial Fibrillation

Mouhannad M. Sadek

Introduction

Catheter ablation for atrial fibrillation (AF) is increasingly the treatment of choice for patients with paroxysmal and persistent AF [1]. Due to the complexity of the procedure and the need for transseptal puncture, AF ablation is traditionally associated with long procedure times and high radiation exposure [2, 3]. There has been growing interest in reducing radiation use during these procedures [4]. In addition, there is concern regarding the musculoskeletal affects of wearing lead apparel for prolonged periods [5].

Non-fluoroscopic catheter ablation of AF has been demonstrated in multiple studies and shown to be feasible and safe [6–9]. The use of electroanatomic mapping systems (EAMS), contact force technology, and intracardiac echocardiography (ICE) imaging has allowed the procedure to be performed with zero or near-zero fluoroscopic radiation [4, 10, 11].

In this chapter, we will describe the procedural aspects of non-fluoroscopic AF ablation and specifically describe the transseptal procedure using ICE imaging only. Please refer also to the catheter placement chapter for details on how to achieve fluoroscopy free access to the venous vasculature and to the right atrium.

Relevant Anatomy

Transseptal Puncture

The transseptal puncture is typically performed at the fossa ovalis by dropping down the transseptal apparatus from the superior vena cava (SVC) to engage the fossa. Fluoroscopic imaging is usually used to safely advance the apparatus into the SVC prior to the drop. While pulling back the apparatus, fluoroscopy is used to observe for a sudden drop from the SVC-right atrium (RA) junction onto the fossa ovalis. Multiple fluoroscopic views are used to confirm exact positioning, with a typical right anterior oblique (RAO) view showing the apparatus positioned in the middle between the posterior wall of the atrium and tricuspid annulus, and a typical left anterior oblique (LAO) view showing the apparatus facing the left side. At this point a needle is advanced through the fossa into the left atrium (LA), which is followed by the rest of the apparatus (dilator and sheath). In many centers, either transesophageal echocardiography (TEE) or ICE imaging is used to complement fluoroscopy and ensure engagement of the fossa prior to performing the puncture.

M. M. Sadek (✉)
Arrhythmia Service, Division of Cardiology, University of Ottawa Heart Institute, Ottawa, ON, Canada
e-mail: msadek@ottawaheart.ca

R. Proietti et al. (eds.), *Cardiac Electrophysiology Without Fluoroscopy*, https://doi.org/10.1007/978-3-030-16992-3_11

Left Atrial Anatomy

Typically there are four pulmonary veins (PVs) that drain blood from the lungs into the LA. However in some patients there is variation in anatomy, with the most common being a common ostium for the left PVs. In addition, many patients have a right middle PV present [12].

The standard of care for AF ablation is wide-antral pulmonary vein isolation (PVI) by creating ablation lesions (either by radiofrequency ablation or by cryoablation) around the PV ostia [1]. Multiple anatomical considerations need to be taken into account while performing the ablation. The esophagus runs in close proximity to the posterior wall of the LA, and can be present either in the middle of the posterior wall, closer to the right PVs or closer to the left PVs [13]. The variable location and close proximity factor in the risk of atrio-esophageal fistula formation post procedure. In addition, the right phrenic nerve usually courses anterior to the right PV ostia, and ablation in that area can lead to phrenic nerve paralysis [14].

Finally, the risk of PV stenosis post procedure is higher when ablation lesions are placed closer to the PV ostia, and can be avoided by placing ablation lesions away from the PVs. Hence, wide-area PVI has become the standard of care for AF ablation [1].

Non-fluoroscopic Ablation Approach

Patient Preparation

Patients are all maintained on oral anticoagulation for a minimum of 4 weeks prior to the procedure. Those at particularly high risk of left atrial appendage (LAA) thrombus undergo TEE within 48 h of the procedure to ensure the absence of LAA thrombus. These procedures are commonly performed under general anesthesia or deep conscious sedation.

Advancing the ICE Catheter to the Heart (Fig. 11.1)

After gaining femoral access (please refer to the chapter on catheter placement for further details), which can be guided by vascular ultrasound, the ICE catheter is then advanced into the RA. In our institution, ICE is performed using an 8-French phased-array AcuNav probe at 7.5 MHz (Siemens Medical Solutions distributed by Biosense Webster, Diamond Bar, California). The ICE monitor is connected to the dedicated monitor boom.

In order to place the ICE catheter in the heart safely without fluoroscopy, the probe is advanced

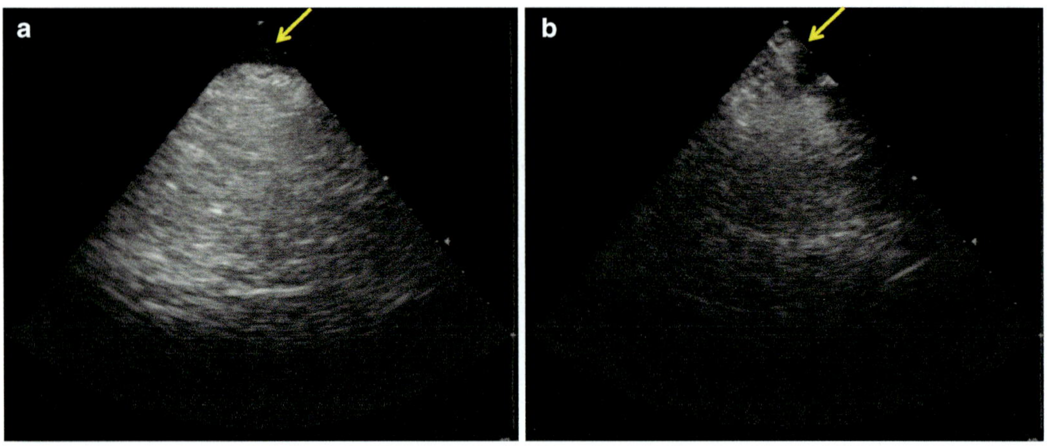

Fig. 11.1 (Panel **a**) Arrow showing lumen in the path of the ICE catheter, which allows safe advancement forwards towards the right atrium. (Panel **b**) Arrow showing soft tissue in the path of the ICE catheter. In this situation, clockwise or counterclockwise torque is needed to show lumen prior to advancing the ICE catheter

from the femoral vein to the RA while ensuring that lumen is present in the path of the probe. This is done by visualizing "black lumen" on the top right of the ICE display (i.e., in front of the probe). If tissue is encountered, the probe can be gently withdrawn and a clockwise or counter-clockwise torque can be applied to show lumen, and the probe can be advanced again.

In some instances, a branching point is identified, and the probe can be anteriorly-flexed towards the main branch of the vein to allow it to pass towards the heart. Care should be taken not to advance the probe against resistance.

Baseline ICE Study (Fig. 11.2)

The ICE probe is positioned in the RA, right ventricle (RV), and SVC where visualization of the cardiac structures is performed. Pre-ablation, ICE imaging is used to document baseline ventricular function, valvular function, PV flows, and the absence of a baseline pericardial effusion. In the presence of a cardiac implantable electronic device (CIED), ICE is used to visualize lead position and assess the insertion sites. Following this, further intra-procedural imaging is performed to monitor catheter position, catheter contact, and monitor for complications.

Coronary Sinus Cannulation (Fig. 11.3)

Once the ICE probe is positioned in the RA, the coronary sinus ostium can be visualized just posterior to the tricuspid valve by applying clockwise torque on the ICE probe. Following this, a decapolar catheter is advanced into the RA and, by using the EAMS and intracardiac electrograms, advanced into the coronary sinus.

In the case of difficult coronary sinus cannulation, multiple steps are taken in sequence. These include electroanatomic mapping of the coronary sinus using the mapping/ablation catheter and long sheath (thus providing an anatomical "road map" for the decapolar catheter), and utilizing

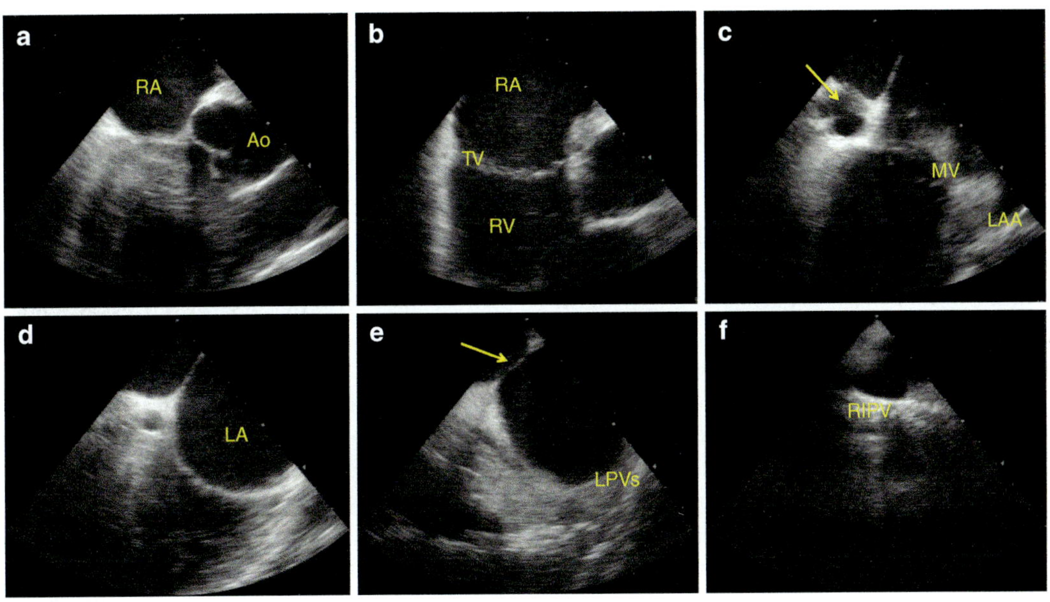

Fig. 11.2 ICE views from the right atrium (RA): clockwise torque is applied to the ICE catheter to move from Panel **a** through **f**. (Panel **a**) RA view showing the aortic root (Ao). (Panel **b**) RA view showing the tricuspid valve (TV) and right ventricle (RV). (Panel **c**) Coronary sinus ostium (arrow), mitral valve (MV), and left atrial appendage (LAA). (Panel **d**) Further clockwise torque showing the left atrium (LA). (Panel **e**) The fossa ovalis (arrow) where the transseptal puncture would be performed, across from the left pulmonary veins (LPVs) common ostium. (Panel **f**) Right inferior pulmonary vein (RIPV) ostium shown

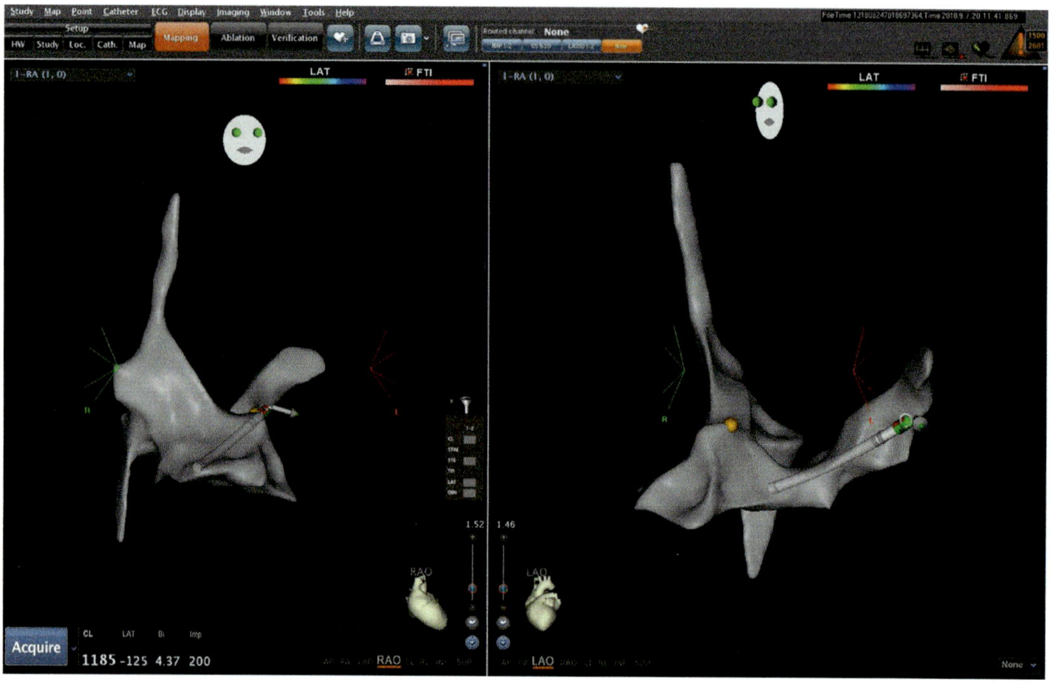

Fig. 11.3 A simple anatomical map of the right atrium. The ablation catheter is shown in both right anterior oblique and left anterior oblique views in the coronary sinus, providing a road map for entry of a decapolar catheter

a long pre-shaped Swartz SL3 sheath (St. Jude Medical, St Paul, Minnesota). The SL3 sheath is advanced into the RA utilizing the same technique used to advance the steerable sheath into the SVC prior to transseptal access (see below).

Transseptal Access (Fig. 11.4)

The ICE catheter is advanced into the RA, following which a posterior and right-sided tilt of the ICE catheter is applied to visualize the SVC.

A long J-wire is passed from the right femoral vein to the SVC, followed by advancement of a long steerable sheath (Agilis NxT, St. Jude Medical, St. Paul, MN) over the wire into the SVC (under ICE visualization). A Brockenbrough (BRK) needle (St. Jude Medical, St. Paul, MN) is advanced into the sheath and the apparatus is then pulled back to the fossa ovalis, following which the transseptal puncture is performed under ICE guidance. At this point, saline contrast can be injected to show LA filling and confirming the LA location of the needle tip. The dilator and sheath are carefully advanced over the needle, and once the sheath is in good position, the needle and dilator are withdrawn.

Challenging Transseptal Access Scenarios

Some challenges can be encountered during non-fluoroscopic transseptal access. One of these scenarios is the inability to advance the wire from the groin into the SVC (due to either coiling in the RA or advancing into the RV). In this case, the J-wire can be advanced into the RA (as confirmed by ICE). Next, the transseptal sheath-dilator assembly is advanced over the wire so that the tip is estimated to be in the mid-IVC region. The dilator and J-wire are then withdrawn, and the ablation catheter is advanced through the sheath. The ablation catheter's location could be tracked on the EAMS system and then advanced into the SVC as guided by both ICE imaging and the electroanatomical map. Once the ablation catheter is in the SVC, the sheath can be

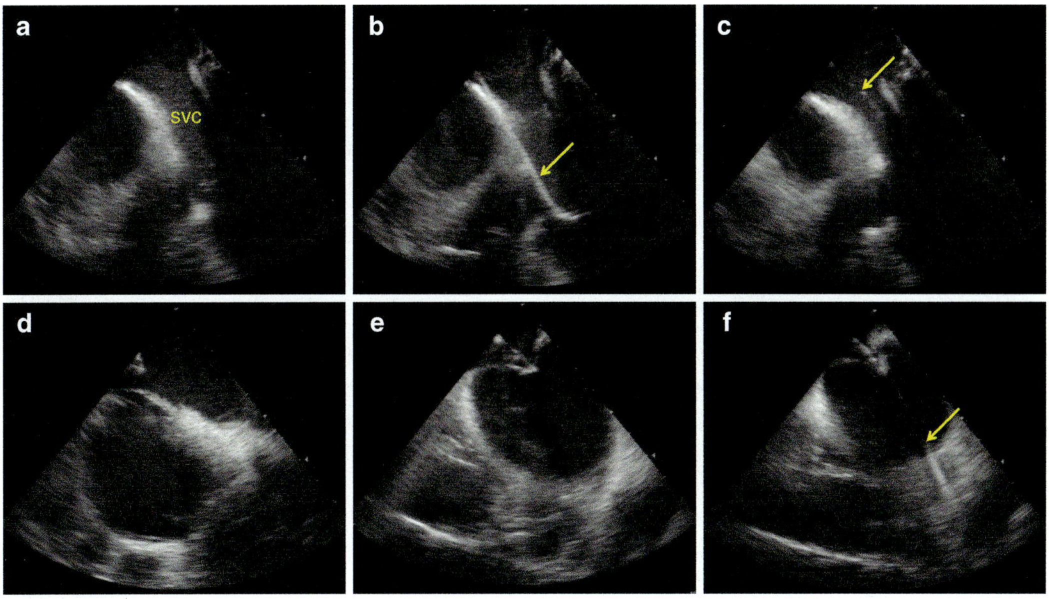

Fig. 11.4 (Panel **a**) From the right atrial view, posterior and right-ward tilt is applied to the ICE catheter, and the SVC is visualized. (Panel **b**) A wire (arrow) is advanced into the SVC. (Panel **c**) A long sheath/dilator assembly (arrow) is advanced over the wire into the SVC. (Panel **d**) The wire is interchanged for the transseptal needle, and the apparatus is pulled back onto the fossa ovalis. (Panel **e**) Torque is removed off the ICE catheter to allow for direct visualization of the fossa ovalis and to guide the transseptal puncture. (Panel **f**) In cases where the dilator/needle assembly crosses the septum but the sheath does not due to resistance at the septum, a wire (arrow) can be advanced into the left pulmonary veins to serve as a "rail" to push the dilator and sheath assembly further into the left atrium in a safe fashion

advanced over it into the SVC, and the ablation catheter can be again interchanged for the wire and dilator. At this point, the transseptal drop can be performed in a standard fashion.

Another scenario that can occur after successful transseptal puncture is the inability to advance the sheath over the dilator into the LA due to a thickened septum. One possible solution is to advance a wire through the dilator and into the left PVs. The location of the wire within the left PVs can be confirmed by advancing the ICE probe into the RV outflow tract and clocking the catheter to show the LAA-PV ridge, and the wire can be steered safely into the left PVs and not into the LAA. At this point, the wire can serve as a "rail" to advance the sheath and dilator further into the LA safely.

An additional scenario that can be encountered is the inability to drop the apparatus onto the fossa ovalis. In this situation, the ablation catheter can be inserted through the steerable sheath and be guided onto the fossa ovalis by ICE imaging. The sheath is then advanced over the ablation catheter so it can be in contact with the fossa, and the ablation catheter is removed. Now, the dilator (and BRK needle within it) is advanced through the sheath and directly onto the fossa ovalis, and the transseptal puncture is performed in a standard fashion.

Left Atrial Mapping

Following transseptal puncture, the LA is mapped using an EAMS. A steerable multi-electrode mapping catheter is used to form a map of the LA, particularly focusing on the PVs, LAA, and the mitral valve annulus (Fig. 11.5). Careful attention is paid to the PV ostia, which are identified while positioning the multi-electrode catheter via ICE imaging.

Following this, the multi-electrode catheter is interchanged for the ablation catheter and ablation is started. In our institution, a single transseptal

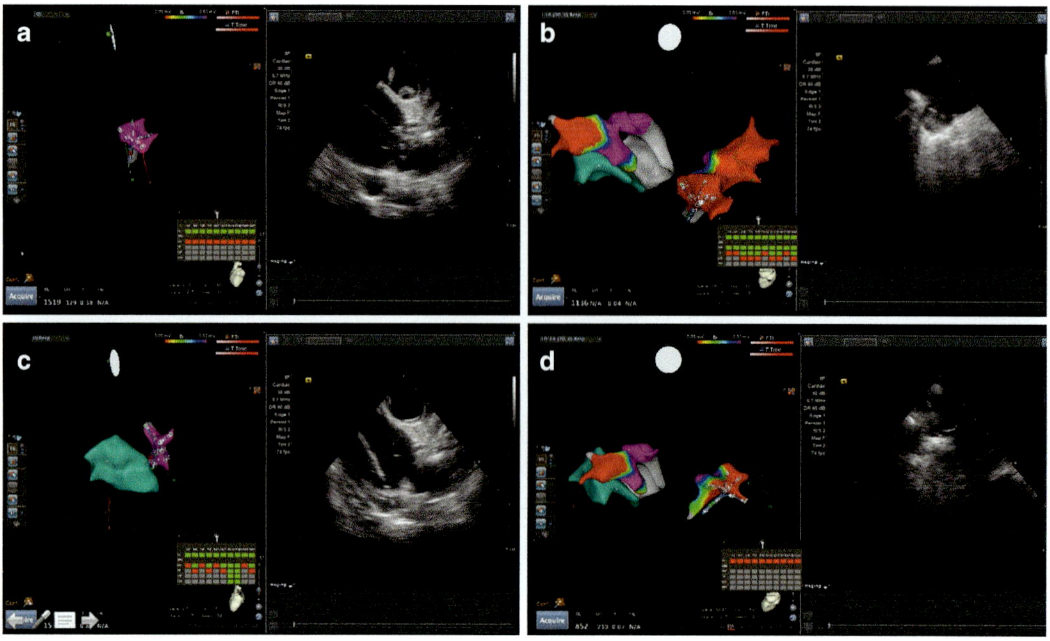

Fig. 11.5 Using ICE imaging to anatomically localize the left atrial appendage (LAA) and pulmonary vein ostia on the electroanatomic mapping system. (Panel **a**) The multi-electrode catheter is placed at the LAA ostium. (Panel **b**) The multi-electrode catheter is placed at the right inferior pulmonary vein ostium. (Panel **c**) The multi-electrode catheter is placed at the left pulmonary veins common ostium. (Panel **d**) The multi-electrode catheter is placed at the right superior pulmonary vein ostium

puncture is performed during non-fluoroscopic ablation; however, a double transseptal puncture to allow the use of both the ablation and multi-electrode catheter simultaneously is also feasible. The most frequently used ablation strategies for PVI include point-by-point ablation using radiofrequency energy delivered through an irrigated catheter or cryoablation technology.

Following ablation, the multi-electrode catheter is used to confirm elimination of all PV potentials and, in the presence of ablation lines, persistent bidirectional block as the procedural endpoint. Intravenous adenosine can also be administered to assess dormant conduction, and additional ablation can be applied if this is present.

Results of Non-fluoroscopic Atrial Fibrillation Ablation

Non-fluoroscopic PVI for paroxysmal AF has been reported utilizing ICE imaging, intracardiac electrograms, and electroanatomic mapping. Ferguson et al. demonstrated that non-fluoroscopic ablation of AF was feasible and safe in 21 cases; however they required fluoroscopic rescue for two cases to aid with transseptal puncture [6]. One possible reason for this may be the use of rotational ICE in their study, which differs from standard phased-array ICE used in most electrophysiologic procedures.

Reddy et al., Bulava et al., and Lyan et al. published three case series of non-fluoroscopic ablation in patients with paroxysmal AF [7–9]. In the first series [7], which included 20 patients, prolonged procedure times were noted with non-fluoroscopic ablation and there was no comparison to standard fluoroscopic ablation. There were no complications in this series.

In the second series [8], there were 40 patients with paroxysmal AF randomized to a fluoroscopic and non-fluoroscopic approach. In the non-fluoroscopic arm, one patient required fluoroscopic rescue for confirmation of femoral access. All non-fluoroscopic cases were performed safely with no increase in procedure time. There were no serious procedure-related complications, and no difference in arrhythmia-free survival at 12 months between the two groups.

In the third series [9], which included 245 patients with paroxysmal AF randomized to a fluoroscopic and non-fluoroscopic approach, comparable safety profiles and procedure durations to fluoroscopic ablation were observed. Three patients in the non-fluoroscopic ablation group required fluoroscopy to guide pericardial access during drain insertion for iatrogenic effusion, and there were two patients in the fluoroscopic arm that also required drain insertion. AF ablation without fluoroscopy did not affect procedure duration or procedural long-term efficacy.

More recently, at our own institution, we have performed 70 consecutive non-fluoroscopic LA ablation procedures (31 paroxysmal AF, 33 persistent AF and 6 LA flutters), all of which were completed without the need for rescue fluoroscopy [15]. There was an initial increase in procedural time for ablation of LA arrhythmias upon transitioning to non-fluoroscopic ablation. However, after excluding the first 20 cases to allow for operator learning, the transition to non-fluoroscopic ablation was not associated with an increase in mean procedural time. All procedures were completed successfully with no complications.

Finally, a small case series by Razminia et al. showed the feasibility of balloon cryoablation by an ICE-guided non-fluoroscopic approach [16]. Five consecutive patients with paroxysmal AF underwent the procedure. Hemodynamic pressure monitoring was used to confirm venous occlusion by the balloon, and 20 PVs were successfully isolated. There were no major complications during the study.

Limitations of Non-fluoroscopic Atrial Fibrillation Ablation

There are important limitations to performing non-fluoroscopic catheter ablation of AF. Possible limitations include patients with CIEDs. In the case of single or dual chamber devices, the atrial and ventricular leads can be visualized with ICE, avoided with catheters, and checked at the end of the procedure to ensure no dislodgement [15]. However, in patients with coronary sinus leads as part of cardiac resynchronization therapy, although the coronary sinus lead body can be visualized, its course along the coronary sinus venous system and the tip cannot be seen without fluoroscopy. Hence, there is a risk of coronary sinus lead dislodgement if fluoroscopy is not used, and this would likely be identified at device interrogation or radiological imaging post-procedure.

Another limitation is the potential need for fluoroscopy in the case of a complication. For example, if a pericardial effusion develops during the procedure, the use of fluoroscopy can easily confirm the presence of the wire in the epicardial space prior to drain insertion. Although this can also be performed with echocardiography, fluoroscopy does have the advantage of ease of use and efficiency in such a scenario.

Finally, non-fluoroscopic AF ablation relies heavily on the operators' skill in ICE image guidance and interpretation. Thus, familiarity and experience with ICE imaging is very important, especially to trouble-shoot difficult transseptal access scenarios.

Conclusion

Non-fluoroscopic ablation of AF is safe and feasible. There is a learning curve to consider, and procedural duration does improve with increasing operator experience. Challenges can be overcome with the use of ICE imaging and electroanatomic mapping.

References

1. Calkins H, Kuck KH, Cappato R, et al. 2012 HRS/EHRA/ECAS expert consensus statement on catheter and surgical ablation of atrial fibrillation: recommendations for patient selection, procedural techniques, patient management and follow-up, definitions, endpoints, and research trial design: a report of the Heart Rhythm Society (HRS) Task Force on Catheter and Surgical Ablation of Atrial Fibrillation. Developed in partnership with the European Heart Rhythm Association (EHRA), a registered branch of the European Society of Cardiology (ESC) and the European Cardiac Arrhythmia Society (ECAS); and in collaboration with the American College of Cardiology (ACC), American Heart Association (AHA), the Asia Pacific Heart Rhythm Society (APHRS), and the Society of Thoracic Surgeons (STS). Endorsed by the governing bodies of the American College of Cardiology Foundation, the American Heart Association, the European Cardiac Arrhythmia Society, the European Heart Rhythm Association, the Society of Thoracic Surgeons, the Asia Pacific Heart Rhythm Society, and the Heart Rhythm Society. Heart Rhythm. 2012;9:632–696.e21.

2. Macle L, Weerasooriya R, Jais P, et al. Radiation exposure during radiofrequency catheter ablation for atrial fibrillation. Pacing Clin Electrophysiol. 2003;26:288–91.
3. Lickfett L, Mahesh M, Vasamreddy C, et al. Radiation exposure during catheter ablation of atrial fibrillation. Circulation. 2004;110:3003–10.
4. Voskoboinik A, Kalman ES, Savicky Y, et al. Reduction in radiation dose for atrial fibrillation ablation over time: a 12-year single-center experience of 2344 patients. Heart Rhythm. 2017;14:810–6.
5. Birnie D, Healey JS, Krahn AD, et al. Prevalence and risk factors for cervical and lumbar spondylosis in interventional electrophysiologists. J Cardiovasc Electrophysiol. 2011;22:957–60.
6. Ferguson JD, Helms A, Mangrum JM, et al. Catheter ablation of atrial fibrillation without fluoroscopy using intracardiac echocardiography and electroanatomic mapping. Circ Arrhythm Electrophysiol. 2009;2:611–9.
7. Reddy VY, Morales G, Ahmed H, et al. Catheter ablation of atrial fibrillation without the use of fluoroscopy. Heart Rhythm. 2010;7:1644–53.
8. Bulava A, Hanis J, Eisenberger M. Catheter ablation of atrial fibrillation using zero-fluoroscopy technique: a randomized trial. Pacing Clin Electrophysiol. 2015;38:797–806.
9. Lyan E, Tsyganov A, Abdrahmanov A, et al. Nonfluoroscopic catheter ablation of paroxysmal atrial fibrillation. Pacing Clin Electrophysiol. 2018;41:611–9.
10. Sommer P, Bertagnolli L, Kircher S, et al. Safety profile of near-zero fluoroscopy atrial fibrillation ablation with non-fluoroscopic catheter visualization: experience from 1000 consecutive procedures. Europace. 2018;20:1952–8.
11. Lee G, Hunter RJ, Lovell MJ, et al. Use of a contact force-sensing ablation catheter with advanced catheter location significantly reduces fluoroscopy time and radiation dose in catheter ablation of atrial fibrillation. Europace. 2016;18:211–8.
12. Wannasopha Y, Oilmungmool N, Euathrongchit J. Anatomical variations of pulmonary venous drainage in Thai people: multidetector CT study. Biomed Imaging Interv J. 2012;8:e4.
13. Nair GM, Nery PB, Redpath CJ, Lam B-K, Birnie DH. Atrioesophageal fistula in the era of atrial fibrillation ablation: a review. Can J Cardiol. 2014;30:388–95.
14. Bai R, Patel D, Di Biase L, et al. Phrenic nerve injury after catheter ablation: should we worry about this complication? J Cardiovasc Electrophysiol. 2006;17:944–8.
15. Sadek MM, Ramirez FD, Nery PB, et al. Completely non-fluoroscopic catheter ablation of left atrial arrhythmias and ventricular tachycardia. J Cardiovasc Electrophysiol. 2018;30:78–88.
16. Razminia M, Demo H, Arrieta-Garcia C, D'Silva OJ, Wang T, Kehoe RF. Nonfluoroscopic ablation of atrial fibrillation using cryoballoon. J Atr Fibrillation. 2014;7:1093.

Non-fluoroscopic Catheter Ablation of Idiopathic Ventricular Arrhythmias

12

Santiago Rivera, Maria de la Paz Ricapito, and Danna Spears

Introduction

Ventricular tachycardia (VT) is usually related to structural heart disease. However, 10–20% of patients with VT present without structural heart disease, metabolic/electrolyte abnormalities or long QT syndrome [1]. We refer to them as idiopathic ventricular arrhythmias. Sudden cardiac death is rare in this patient population and catheter-based ablation has been described as the gold standard treatment if antiarrhythmic drugs are not tolerated, ineffective or not desired by the patient [2]. Ablation is curative in most affected patients, procedural complications are rare and it has been traditionally performed under fluoroscopy guidance [1, 2]. Nevertheless, the use of fluoroscopy during catheter ablation of ventricular arrhythmias can scale up to 60 min [3]. Fluoroscopy has limited spatial resolution and involves ionizing radiation that exposes patients and staff to harmful effects [4–7]. Evidence shows that no safety dose threshold exists, and even low doses can be harmful [8, 9]. Zero fluoroscopy ablation significantly reduces ablation time and radiation dose without compromising success, complication, and recurrence rates.

This chapter will review the most frequent types of idiopathic ventricular arrhythmias and describe the non-fluoroscopic catheter-based ablation approach.

S. Rivera (✉)
Cardiac Electrophisiology Department, Buenos Aires Cardiovascular Institute (ICBA), Buenos Aires, Argentina

M. de la Paz Ricapito
Cardiac Imaging Department, Buenos Aires Cardiovascular Institute (ICBA), Buenos Aires, Argentina

D. Spears
Inherited Arrhythmia Program, Division of Cardiology—Electrophysiology, Pregnancy and Heart Disease Program—Arrhythmia Clinic, University of Toronto, Toronto, ON, Canada

Canadian Working Group on Radiation Reduction in Arrhythmia Management, University Health Network–Toronto General Hospital, Toronto, ON, Canada
e-mail: danna.spears@uhn.ca

Relevant Anatomy

Outflow Tracts

The right ventricular outflow tract (RVOT) or infundibulum is a muscular tube that provides support to the pulmonary valve [10]. It is located anteriorly and slightly superior to the aortic valve. The posterior septal aspect of the superior RVOT lies adjacent to the right coronary cusp, whereas the anterior septal aspect tends to be situated at the junction of the right and left cusp [10, 11]. It is located to the left of the right atrial appendage also anterior and superior to the supraventricular crest and the bundle of His. The supraventricular

R. Proietti et al. (eds.), *Cardiac Electrophysiology Without Fluoroscopy*,
https://doi.org/10.1007/978-3-030-16992-3_12

crest is a prominent muscular band with a parietal part formed by the superior right ventricular free wall and a medial part merging with the ventricular septum, which separates the outflow tract from the inflow tract of the right ventricle (RV) [12]. Caudally, the posterior aspect of the right ventricular outflow tract is in continuity with the superior segments of the left ventricle (LV) [10–12].

The aortic left sinus of Valsalva is more cranially located than the right sinus [13, 14]. It is related to the superior LV wall, whereas the aortic right sinus of Valsalva is close to the epicardial aspect of the paraseptal superior left ventricular wall. It's worth mentioning that the noncoronary sinus of Valsalva is unrelated to either the right or left ventricular myocardium but is related to the Bachmann bundle and the interatrial groove from which the terminal crest originates [10, 14]. This explains why pacing from the noncoronary aortic sinus results in atrial capture.

The RVOT is related posteriorly and inferiorly to the aortic root and to the left ventricular Summit (LVS). Most RVOT tachycardias are originated at the anterior septal aspect, under the pulmonic valve (Position 3) (Fig. 12.1), whereas LVOT tachycardias predominantly originate at the medial aspect of the basal LV (septal-paraHisian region, aorto-mitral continuity, and superior mitral annulus), the LVS and the left and right aortic cusps [15]. Myocardial fibres may extend above the right coronary cusp into the aortic sinus [16]. Although the non-coronary and left coronary cusps usually lack ventricular myocardial extensions, myocardial extensions may occur into all three cusps, and above the pulmonic valve as well [10, 14]. Most outflow tract arrhythmias originate in perivalvular tissue, which is anatomically predisposed to fibre disruption, which may predispose the tissue to triggered activity and arrhythmogenesis [10–16].

The left ventricle differs from the right ventricle in four major anatomic details: (1) thicker ventricular wall; (2) no muscular separation between the inflow and outflow valves, and the aorto-mitral

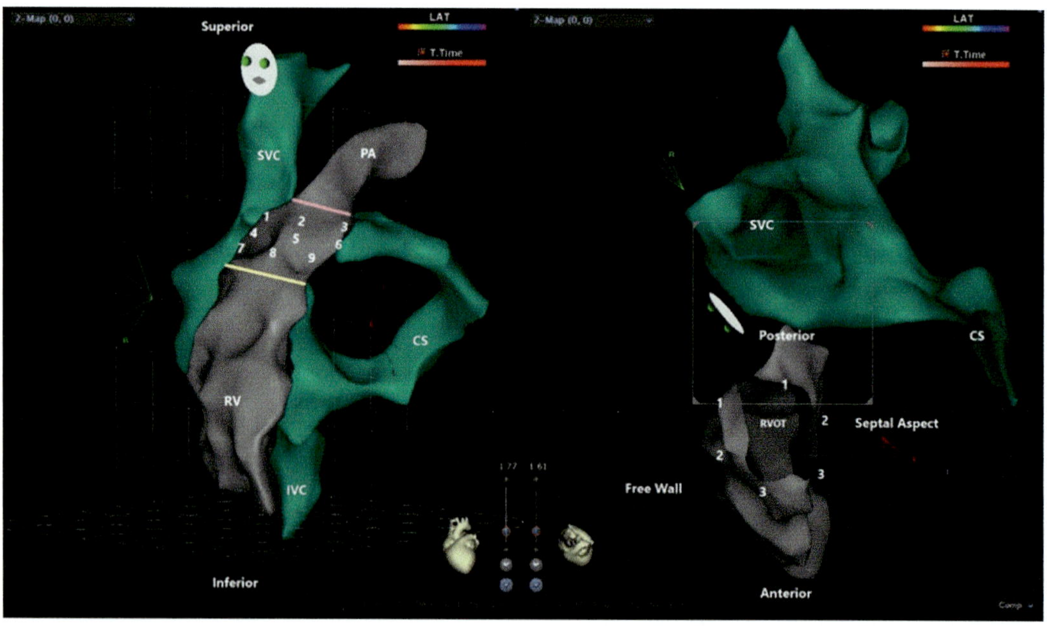

Fig. 12.1 Left panel: Left anterior oblique view of the right ventricle and right ventricular outflow tract (RVOT) (grey) and right atrium and coronary sinus (CS) system (green). The superior and inferior vena cava are demarcated as SVC and IVC. The yellow and pink lines correspond to the supraventricular crest and pulmonic valve planes, respectively. Numbers 1-2-3 are consistent with superior sites of origin of RVOT arrhythmias, 4-5-6 represent mid-locations, and 7-8-9 correspond to inferior origins. Right panel: Superior view of the RVOT. The pulmonary artery (PA) has been clipped to obtain an endoscopic view. Notice sites 1-2-3 are repeated at the septal and free wall. These represent posterior (1), middle (2) and anterior (3) locations of ventricular arrhythmias at both medial and lateral aspects of the RVOT

continuity; (3) the mitral valve is positioned cranially relative to the tricuspid valve; (4) the right and left AV junctions diverge when viewed in the RAO projection, merging anterosuperiorly but separating inferoposteriorly [14].

Posterior Superior Process of the Left Ventricle

The AV annuli are not positioned in parallel planes [14]. The tricuspid annular plane is inferiorly and apically displaced by ≈0.5–1 cm relative to the plane of the mitral annulus. Because of this, part of the basal inferoseptal aspect of the LV wall is directly opposed to right atrial tissue rather than RV tissue or epicardium. The posteroseptal process of the left ventricle (PSP-LV) is the promontory of LV between the attachment of the septal leaflet of the tricuspid valve to the AV unit, the ostium of the LV, and a line drawn from the latter to the upper end of the posterior interventricular groove [17]. Superiorly, at the apex of the triangle lies the right fibrous trigone and the posterior aspect of the atrioventricular membranous septum [10]. The inferior wall of the right atrium lies above and lateral to the PSP-LV adjacent to the pyramidal space. The CS orifice is medial to this area. In addition, the atrioventricular node artery and the septal artery ascend onto the PSP-LV crossing within the fat of the pyramidal space. Santangeli et al. first described successful catheter ablation of ventricular arrhythmias arising from the PSP-LV, performed through the right atrium [17].

Papillary Muscles

The LV papillary muscles (PMs) are myocardial ingrowths presenting conical projections into the left ventricular cavity and, like the neighbouring tissue, are made up of myocardium and conduction tissue. Myocardial strands are irregularly distributed between the most apical and basal aspect of the PM anatomy, and Purkinje-ventricular junctions are preferentially located towards the base of the PMs [10]. Typically, the LV presents the posteromedial PM and the anterolateral PM (Fig. 12.2). The RV usually exhibit three PMs (Fig. 12.3): (1) the septal PM, where the right bundle branch (RBBB) becomes subendocardial; (2) anterior PM, which emerges in close anatomi-

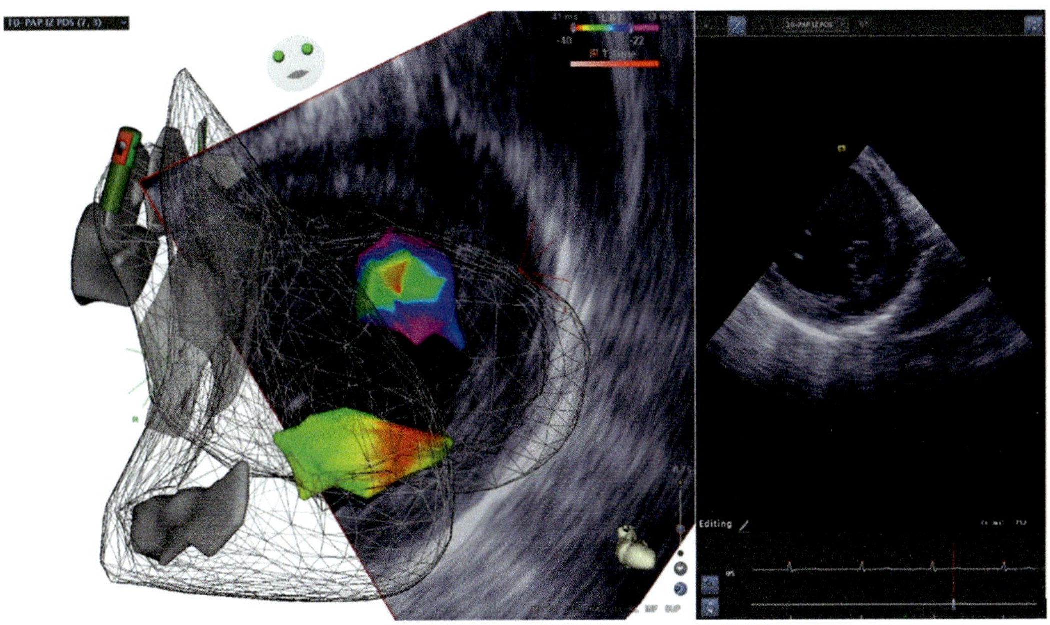

Fig. 12.2 Non-fluoroscopic intracardiac echo-facilitated 3D electroanatomical map of both ventricles and papillary muscles. An activation map shows two arrhythmia foci located at both papillary muscles (PM) of the left ventricle (LV). On the right, an ICE 2D clip of the LV and anterolateral PM

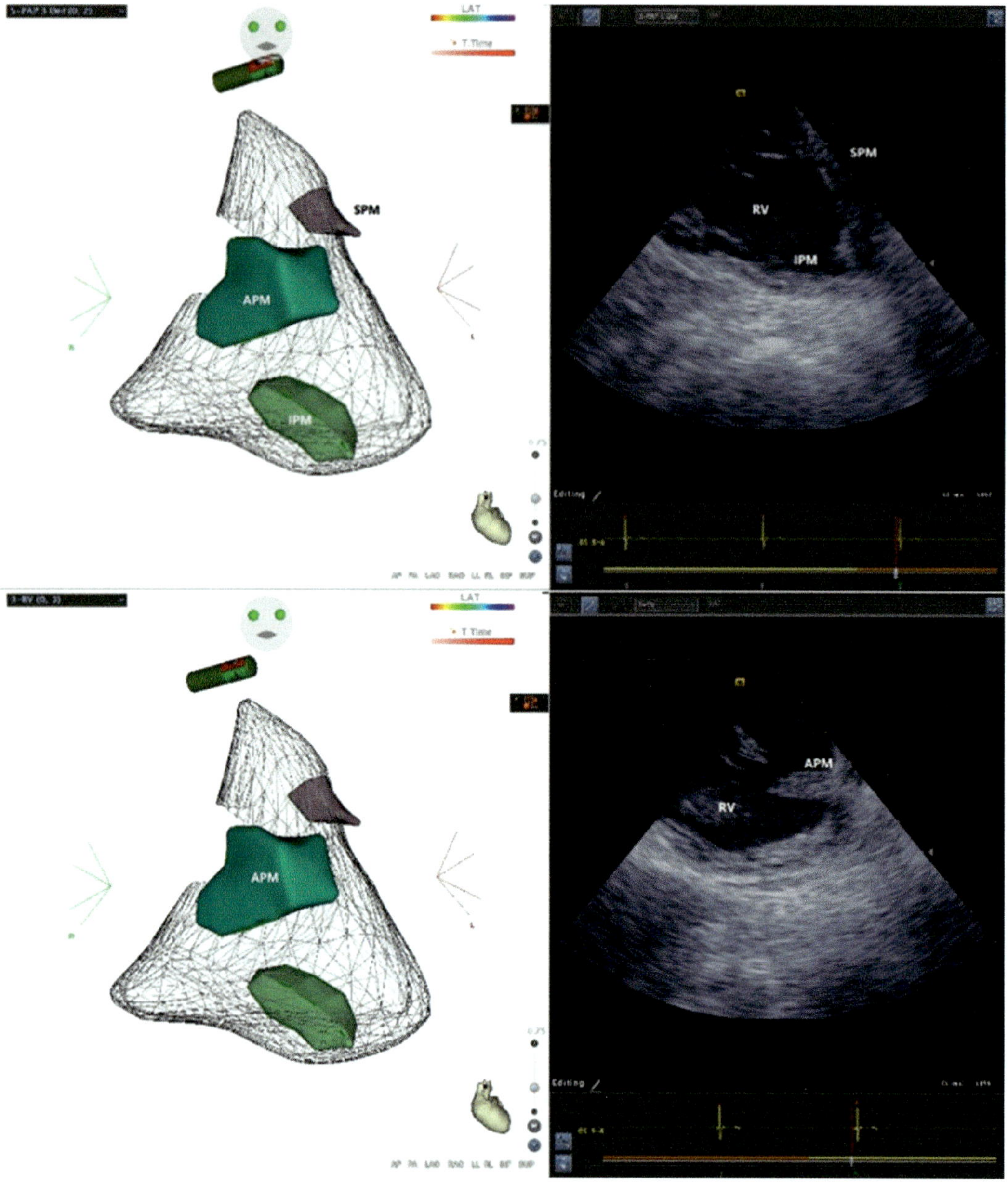

Fig. 12.3 On the left, intracardiac echo-facilitated 3D maps of the right ventricle and RV PMs. On the left, ICE 2D clips of the RV PMs: *SPM* septal papillary muscle, *APM* anterior papillary muscle, *IPM* inferior papillary muscle

cal relation to the moderator band, which is also traversed by the RBBB; and (3) the posterior PM, located at the inferior wall of the RV. The RV is prone to high anatomical variability regarding PM distribution, and sometimes is difficult to discriminate between the presence of PMs or direct insertion of the cords into the myocardium [10–16].

Summit of the Left Ventricle

McAlpine described this portion of the epicardium of the left ventricular outflow tract as a triangular region formed by the left main coronary artery bifurcation that is bounded by the left anterior descending coronary artery superior to the first septal perforating branch anteriorly

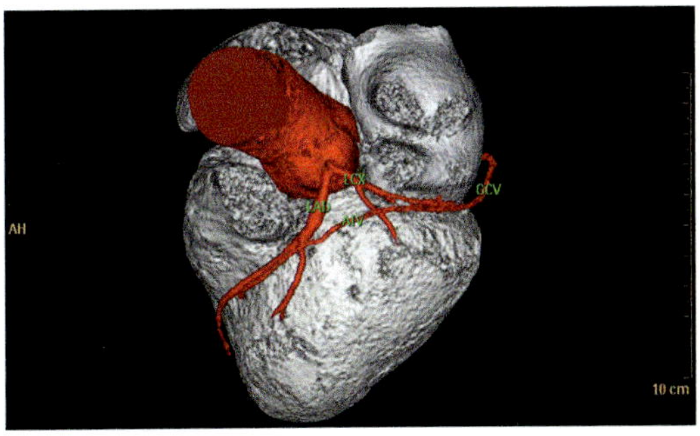

Fig. 12.4 Multi-detector cardiac tomography showing the boundaries of the Summit of the left ventricle: *LCX* left circumflex artery, *AIV* anterior interventricular vein, *LAD* left anterior descendant artery, *GCV* great cardiac vein

and left circumflex coronary artery laterally, which lies superior to the aortic portion of the LV ostium [18]. The LVS is bisected by the cardiac vein into an area lateral to this structure (Apical LVS), which is accessible to epicardial catheter ablation and a superior region (Basal LVS), that is inaccessible to catheter ablation because of the proximity of the left proximal coronary arteries and the thick layer of epicardial fat that overlies the proximal portion of these vessels (Fig. 12.4) [19, 20].

Classification of Ventricular Arrhythmias Without Structural Heart Disease

Polymorphic Arrhythmias

1. Drug related. These include primarily the antiarrhythmic drugs (IA, IC, sotalol and bepridil), digitalis, sympathomimetics and phosphodiesterase inhibitors. Other drugs such as vasodilators and anti-anginal drugs (lidoflazine, vincamine, fenoxedil), psychotropic agents (phenothiazine and imipramine), antimitotics, antimalarials (chloroquine) or antibiotics (erythromycin, pentamidine) may also cause VT.
2. Myocardial ischaemia.
3. Channelopathies (Brugada syndrome; Long QT and short QT syndromes; catecholaminergic polymorphic ventricular tachycardia).

Monomorphic Arrhythmias

1. Outflow tract tachycardias: Clinical presentation consists of PVCs and non-sustained VT. Sustained tachycardia is not uncommon. Symptoms include palpitations (48–80%) and Presyncope (28–50%), although syncope is uncommon (10%) [21]. RVOT PVCs have been shown to consistently initiate ventricular fibrillation in a selected group of patients with Brugada and long QT syndromes [22].

   The most frequent trigger is exercise, and treadmill testing can reproduce the clinical VT in most patients. Other triggers include stress, anxiety, and stimulants such as caffeine. Outflow tract arrhythmias are modulated by hormonal influence in females, as they are more often observed during premenstrual and perimenopausal periods and with gestation [23].

   The ECG can predict the site of origin of the arrhythmia [22, 24–27]. RVOT arrhythmias usually exhibit a left bundle branch block configuration, with late precordial S to R wave transition (>lead V3) and inferior QRS axis. It is possible to differentiate between septal and free wall location, as QRS notching and the lack of r waves in lead V1 usually suggest a free wall origin. Lead I can be used to determining whether the foci are located anteriorly (Position 3), posteriorly (Position 1), or at mid-portions (Position 2) whenever the QRS is negative, positive or presents an M shape, respectively (Fig. 12.1). It is also possible to discriminate between RVOT and LVOT origins: an r wav e in lead V1 exhibiting >40 ms duration or a dome-like shape suggests that the foci is located at the LVOT. Early precordial transition (<V3) is also consistent with an LVOT or aortic cusps origin. Left coronary cusps foci usually exhibit an M or W shape in lead V1, while a QS or QR pattern suggests an origin at the right cusp.
2. Summit of the left ventricle arrhythmias: The LVS is a major source of ventricular arrhythmias (VAs) and the most common site of origin of epicardial idiopathic VAs [3]. Catheter ablation can eliminate LVS VAs. However, ablation of VAs originating from the basal

portion of the LV summit near the left main coronary artery is challenging due to proximity of the coronary arteries and the thick epicardial fat pad that covers that region [28]. Epicardial catheter ablation of LVS arrhythmias has been associated with poor results, mainly due to a high prevalence of arrhythmias originating at the inaccessible area and fat tissue surrounding this area [29]. Around 50% of the basal LV summit VAs could be eliminated by a direct approach through a great cardiac vein (GCV) branch running below the proximal left coronary arteries and a remote approach from endocardial sites such as the aortic-mitral continuity and left coronary cusps [3, 28, 29].

The prevalence of LV summit VA is much higher within the great cardiac vein and anterior interventricular vein (AIVV) than on the epicardial surface of either side of these veins. LVS VAs with an origin superior to the GCV are in the inaccessible area bounded by the left coronary arteries, GCV, and AIVV. In this region, catheter ablation is unlikely to be successful because of a thick layer of epicardial fat overlying the proximal coronary arteries and may be potentially hazardous to these vessels [30]. Adjacent sites such as the endocardial LV/RVOT, coronary cusp region or coronary venous system are successful in eliminating these arrhythmias. Successful ablation of VAs from the inaccessible LVS area can be achieved from the left coronary cusp in 56% of cases, and from the GCV–AIV region in >70% of cases. Yamada et al. described a 100% and 48% success rates for catheter ablation of Apical (including the GCV) and Basal LVS VAs, respectively [3, 28, 29].

Several ECG parameters may be helpful to predict the site of origin of the foci. The ECG features found to be more prevalent in successful cases are Q-wave ratio aVL/aVR >1.85, R/S ratio in V1 > 2, and lack of q wave in V1, which reflect a more lateral site of origin of the VAs, distant from the midline at the apex of the LVS triangle. Patients with successful ablations may present a QS pattern in lead I, which again points to a more lateral (and epicardial) origin of the VAs. When LVS VAs exhibit a III/II amplitude ratio of 1.25 and an aVL/aVR amplitude ratio of 1.75, those VAs are likely to require a pericardial approach for ablation [3, 31, 32].

3. Purkinje Related Arrhythmias
   (a) Fascicular ventricular tachycardia (FVT): Fascicular VT is the most common idiopathic left VT. The diagnostic triad include: (1) atrial pacing induction; (2) right bundle branch block (RBBB) and left-axis configuration; and (3) absence of structural heart disease. It was then demonstrated that the tachycardia was sensitive to verapamil [33]. FVT can be classified into three subgroups: (1) common or left posterior FVT (RBBB configuration and a superior axis) in 90% of cases; (2) uncommon or left anterior fascicular VT (RBBB configuration and right-axis deviation); and (3) rare or upper septal fascicular VT (narrow QRS configuration and normal or right-axis deviation) [34]. Re-entry is the underlying mechanism, as it can be induced, entrained, and terminated by programmed ventricle or atrial stimulation [34, 35]. Two potentials, P1 (mid-diastolic) and P2 (pre-systolic), are recorded during VT at the mid-septum [35]. The activation sequence during sinus rhythm demonstrates first the P2 (normal conduction tissue), which is recorded after the His bundle potential and before the onset of the QRS complex. The P1 (slow-pathway) is usually fused with the VEGM. This sequence is reversed during VT: P1-P2-VEGM. These suggest the presence of a macroreentry involving the normal Purkinje system (P2) and abnormal Purkinje tissue (P1) with decremental properties and verapamil sensitivity, which represents the antegrade limb of the circuit. With left posterior fascicular VT, the earliest ventricular activation is recorded from the apical septum, and diastolic potentials are recorded from the

mid-septum [34]. His activation follows QRS onset by 5–30 ms. During sinus rhythm, recording from the same site demonstrates the Purkinje potentials after the His bundle potential and before the onset of the QRS complex. With left anterior fascicular VT, the earliest ventricular activation is recorded from the anterolateral left ventricle, and diastolic potentials are recorded from the mid-septum [36]. The P2 potential during VT is the ablation target. After successful ablation, and during sinus rhythm, the activation sequence shows P1-VEGM and a late P2 following the VEGM, representing conduction block at P2 [34, 37].

(b) Papillary muscles. The papillary muscles (PMs) of the LV are potential sites of origin of ventricular arrhythmias [38]. Catheter ablation has been described as an effective treatment, although radiofrequency delivery at these regions has been associated with poor catheter stability and high recurrence [39]. Cryo-energy can provide stable contact and lower recurrence rates [40, 41]. It has been reported that almost half of the patients with PM VAs may present with variable QRS morphologies. In this scenario, recurrence after RF ablation can be as high as 60% [42–44]. Spontaneous variable QRS morphologies may respond to preferential conduction to multiple breakout sites, due to an anisotropic mechanism given the complexity of the myocardial strands distribution between the base and apex of the PM [39–43]. Ablation at sites with excellent pace mapping can be unsuccessful, also suggesting that the site of VA origin may be located away from the breakout site [45]. Purkinje potentials can be observed in 45% of PM VAs [43]. They are frequently recorded at the base of the PMs at the Purkinje-fibre-muscular interface, and rarely at a distal aspect, suggesting that the Purkinje network may not extend further towards the chordae insertion site and that VAs may arise from the myocardium itself [43]. Distal Purkinje fibres may be involved in triggering or maintaining PM VAs [46, 47].

Monomorphic ventricular PVCs originating from the PMs have been found to initiate idiopathic ventricular fibrillation or polymorphic VT [48]. Ventricular arrhythmias from the right ventricular papillary muscles are less frequent [49, 50]. Bileaflet mitral valve prolapse (MVP) syndrome is characterized by the myxomatous degeneration of both mitral leaflets, T-wave inversion of the inferolateral ECG leads, and complex ventricular ectopy such as PM, fascicular and outflow tracts VAs [51]. This is most commonly observed in young woman [52]. Ventricular fibrillation is often triggered by PM and fascicular arrhythmias, and there is a transient increased risk of malignant VAs when ablating at a Purkinje target or PM, which usually exhibit Purkinje signals at the site of origin of VA. Papillary muscles that lie within an infarct zone might give rise to ventricular arrhythmias [53].

Although PM-FVT and FVT share many ECG similarities, a superior right axis or horizontal axis deviation in posterior PM-FVT and R/S ratio <1 in leads I, V5, and V6 in anterior PM-FVT will differentiate PM-FVT from common type FVT [47]. PM fascicular VT (PM-FVT) is a distinct entity, caused by a re-entry mechanism involving the Pk network around the PMs which cover the endocardial surface of the ventricles and is largely distributed at the midventricular area and PMs. The QRS morphology may be similar to anterior and left posterior fascicular VT (FVT). They all share RBBB with r<R′ configuration. Nevertheless, a superior right axis or horizontal axis deviation in posterior PM-FVT and R/S ratio <1 in leads I, V5, and V6 in anterior PM-FVT are predictors of PM-FVT. Mid-diastolic potentials (MDP) are recorded around the papillary muscles, in contrast with FVT, whereas MDP are usually recorded at the distal third of the fascicle-Purkinje network on the LV septum. The QRS morphology and VT cycle length may often change after ablation of the left posterior or anterior fascicle, meaning that it does not eliminate a critical limb of the re-entry circuit. Because of the variable distribution of Purkinje fibres, there is the potential for variable recruitment of the Purkinje network at the PMs. The hallmark for PM VA and PM-FVT differentiation are: (1) Patients with PM VAs usually present with PVCs and NSVT; (2) PM VAs are refractory to verapamil; (3) PM-FVT exhibits a re-entry mechanism, while PM VAs responds to triggered activity or abnormal automatism; (4) PM VA are distinguished by longer QRS durations.

(c) Purkinje focal tachycardia: It might be difficult to distinguish FVT from PFT, as ECG characteristics are similar [38]. Nevertheless, faster VT is prone to exhibit wider QRS in contrast to FVT. The mechanism of the arrhythmia is consistent with abnormal automaticity [36]. It is responsible to lidocaine, B-blockers and class I A antiarrhythmic drugs. Verapamil has no effect in FPT. During VT, a negative HV interval is frequently observed [36–38].

4. Mitral annulus VAs: The ECG typically exhibit high amplitude, long QRS duration and positive complexes along all the precordial leads, as the vector is travelling from the base to the apex. Lead I will show a more positive or negative complex depending on whether the arrhythmia is originated at the septal or lateral annulus, respectively. Similarly, a superiorly or inferiorly directed QRS axis will be equally useful determining an inferior or superior origin at the annulus. The right bundle branch block pattern is consistent with PM, fascicular, papillary muscle fascicular VT (PM-FVT) and mitral valve VAs. Although differentiating them by simple ECG analysis may be challenging, they present distinctive characteristics. The QRS duration of PM and MV VAs is significantly longer (>135 ms). Fascicular and PM-FVT have a higher prevalence of r<R′ pattern in V1, with 83% sensitivity and 91% specificity for differentiating fascicular from PM VAs. A positive precordial concordance of the clinical VA shows 87% sensitivity and 71% specificity for differentiating MVA VA from PM VA. Amongst VAs with superior axis, the presence of R>S in lead V5 shows 100% sensitivity and 100% specificity for diagnosing MVA VAs [53]. Differentiation between PM and MV VAs tend to be harder when PM arrhythmias exhibit a distal origin, over the chordal insertion site, near the mitral annulus.

Arrhythmia Mechanism

Abnormal Automaticity

Ventricular non-pacemaker myocardial cells may exhibit automaticity properties under conditions that drive the maximum diastolic potential towards the threshold potential. The intrinsic rate of an automatic abnormal focus depends on the membrane potential; the more positive the membrane potential, the faster the automatic rate. Abnormal automaticity is thought to play a role in cases of elevated extracellular potassium, low intracellular pH, and catecholamine excess [54].

An important distinction between enhanced normal and abnormal induced automaticity is that the latter is less sensitive to overdrive suppression.

Triggered Activity

Triggered activity is caused by afterdepolarizations. These are membrane potential oscillations that occur during or immediately after a preceding action potential (the trigger), and when they reach the threshold potential, a new action potential is generated [55]. There are two types of after depolarizations:

1. Delayed afterdepolarizations (DADs): These oscillations are caused by a variety of conditions that raise the diastolic intracellular Ca^{2+} concentration, causing oscillations that can

trigger a new action potential if they reach the stimulation threshold, during phase 4 of the action potential. The amplitude and rate of the DADs increases as the cycle length decreases. Digitalis toxicity was the first observed cause of DAD, of which bidirectional fascicular tachycardia is an example. This occurs via inhibition of the Na/K pump, which releases Ca^{2+} from the sarcoplasmic reticulum. Catecholamines can cause DADs by causing intracellular Ca^{2+} overload via an increase in ICa-L and the Na^{+}/–Ca^{2+} exchange current. Ischaemia-induced DADs are thought to be mediated by the accumulation of lysophosphoglycerides in the ischaemic tissue, with subsequent elevation in Na^{+} and Ca^{2+}. Mutations in the ryanodine receptor of the sarcoplasmic reticulum can also lead to intracellular Ca^{2+} overload, facilitating clinical arrhythmias such as catecholaminergic polymorphic VT.

Longer APs are associated with more Ca^{2+} overload and facilitate DADs. Therefore, drugs that prolong AP (Class IA antiarrhythmic agents) can occasionally increase DAD amplitude. Triggered arrhythmias induced by DADs may be terminated by single stimuli and should be distinguished from re-entrant tachycardias. In most cases of DAD-induced arrhythmias, the shorter the cycle of stimulation, the shorter the coupling interval to the induced arrhythmia. This contrasts with the inverse relationship seen in re-entrant arrhythmias, where the shorter the coupling intervals of the initiating stimuli, the longer the coupling interval of the first arrhythmia beat.

Adenosine can reduce the Ca^{2+} inward current indirectly by inhibiting adenylate cyclase and cyclic adenosine monophosphate effect. Though it may abolish catecholamine-induced DADs, it does not alter DADs induced by Na^{+}/K^{+} pump inhibition. The interruption of VT by adenosine points towards catecholamine-induced DADs as the underlying mechanism [54, 55].

2. Early Afterdepolarization-Induced Triggered Activity: EADs occur during the phase 2 or 3 of the action potential. Phase 2 EADs appear to be related to Ica-L current, while phase 3 EADs may be the result of low IK1. A fundamental condition underlying the development of EADs is AP prolongation (QT prolongation). Factors involved in prolongation of the AP include drugs, hypokalemia and/or bradycardia. Catecholamines may enhance EADs by increasing Ca^{2+} current; however, the increase in heart rate and K^{+} current may reduce the action potential duration, thus abolishing EADs. Early afterdepolarization-triggered arrhythmias increase at slow rates, so it is not expected to follow premature stimulation, except for a long compensatory pause after a premature stimulus, which can initiate torsades de pointes [54, 55].

Re-entry

It is the most frequent mechanism of cardiac arrhythmias. It refers to a repetitive propagation of the activation wavefront, returning to its site of origin to reactivate that site. Re-entry has been divided in two main groups: (1) anatomical re-entry, where the circuit is determined by anatomical structures, and (2) functional re-entry, which is characterized by a lack of anatomic boundaries as the circuit depends on myocardial tissue at different stages of refractoriness generating electrical gradients, thus predisposing re-entry. Both forms can coexist in the same setting and share biophysical mechanisms [54].

Re-entry usually requires:

1. Substrate: myocardial tissue with different electrophysiological properties, conduction, and refractoriness.
2. Area of block (anatomical, functional, or both): an area of inexcitable tissue around which the wavefront can circulate.
3. Unidirectional conduction block.
4. Path of slowed conduction that allows delay in the conduction of the circulating wavefront to enable the recovery of the refractory tissue proximal to the site of unidirectional block (Exitable Gap). Conduction velocity cannot exceed the circuit length.
5. Critical tissue mass to sustain the circulating re-entrant wavefronts.
6. A trigger.

Favours automaticity	Favours triggered activity	Favours re-entry
Non-inducible by PES	Initiated by PES (continuous stimulation)	Initiated by PES
Initiated by burst pacing	May be terminated by PES	Terminated by PES
Adenosine sensitivity (slowing)	Terminated by adenosine	Not terminated by adenosine
Absence of entrainment	No Entrainment/ no reset with fusion	Reset with fusion
Continuous stimulation: Overdrive suppression	Continuous stimulation: acceleration or termination	Continuous stimulation: entrainment or termination

Non-fluoroscopic Ablation Approach

After obtaining femoral access, usually, an external irrigation radiofrequency ablation catheter is advanced into the inferior vena cava under electroanatomic mapping (EAM) system guidance. The geometric contours of the inferior vena cava (IVC) are created by advancing the catheter tip up to the initial appearance of atrial electrograms that denoted the junction between the IVC and the right atrium (RA). Any difficulties while advancing the catheter can be overcome with a geometric acquisition of the trajectory of the catheter through the venous system. The catheter is then advanced to the RA to delineate its border (Fig. 12.5), tagging the area where a His deflection is recorded and reproducing in detail the tricuspid annulus. Anatomical details are enhanced by contact force sensing. In patients with outflow tract VT the coronary sinus should be reconstructed up to its distal portion.

Once the 3D shell of the RA is obtained, two quadripolar catheters are advanced in the RA and positioned, respectively, in the His bundle region and in the RV using the right and left anterior oblique views of the EAM system. In the same manner, a multipolar deflectable catheter can be introduced in the distal CS (GCV) if required, and advanced into the AIVV as far as possible until the proximal electrode pair recorded an earlier ventricular activation than the most distal electrode pair during the clinical arrhythmia. This is particularly useful when mapping outflow tract or LV Summit arrhythmias.

To integrate ICE into the EAMS, a 10-Fr ICE catheter (Soundstar, Biosense-Webster, Inc., Diamond Bar, CA) could be inserted through the left femoral vein and advanced up to the RA (Homeview). Sequential ICE contours of the right and/or the left ventricle are acquired to create a 3D shell of the chambers using the CartoSound™ module (Biosense-Webster, Inc., Diamond Bar, CA) that allows for intracardiac-echo facilitated 3D EAM. Detailed imaging of the RVOT, pulmonary valve, aortic root, aortic valve, LVOT and papillary muscles can be obtained. The origin of the coronary arteries can also be marked on the reconstructed 3D echo shell when necessary. The anatomical structures are visualized in each 2D clip and manually delineated on the mapping system. A detailed 3D Shell is finally obtained once the 2D clips are merged. ICE integration mapping systems present anatomical advantages over standard EAM systems, allowing for the visualization of solid structures or vascular structures such as the coronary arteries. When ablating LVS related arrhythmias, attention is paid at the LVS area, specially at the basal aspect, were the left coronary artery is visualized, surrounded by a thick layer of adipose tissue and in close contact with the RVOT and pulmonary artery (PA) (Fig. 12.6).

The resulting 3D ICE shells of the ventricles are used for catheter navigation. If required, the left ventricle (LV) can be accessed through a retrograde transaortic approach (Figs. 12.7 and 12.8). A detail 3D shell of the aorta is obtained while advancing the ablation catheter in the vessel from the femoral artery. Once the catheter reaches the aortic arch, its distal portion is looped and then advanced in the aortic root, to avoid the engagement of the left main coronary artery. At this point, the direct visualization of the catheter enabled by ICE is used to safely cross the valve, which will be achieved by prolapsing the catheter through it.

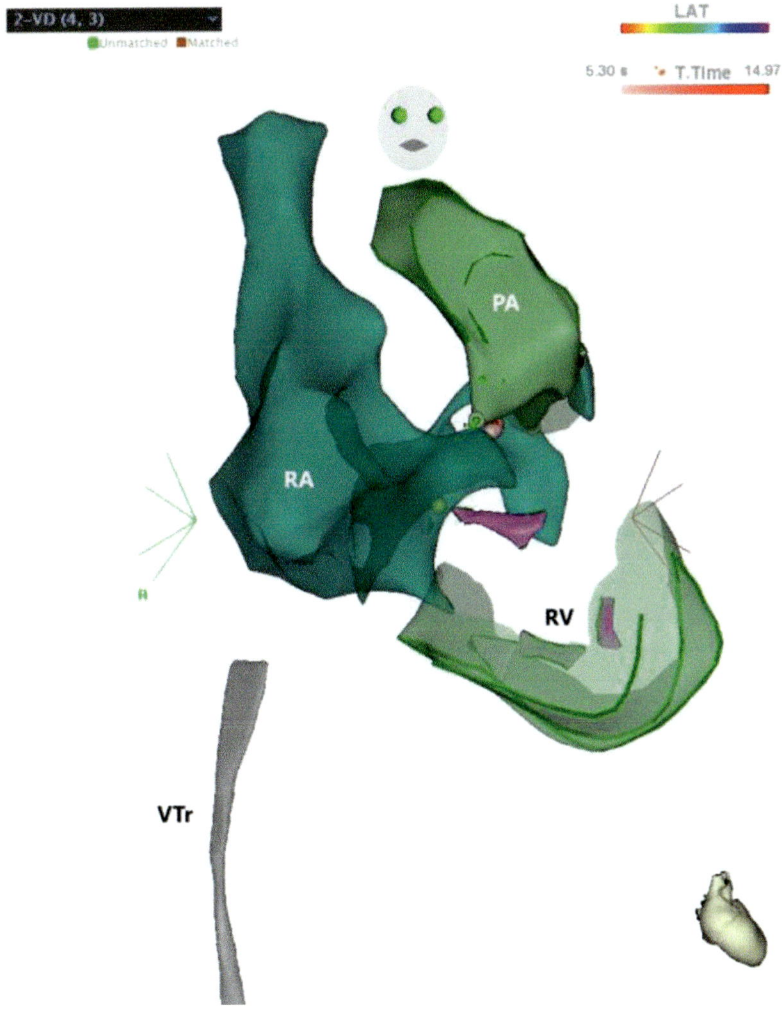

Fig. 12.5 Initial acquisition of the venous trajectory (VTr) of the ablation catheter and anatomic map of the right atrium (RA), ventricle (RV) and pulmonary artery (PA)

Local earliest activation combined with sharp negative deflection (QS) in the unipolar derivation and optimal pace mapping (>11/12 leads; PM Score >22 or >90% QRS match correlation) is used to determine the site of origin of focal arrhythmias. Abnormal Purkinje potentials (PP) in sinus rhythm and/or during ventricular tachycardia re-used to guide ablation of fascicular VT.

For outflow tract arrhythmias, sequential mapping should be performed from the RVOT and pulmonary artery using a trans-tricuspid approach, and Aortic root (Sinuses of Valsalva) and aorto-mitral continuity (AMC) mapping through a transaortic approach (Fig. 12.9). Simultaneous GCV and AIVV recording should be obtained using a multipolar catheter placed at the CS. The earliest activation site is determined by the longest VEGM to QRS interval.

Pace mapping should be performed at fix pacing cycle and stimulus amplitude of 1 mA greater than the late diastolic threshold. In patients without spontaneous arrhythmia's, induction can be attempted by programmed electrical stimulation from the RVOT and CS, with 1, 2 and 3 extrastimuli introduced after an 8-beat drive train, if necessary, with the addition of an isoproterenol infusion. Intravenous heparin must be administered to maintain an activated clotting time of ≥300 s during left-sided procedures.

To ensure the location of the ablation catheter relative to the left coronary arteries and to minimize the risk of thermal injury, a 3D recon-

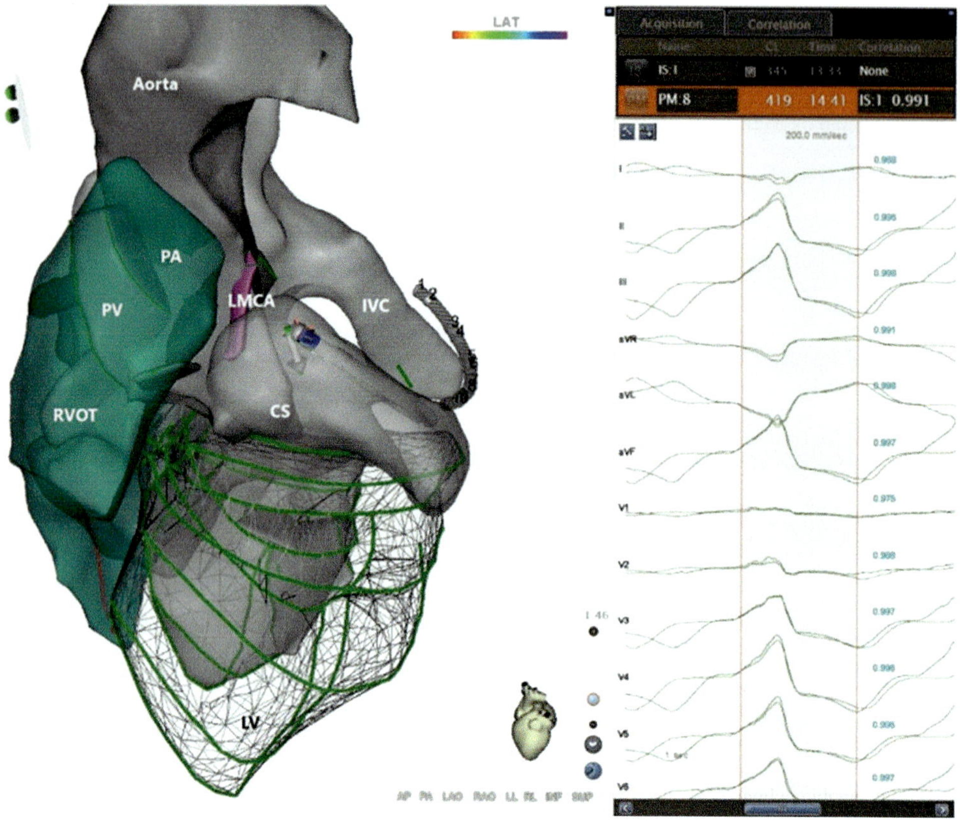

Fig. 12.6 Intracardiac echo-facilitated 3D map of the right ventricular outflow tract (RVOT), pulmonic valve (PV), pulmonary artery (PA), left ventricle (LV), distal coronary sinus (CS), Aorta and left main coronary artery (LMCA). On the right panel: Pacemapping 99% correlation to the clinical arrhythmia located at the Summit of the left ventricle

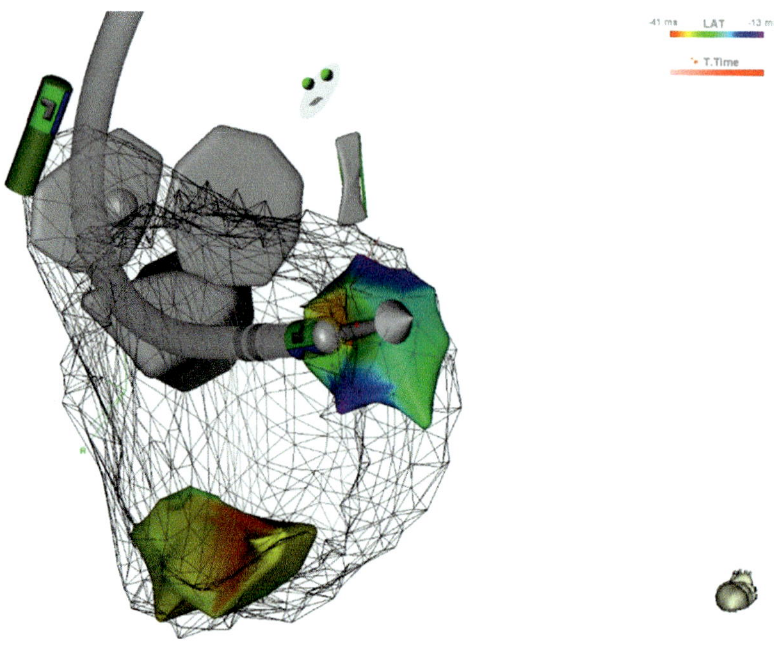

Fig. 12.7 Intracardiac echo-facilitated 3D map of the left ventricle, papillary muscles and aortic valve. Notice the ablation catheter accessing the LV through a transaortic approach after being prolapsed through the aortic valve

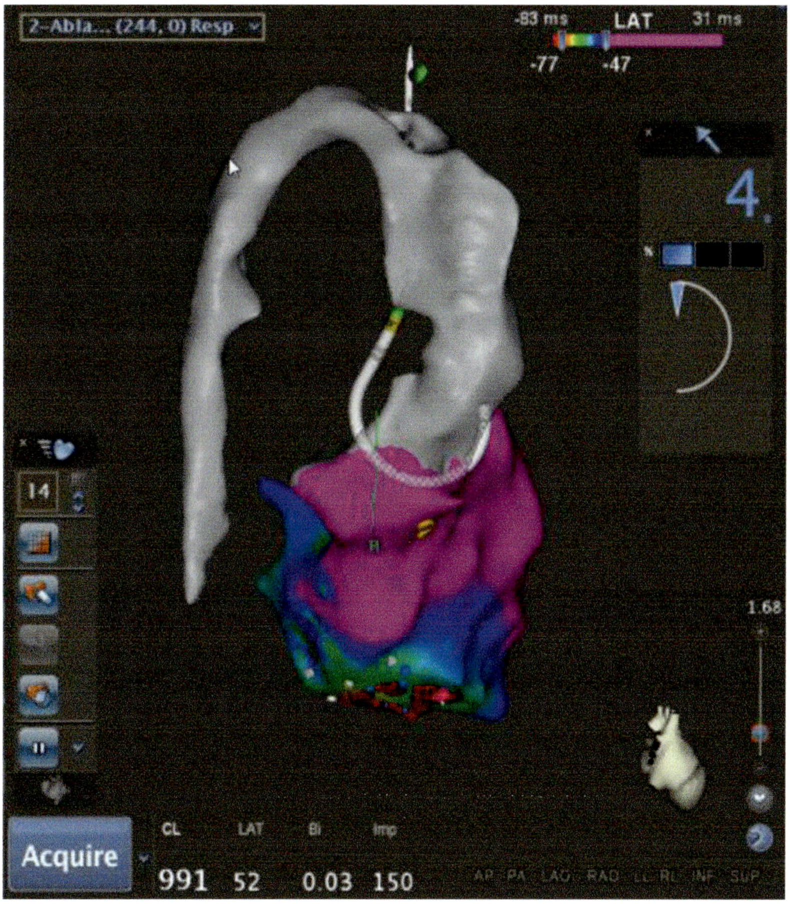

Fig. 12.8 3D map of descending aorta, aortic root, and retrograde passage of mapping catheter into the left ventricle

struction of the left coronary main trunk and left anterior descendant artery can be obtained in all patients with ventricular arrhythmias located near the coronary arteries (Fig. 12.10).

We suggest that RF energy is delivered at these locations only if all the following criteria are achieved: (1)effective lesion location >5 mm away from the coronary artery; (2) maximum power of 30 W if ablation was performed within the coronary sinus system or pulmonary artery, and up to 40 W at the endocardium; 3-Contact force vector should always point towards the epicardium (Downwards), opposing the epicardial arteries (Fig. 12.11).

If myocardial sites exhibiting the earliest bipolar activity or local unipolar QS pattern are located >5 mm away from the coronary artery, RF-energy should be delivered at locations with an early activity preceding the QRS onset for ≥25 ms during the VA, or at pace mapping areas exhibiting QRS match ≥90% (PASO Module, CARTO 3 System) (Fig. 12.6). Irrigated RF ablation should be titrated in the power-control mode from 10 to 30 W and with irrigation flow rates of 24 mL/min, if the arrhythmia was mapped within the GCV or pulmonary artery, and up to 40 W (irrigation flow rates of 16 mL/min) at endocardial sites. An RF application should be avoided whenever the ablation catheter is positioned at <5 mm or overlapping a coronary artery. In those cases, an alternative ablation site, near the earliest activation site, can be selected (Fig. 12.12). When a reduction in the incidence of VT or PVCs is observed RF should be delivered for up to 90 s; otherwise, RF delivery must be terminated, and the catheter repositioned.

Fascicular and Focal Purkinje VT approach: The target of ablation for FVT is the P2 potential during VT, located at the mid-septum in its common form. For focal Purkinje VT, the

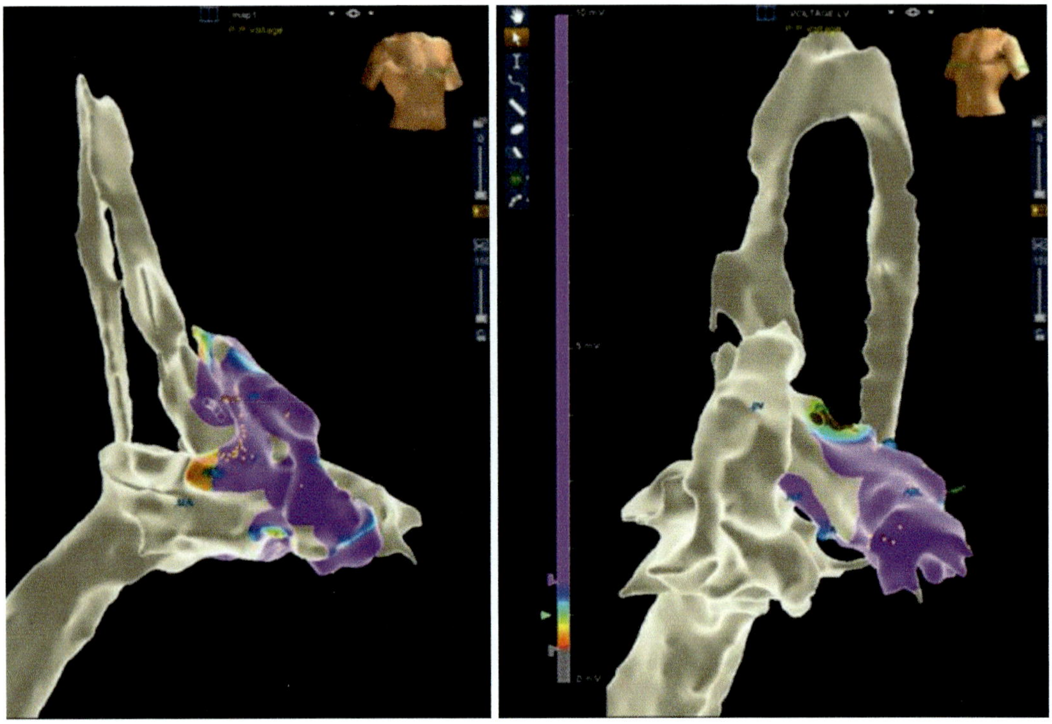

Fig. 12.9 3D Map construction of the aortic arch, aortic root, RV outflow tract, and LV outflow tract for PVC ablation in the LVOT

ablation target is the earliest Purkinje potential during the clinical arrhythmia. For this, the LV can be accessed from either a transaortic or transseptal approach, without the use of fluoroscopy. In the first case, ICE can be used to achieve a real-time beat-to-beat visualization of the aortic valve while prolapsing the catheter through it, although aortic retrograde access can also be performed without ICE. In the second scenario, we strongly suggest performing transseptal access with ICE guidance. The transseptal puncture is performed by advancing a guide wire into the superior vena cava (SVC). A transseptal deflectable sheath and dilator (Agilis, St Jude Medical INC) are advanced over the wire into the SVC and the guide wire is removed for the transseptal needle to be inserted. The system is then pulled back as a unit from the SVC to the fossa ovalis, up to when the dilator tip can be seen tenting the fossa and aiming posterior towards the left pulmonary veins, to confirm that the puncture point was neither too anterior nor posterior. The transseptal needle is then advanced out of the dilator to perforate the fossa towards the left atrium. The dilator and sheath are carefully advanced over the needle, into the left atrium. The dilator is then removed, and the ablation catheter placed towards the LV.

The end-point of catheter ablation should be the elimination and non-inducibility of the clinical arrhythmia, spontaneously and/or during isoproterenol infusion (2–10 μg/min), programmed electrical stimulation from both the atrium and ventricles, or burst pacing from the RV to a cycle length as short as 300 ms.

Intracardiac echography facilitates navigation by allowing the direct visualization of solid endocavitary structures and granting detailed anatomical landmarks (Fig. 12.13); monitoring contact at the electrode-myocardium interface during pace mapping, activation mapping, and ablation; and the possibility of real-time assessment of the location of the ablation electrode relative to the coronary arteries, without the use of fluoroscopy. A strong association was detected between the use of

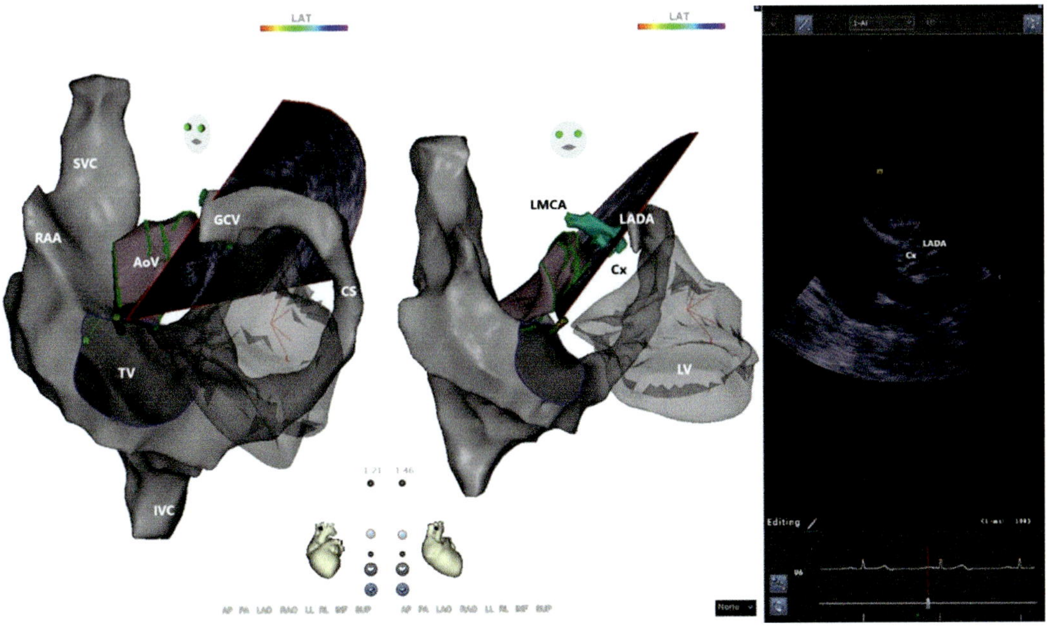

Fig. 12.10 Right atrial anatomy and aortic valve plane (AoV). The left main coronary artery (LMCA), circumflex artery (Cx) and left anterior descendant coronary artery (LADA) have been 3D reconstructed through 2D ICE clips, as observed in the right panel

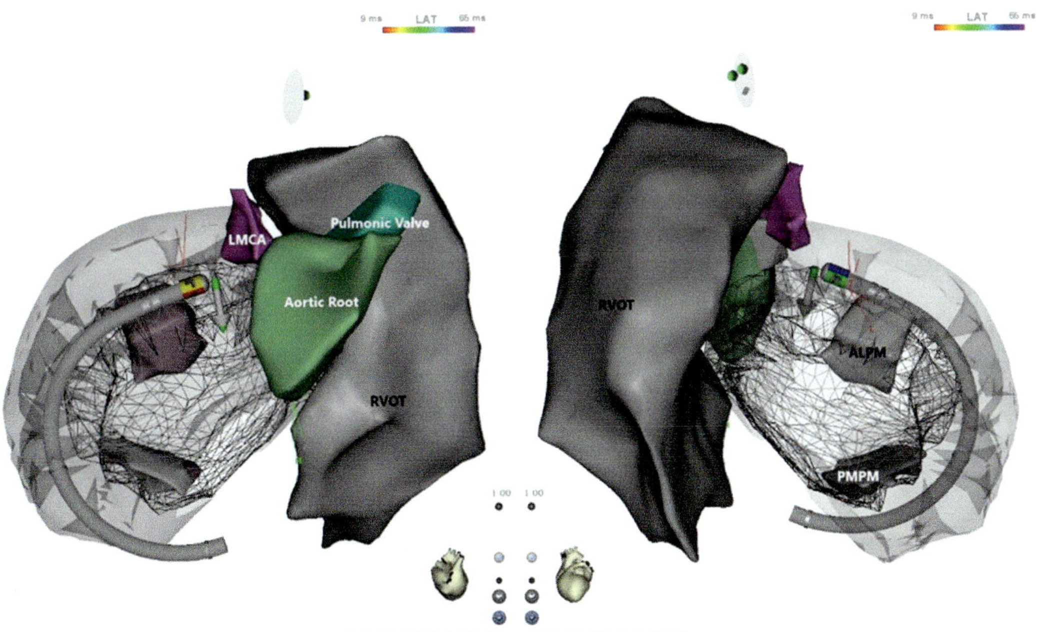

Fig. 12.11 The ablation catheter is placed inside the coronary sinus, at the distal great cardiac vein, over the earliest activation site of a LV Summit arrhythmia. Notice the contact force vector (arrow) pointing downwards, to the epicardium and away from the left coronary artery (LMCA)

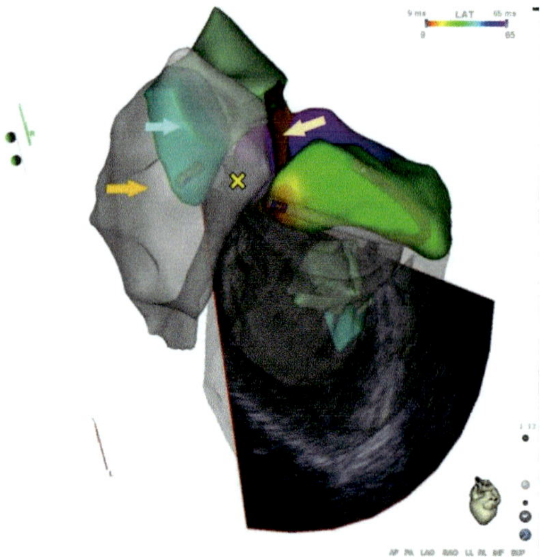

Fig. 12.12 The ablation catheter is placed at the earliest activation site at the great cardiac vein, which overlaps the left anterior descending coronary artery (yellow arrow). An alternative successful ablation site was located at the pulmonary artery (X), immediately after the pulmonic valve (blue arrow) >5 mm away from the vessel. The orange arrow points towards the RVOT

ICE3D and success of the procedure. The risk of recurrence of VT can be 20 times higher in patients who undergo ablation without ICE3D [40].

Results of Non-fluoroscopic VT Ablation

Although limited, current data provides interesting results. Recently, Lamberti et al. [56] described results of non-fluoroscopic catheter ablation of ventricular tachycardia in 19 patients who underwent ablation for idiopathic VT. Twelve had outflow-tract VT, three FVT, two peri-tricuspid VT, one peri-mitral VT, and one lateral left free-wall VT. Acute success rate was 100% and no complication was reported. Recurrence of the clinical arrhythmia occurred only in two patients. Koźluk et al. [57] described catheter ablation of ventricular arrhythmias without the use of fluoroscopy in 55 patients with RV and 24 patients with LV arrhythmias. No complications were reported in the study.

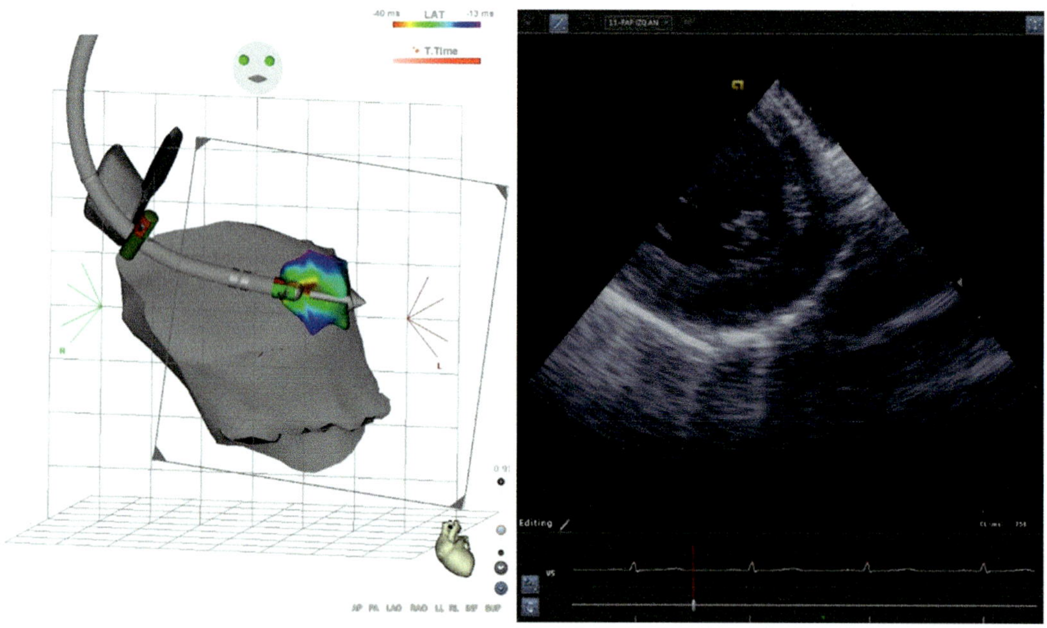

Fig. 12.13 Intracardiac echo-facilitated electroanatomical map of the LV. An activation map of the anterolateral PM was created, locating the earliest activation site of the clinical arrhythmia

Finally, a comparative study of fluoro versus non-fluoro approach performed in seven centres in China showed that ablation of different ventricular arrhythmia substrates was feasible without fluoroscopy in 94.4% of patients (the need of coronary angiography in 9 cases preclude a 100% of fluoro free cases when patients were assigned to this approach), with same efficacy, same time and same complication rates when compared to standard fluoroscopy approach [58].

It is feasible to perform ablations within both right and left sides of the heart without fluoroscopy, with excellent results. Nevertheless, the number and type of non-fluoroscopic procedures depend on the operator's experience. Pregnant patients, those with malignancy history or with hematologic diseases will benefit most from a non-fluoroscopy ablation approach.

Limitations

One major limitation of non-fluoroscopic ventricular arrhythmia ablation approach is that to perform safe epicardial access through pericardial puncture, fluoroscopy may still be needed to avoid complications. Nevertheless, fluoroscopy may be avoided if performing a mini-invasive surgical approach of the pericardial space.

Conclusion

Non-fluoroscopic procedures can reduce the risk of cancer incidence and mortality by 96% compared to those for a conventional fluoroscopic procedure, without increasing the risk of complications or compromising ablation success. Advanced mapping technologies such as intracardiac echo-facilitated 3D electroanatomical mapping or image integration can provide more detailed anatomical information, allowing for the suppression of fluoroscopy as guiding method for treating idiopathic ventricular arrhythmia substrates.

References

1. Al-Khatib SM, Stevenson WG, Ackerman MJ, Bryant WJ, Callans DJ, Curtis AB, Deal BJ, Dickfeld T, Field ME, Fonarow GC, Gillis AM, Hlatky MA, Granger CB, Hammill SC, Joglar JA, Kay GN, Matlock DD, Myerburg RJ, Page RL. 2017 AHA/ACC/HRS guideline for management of patients with ventricular arrhythmias and the prevention of sudden cardiac death: a report of the American College of Cardiology/American Heart Association task force on clinical practice guidelines and the Heart Rhythm Society. J Am Coll Cardiol. 2018;72(14):1677–749.
2. Priori SG, Blomström-Lundqvist C, Mazzanti A, Blom N, Borggrefe M, Camm J, Elliott PM, Fitzsimons D, Hatala R, Hindricks G, Kirchhof P, Kjeldsen K, Kuck KH, Hernandez-Madrid A, Nikolaou N, Norekvål TM, Spaulding C, Van Veldhuisen DJ, ESC Scientific Document Group. 2015 ESC Guidelines for the management of patients with ventricular arrhythmias and the prevention of sudden cardiac death: the task force for the management of patients with Ventricular Arrhythmias and the Prevention of Sudden Cardiac Death of the European Society of Cardiology (ESC). endorsed by: Association for European Paediatric and Congenital Cardiology (AEPC). Eur Heart J. 2015;36(41):2793–867.
3. Yamada T, Doppalapudi H, Litovsky SH, McElderry T, Neal Kay G. Challenging radiofrequency catheter ablation of idiopathic ventricular arrhythmias originating from the left ventricular summit near the left main coronary artery. Circ Arrhythm Electrophysiol. 2016;9:e004202.
4. Yang L, Sun G, Chen X, et al. Meta-analysis of zero or near-zero fluoroscopy use during ablation of cardiac arrhythmias. Am J Cardiol. 2016;118:1511–8.
5. Gaita F, Guerra PG, Battaglia A, Anselmino M. The dream of near-zero X-rays ablation comes true. Eur Heart J. 2016;37:2749–55.
6. Casella M, Dello Russo A, Pelargonio G, Del Greco M, Zingarini G, Piacenti M, Di Cori A, Casula V, et al. Near zero fluoroscopic exposure during catheter ablation of supraventricular arrhythmias: the NO-PARTY multicentre randomized trial. Europace. 2016;18:1565–72.
7. Anselmino M, Sillano D, Casolati D, Ferraris F, Scaglione M, Gaita F. A new electrophysiology era: zero fluoroscopy. J Cardiovasc Med (Hagerstown). 2013;14:221–7.
8. Casella M, Dello Russo A, Russo E, Catto V, Pizzamiglio F, Zucchetti M, Majocchi B, et al. X-ray exposure in cardiac electrophysiology: a retrospective analysis in 8150 patients over 7 years of activity in a modern, large-volume laboratory. J Am Heart Assoc. 2018;7:e008233.

9. Razminia M, Manankil MF, Eryazici PL, Arrieta-Garcia C, Wang T, D'Silva OJ, Lopez CS, et al. Nonfluoroscopic catheter ablation of cardiac arrhythmias in adults: feasibility, safety, and efficacy. J Cardiovasc Electrophysiol. 2012;23:1078–86.
10. Cabrera JA, Sánchez-Quintana D. Cardiac anatomy: what the electrophysiologist needs to know. Heart. 2013;99(6):417–31.
11. Buckberg GD, Nanda NC, Nguyen C, Kocica MJ. What Is the heart? anatomy, function, pathophysiology, and misconceptions. J Cardiovasc Dev Dis. 2018;5(2):E33.
12. Enriquez A, Saenz LC, Rosso R, Silvestry FE, Callans D, Marchlinski FE, Garcia F. Use of intracardiac echocardiography in interventional cardiology: working with the anatomy rather than fighting it. Circulation. 2018;137:2278–94.
13. Movsowitz C, Schwartzman DS, Callans DJ, et al. Idiopathic right ventricular outflow tract tachycardia: narrowing the anatomic location for successful ablation. Am Heart J. 1996;131:930–6.
14. Rice K, Simpson J. Three-dimensional echocardiography of congenital abnormalities of the left atrioventricular valve. Echo Res Pract. 2015;2(1):R13–24. https://doi.org/10.1530/ERP-15-0003.
15. Ho SY. Structure and anatomy of the aortic root. Eur J Echocardiogr. 2009;10(1):i3–10. https://doi.org/10.1093/ejechocard/jen243.
16. Sulieman M, Asirvatham SJ. Ablation above the semilunar valves: when, why and how? Part I. Heart Rhythm. 2008;5:1485–92.
17. Santangeli P, Hutchinson MD, Supple GE, Callans DJ, Marchlinski FE, Garcia FC. Right atrial approach for ablation of ventricular arrhythmias arising from the left posterior-superior process of the left ventricle. Circ Arrhythm Electrophysiol. 2016;9:e004048.
18. McAlpine WA. Heart and coronary arteries. New York: Springer-Verlag; 1975.
19. Yamada T, McElderry HT, Doppalapudi H, Okada T, Murakami Y, Yoshida Y, Yoshida N, et al. Idiopathic ventricular arrhythmias originating from the left ventricular summit: anatomic concepts relevant to ablation. Circ Arrhythm Electrophysiol. 2010;3:616–23.
20. Lin CY, Chung FP, Lin YJ, Chong E, Chang SL, Lo LW, Hu YF, et al. Radiofrequency catheter ablation of ventricular arrhythmias originating from the continuum between the aortic sinus of Valsalva and the left ventricular summit: electrocardiographic characteristics and correlative anatomy. Heart Rhythm. 2016;13:111–21.
21. Dixit S, Marchlinski FE. Clinical characteristics and catheter ablation of left ventricular outflow tract tachycardia. Curr Cardiol Rep. 2001;3:305–13.
22. Van Herendael H, Zado ES, Haqqani H, Tschabrunn CM, Callans DJ, Frankel DS, Lin D, et al. Catheter ablation of ventricular fibrillation: importance of left ventricular outflow tract and papillary muscle triggers. Heart Rhythm. 2014;11:566–73.
23. Jadonath RL, Schwartzman DS, Preminger MW, et al. Utility of 12-lead electrocardiogram in localizing the origin of right ventricular outflow tract tachycardia. Am Heart J. 1995;130:1107–13.
24. Sekiguchi Y, Aonuma K, Takahashi A, et al. Electrocardiographic and electrophysiologic characteristics of ventricular tachycardia originating within the pulmonary artery. J Am Coll Cardiol. 2005;45:887–95.
25. Callans DJ, Menz V, Schwartzman D, et al. Repetitive monomorphic tachycardia from the left ventricular outflow tract: electrocardiographic patterns consistent with a left ventricular site of origin. J Am Coll Cardiol. 1997;29:1023–7.
26. Yamada T, Litovsky SH, Kay GN. The left ventricular ostium: an anatomic concept relevant to idiopathic ventricular arrhythmias. Circ Arrhythmia Electrophysiol. 2008;1:396–404.
27. Yamada T, Lau YR, Litovsky SH, Thomas McElderry H, Doppalapudi H, Osorio J, Plumb VJ, Neal Kay G. Idiopathic ventricular arrhythmias originating from the aortic root: prevalence, electrocardiographic and electrophysiological characteristics, and results of the radiofrequency catheter ablation. J Am Coll Cardiol. 2008;52:139–47.
28. Santangeli P, Marchlinski FE, Zado ES, Benhayon D, Hutchinson MD, Lin D, Frankel DS, et al. Percutaneous epicardial ablation of ventricular arrhythmias arising from the left ventricular summit: outcomes and electrocardiogram correlates of success. Circ Arrhythm Electrophysiol. 2015;8:337–43.
29. Jauregui Abularach ME, Campos B, Park KM, Tschabrunn CM, Frankel DS, Park RE, Gerstenfeld EP, et al. Ablation of ventricular arrhythmias arising near the anterior epicardial veins from the left sinus of Valsalva region: ECG features, anatomic distance, and outcome. Heart Rhythm. 2012;9:865–73.
30. Nagashima K, Choi EK, Lin KY, Kumar S, Tedrow UB, Koplan BA, Michaud GF, et al. Ventricular arrhythmias near the distal great cardiac vein: challenging arrhythmia for ablation. Circ Arrhythm Electrophysiol. 2014;7:906–12.
31. Kumagai K, Fukuda K, Wakayama Y, Sugai Y, Hirose M, Yamaguchi N, Takase K, et al. Electrocardiographic characteristics of the variants of idiopathic left ventricular outflow tract ventricular tachyarrhythmias. J Cardiovasc Electrophysiol. 2008;19:495–501.
32. Vallès E, Bazan V, Marchlinski FE. ECG criteria to identify epicardial ventricular tachycardia in nonischemic cardiomyopathy. Circ Arrhythm Electrophysiol. 2010;3:63–71.
33. Belhassen B, Rotmensch HH, Laniado S. Response of recurrent sustained ventricular tachycardia to verapamil. Br Heart J. 1981;46(6):679–82.
34. Lerman BB, Stein KM, Markowitz SM. Mechanisms of idiopathic left ventricular tachycardia. J Cardiovasc Electrophysiol. 1997;8(5):571–83.
35. Sung RJ, Shapiro WA, Shen EN, Morady F, Davis J. Effects of verapamil on ventricular tachycardias possibly caused by reentry, automaticity, and triggered activity. J Clin Invest. 1983;72:350–60.
36. Kawamura M, Hsu JC, Vedantham V, Marcus GM, Hsia HH, Gerstenfeld EP, Scheinman MM, et al.

Clinical and electrocardiographic characteristics of idiopathic ventricular arrhythmias with right bundle branch block and superior axis: comparison of apical crux area and posterior septal left ventricle. Heart Rhythm. 2015;12:1137–44.
37. Delacey WA, Nath S, Haines DE, et al. Adenosine and verapamil sensitive tachycardia originating from the left ventricle: radiofrequency catheter ablation. Pacing Clin Electrophysiol. 1992;15:2240–4.
38. Yamada T, Doppalapudi H, McElderry T, Okada T, Murakami Y, Inden Y, Yoshida Y, et al. Electrocardiographic and electrophysiological characteristics in idiopathic ventricular arrhythmias originating from the papillary muscles in left the left ventricle: relevance for catheter ablation. Circ Arrhythm Electrophysiol. 2010;3:324–31.
39. Yamada T, McElderry T, Doppalapudi H, Kay N. Ventricular far-field activity may provide a diagnostic challenge in identifying an origin of ventricular tachycardia arising from the left ventricular papillary muscle. Europace. 2009;11:1403–5.
40. Rivera S, Ricapito MP, Espinoza J, Belardi D, Albina G, Giniger A, Roux JF, et al. Cryoablation for ventricular arrhythmias arising from the papillary muscles of the left ventricle guided by intracardiac echocardiography and image integration. JACC Clin Electrophysiol. 2015;1:509–16.
41. Rivera S, Ricapito MP, Tomas L, Parodi J, Bardera Milina G, Banegas R, Bueti P, et al. Results of cryoenergy and radiofrequency-based catheter ablation for treating ventricular arrhythmias arising from the papillary muscles of the left ventricle, guided by intracardiac echocardiography and image integration. Circ Arrhythm Electrophysiol. 2016;9:e003874.
42. Good E, Desjardins B, Jongnarangsin K, Oral H, Chugh A, Ebinger M, Pelosi F, et al. Ventricular arrhythmias originating from a papillary muscle in patients without prior infarction: a comparison with fascicular arrhythmias. Heart Rhythm. 2008;5:1530–7.
43. Doppalapudi H, Yamada T, McElderry T, Plumb VJ, Epstein A, Kay N. Ventricular tachycardia originating from the posterior papillary muscle in the left ventricle. A distinct clinical syndrome. Circ Arrhythm Electrophysiol. 2008;1:23–9.
44. Naksuk N, Kapa S, Asirvatham SJ. Spectrum of ventricular arrhythmias arising from papillary muscle in the structurally normal heart. Card Electrophysiol Clin. 2016;8:555–65.
45. Enriquez A, Supple GE, Marchlinski FE, Garcia FC. How to map and ablate papillary muscle ventricular arrhythmias. Heart Rhythm. 2017;14:1721–8.
46. Wo HT, Liao FC, Chang PC, Chou CC, Wen MS, Wang CC, Yeh SJ. Circumferential ablation at the base of the left ventricular papillary muscles: a highly effective approach for ventricular arrhythmias originating from the papillary muscles. Int J Cardiol. 2016;220:876–82.
47. Komatsu Y, Nogami A, Kurosaki K, Morishima I, Masuda K, Ozawa T, Kaneshiro T, et al. Fascicular ventricular tachycardia originating from papillary muscles: purkinje network involvement in the reentrant circuit. Circ Arrhythm Electrophysiol. 2017;10:e004549.
48. Santoro F, Di Biase L, Hranitzky P, Sanchez JE, Santangeli P, Perini AP, Burkhardt JD, et al. Ventricular fibrillation triggered by PVCs from papillary muscles: clinical features and ablation. J Cardiovasc Electrophysiol. 2014;25:1158–64.
49. Crawford T, Mueller G, Good E, Jongnarangsin K, Chugh A, Pelosi F Jr, Ebinger M, et al. Ventricular arrhythmias originating from the papillary muscles in the right ventricle. Heart Rhythm. 2010;7:725–30.
50. Santoro F, Di Biase L, Hranitzky P, Sanchez JE, Santangeli P, Perini AP, Burkhardt JD, et al. Ventricular tachycardia originating from the septal papillary muscle of the right ventricle: electrocardiographic and electrophysiological characteristics. J Cardiovasc Electrophysiol. 2015;26:145–50.
51. Syed FF, Ackerman MJ, McLeod CJ, Kapa S, Mulpuru SK, Sriram CS, Cannon BC, et al. Sites of successful ventricular fibrillation ablation in bileaflet mitral valve prolapse syndrome. Circ Arrhythm Electrophysiol. 2016;9:e004005.
52. Bogun F, Desjardins B, Crawford T, Good E, Jongnarangsin K, Oral H, Chugh A, et al. Post-infarction ventricular arrhythmias originating in papillary muscles. J Am Coll Cardiol. 2008;51:1794–802.
53. Al'Aref SJ, Ip JE, Markowitz SM, Liu CF, Thomas G, Frenkel D, Panda NC, et al. Differentiation of papillary muscle from fascicular and mitral annular ventricular arrhythmias in patients with and without structural heart disease. Circ Arrhythm Electrophysiol. 2015;8:616–24.
54. Gaztañaga L, Marchlinski FE, Betensky BP. Mechanisms of cardiac arrhythmias. Rev Esp Cardiol (Engl Ed). 2012;65:174–85.
55. Lerman BB, Kenneth SM, Markovitz SM. Mechanisms of idiopathic left ventricular tachycardia. J Cardiovasc Electrophysiol. 1997;8:571–83.
56. Lamberti F, Di Clemente F, Remoli R, Bellini C, De Santis A, Mercurio M, Dottori S, Gaspardone A. Catheter ablation of idiopathic ventricular tachycardia without the use of fluoroscopy. Int J Cardiol. 2015;190:338–43.
57. Koźluk E, Gawrysiak M, Piątkowska A, Lodziński P, Kiliszek M, Małkowska S, Zaczek R, Piątkowski R, Opolski G, Kozłowski D. Radiofrequency ablation without the use of fluoroscopy—in what kind of patients is it feasible? Arch Med Sci. 2013;9:821–5.
58. Wang Y, Chen GZ, Yao Y, Bai Y, Chu HM, Ma KZ, Liew R, Liu H, Zhong GQ, Xue YM, Wu SL, Li YF, Zhao CX, Liu QG, Wang L Wang DW. Ablation of idiopathic ventricular arrhythmia using zero-fluoroscopy approach with equivalent efficacy and less fatigue: a multicenter comparative study. Medicine (Baltimore). 2017;96:e6080.

13 Ventricular Tachycardia with Structural Heart Disease

Ligang Ding and Yan Yao

Ventricular tachycardia (VT) is a major cause of sudden cardiac death. The majority of malignant VTs which carry an elevated risk for sudden cardiac death (SCD) occur in patients with structural heart disease (SHD), and implantable cardioverter defibrillators (ICDs) are the mainstay of therapy [1]. In these individuals, catheter ablation is being increasingly performed as adjunctive therapy to prevent or reduce ICD therapies when antiarrhythmic drugs are ineffective or not desired. In addition, in developing countries, some VT patients with structural heart disease cannot afford the expense of ICD; antiarrhythmic drugs and catheter ablation may become the ultimate therapy to prevent VTs and the onset of SCD.

Electrophysiology (EP) procedures in patients with SHD, including catheter ablation, are traditionally performed under fluoroscopic guidance and are often complex and prolonged enough to involve a non-negligible radiation exposure, which may increase the risk of cancer and genetic anomaly [2]. In recent years, non-fluoroscopic three-dimensional (3D) mapping systems have been developed to guide ablation during EP procedures [3, 4]. Their use has certainly allowed to better understand and ablate complex arrhythmias, but they have been proven to confer the additional benefit of significantly reducing radiation exposure. In this chapter, we will discuss the mechanisms and management of VT in the setting of structural heart disease and discuss the role of catheter ablation and patient populations who are most likely to benefit from this treatment modality. Furthermore, the role of three-dimensional mapping systems in EP procedure is also been discussed.

Mechanism

In patients with SHD, the main challenge for catheter ablation of VT is the complex arrhythmogenicity of the myocardial scar. Electroanatomical remodeling of the scar that occurs in either ischemic or nonischemic SHD may prompt arrhythmias through different mechanisms: enhanced normal automaticity, abnormal automaticity, triggered activity induced by early or late afterdepolarizations, and various forms of reentry [5, 6].

Ectopic automaticity and ***triggered activity*** are likely causes of focal origin VTs, although small reentry circuits can often not be excluded. Automatic VTs can occur in structural heart disease, and automatic premature beats may initiate reentrant VTs. Triggered activity by delayed after depolarizations is the underlying mechanism for

L. Ding · Y. Yao (✉)
State Key Laboratory of Cardiovascular Disease, Cardiac Arrhythmia Center, Fuwai Hospital, National Center for Cardiovascular Diseases, Chinese Academy of Medical Sciences and Peking Union Medical College, Beijing, China
e-mail: ianyao@263.net.cn

R. Proietti et al. (eds.), *Cardiac Electrophysiology Without Fluoroscopy*,
https://doi.org/10.1007/978-3-030-16992-3_13

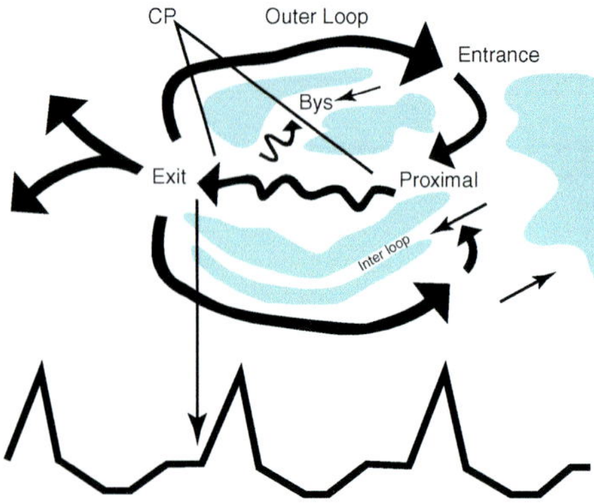

Fig. 13.1 Schematic reentry circuit of ventricular tachycardia (and its components). Conduction pathways can be seen surrounded by areas of scar

VT in the setting of digoxin toxicity, catecholaminergic polymorphic VT, idiopathic outflow tract ventricular arrhythmia (VA), and heart failure [7]. Unlike automaticity, triggered activity is not a self-generating rhythm. Instead, triggered activity occurs as a response to a preceding impulse (the trigger).

Reentry is the underlying mechanism for most sustained VA in the presence of structural heart disease (Fig. 13.1). The existence of structural reentrant substrates provides the rationale for VT ablation in scar-related VTs (Fig. 13.2) [8, 9]. Functional reentry around areas of functional block without anatomical obstacles can also occur. The mechanisms for functionally determined reentrant circuits include the leading circle type of reentry, anisotropic reentry, and spiral wave reentry [6, 10].

Assessment and Preparation Before RFCA

Before the procedure, patients should undergo a comprehensive clinical evaluation and a series of examinations to determine the underlying etiology and prognostic significance of VT. Analysis of the ***12-lead VT electrocardiogram (ECG)*** is essential for diagnosis. Clinical VT morphology helps to localize the exit site of the reentrant circuit from the protected isthmus, and helps with procedural planning [10].

Cardiac imaging plays a potentially important role for preprocedural assessment of cardiac anatomy and myocardial scar, intraprocedural integration of the structural and electrophysiological VT substrate, and post procedural assessment of the efficacy of ablation. Firstly, cardiac imaging could help to make preprocedural determination of the optimal access route. A priori information on cardiac anatomy and 3-dimensional scar architecture has an important influence on planning the access route for VT ablation. **Late gadolinium enhancement-CMR** accurately defines epicardial and intramural scar. Among patients with epicardial substrates, success rates are enhanced by epicardial ablation. Identification of the subset of patients who benefit from first-line epicardial ablation using LGE-CMR has been reported to significantly improve outcomes [11]. Secondly, cardiac imaging could be used as preprocedural exclusion of intracardiac thrombus. ***Transthoracic echocardiography (TTE)*** represents a readily available and inexpensive tool for the assessment of cardiac structure, valve function, the presence of mobile left ventricular thrombus (Fig. 13.3). In recent years, CMR and multidetector cardiac computed tomography (MDCT) have emerged as superior imaging modalities for detailed assessment of left ventricular thrombi. Thirdly, the most important role of cardiac imaging is used as guidance of VT ablation [12–14]. Integrating information on the structural VT substrate, as defined by noninvasive imaging, and the electrophysiological substrate, as defined by invasive electroanatomic mapping (EAM), has the potential to enhance safety and efficacy of ablation procedures (Fig. 13.4a, b). For example, coronary arteries could be localized by introducing MDCT/LGE-CMR data into the navigation system and their fusion with the EAM [15].

Cardiac Imaging Merging with 3-D Mapping Systems Process

EAM was performed during sinus rhythm using CartoV3 (Biosense-Webster, Diamond Bar, CA) or NavX (Ensite NavX, St Jude Medical, St. Paul,

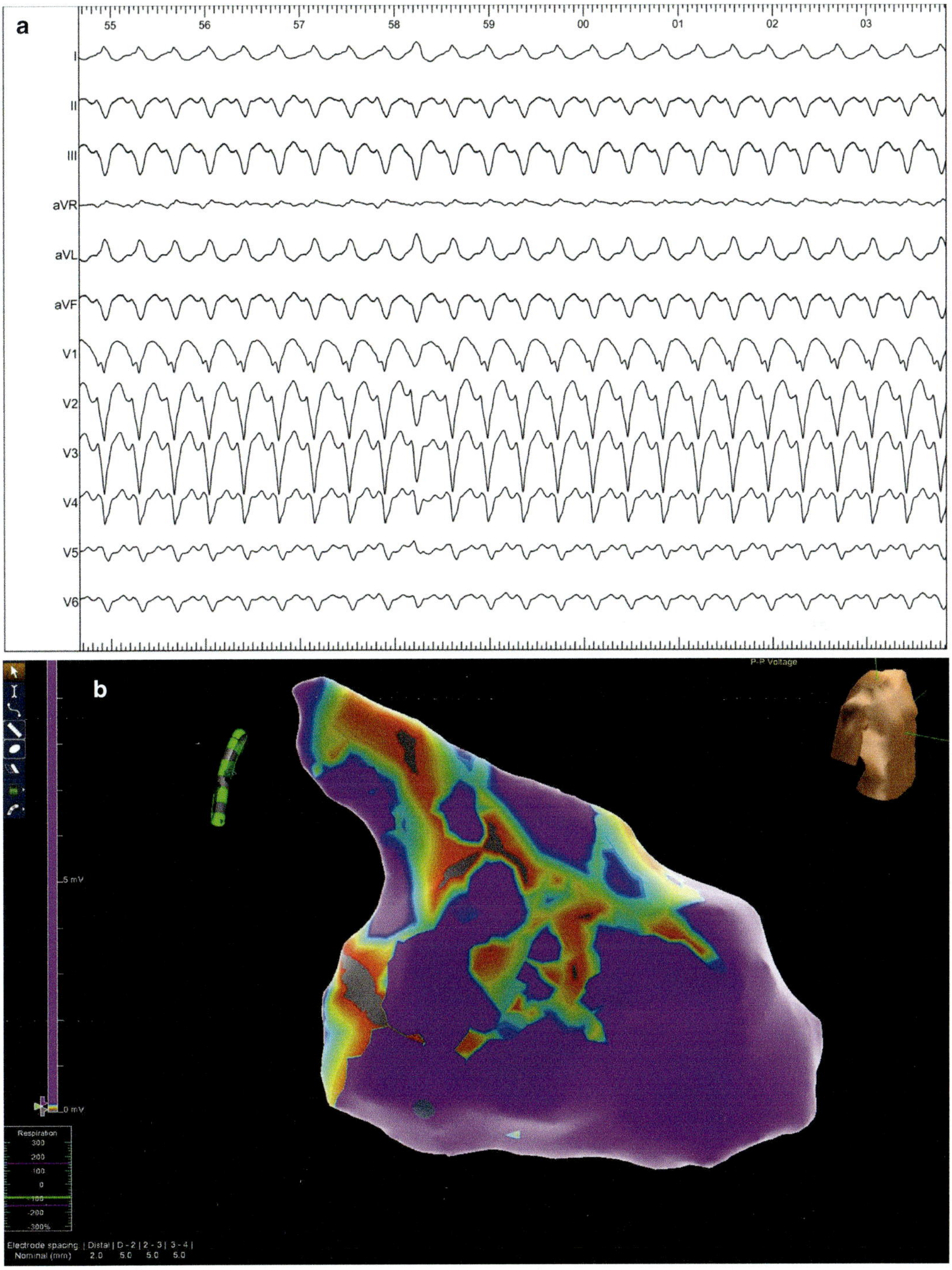

Fig. 13.2 (**a**) Ventricular tachycardia in patient with repaired tetralogy of Fallot. (**b**) Voltage mapping shows scar in the free wall of right ventricular outflow tract. (**c**) Activation mapping shows the central isthmus with mid-diastolic potentials in the free wall of right ventricular outflow tract. (**d**) Ablation terminated the VT at the free wall of right ventricular outflow tract. (**e**) Impulse propagation of VT in RVOT

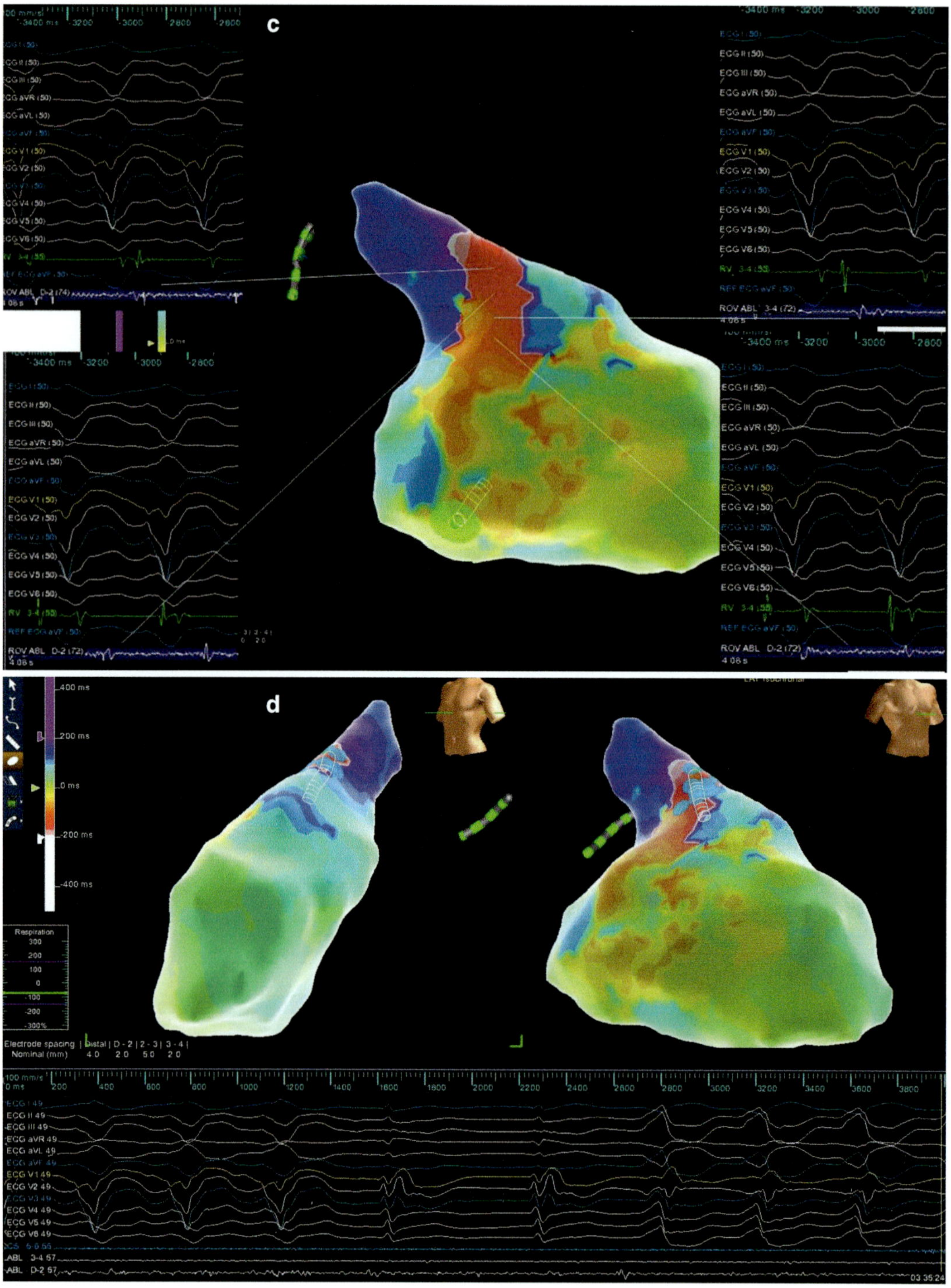

Fig. 13.2 (continued)

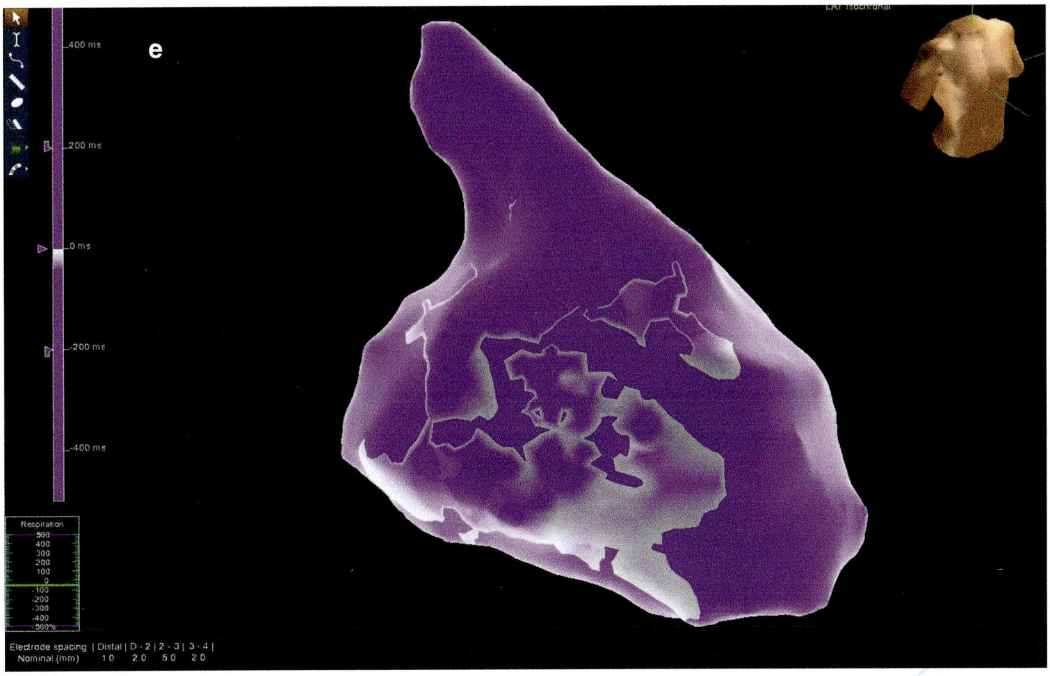

Fig. 13.2 (continued)

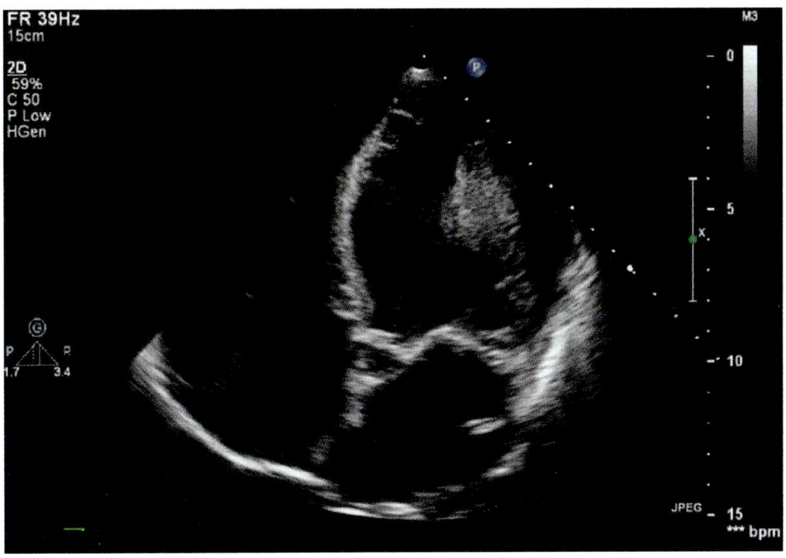

Fig. 13.3 Thrombus formation in left ventricular lateral wall in patient with dilated cardiomyopathy (Thanks Dr. Zhenhui Zhu of Fuwai Hospital who provided the echo image of this patient)

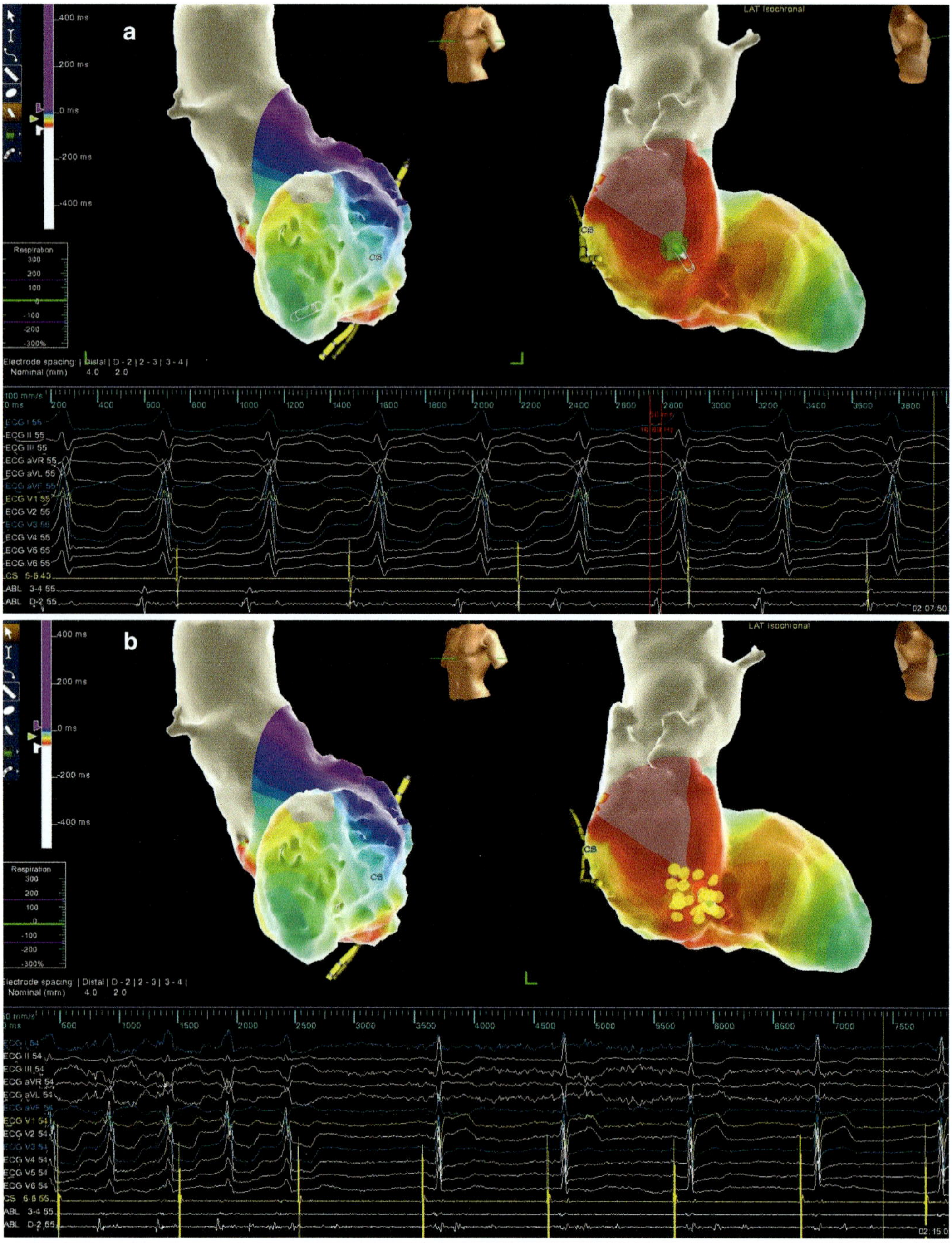

Fig. 13.4 (**a**) Ablation under the guidance of NavX mapping immerging with CT imaging in a 54-year-old male with inferior wall myocardial infarction. (**b**) Ablation at the inferior-septal wall of LV terminated the VT. Note the late potential at the ablation catheter during sinus rhythm. Extensive ablation at the area after termination of VT

MN) system. Mapping was performed with a multipolar high-density mapping catheter (such as PentaRayNav, Biosense Webster; or duodeca polar mapping catheter, St. Paul, MN). A peak-to-peak bipolar amplitude of <1.5 mV is defined as the bipolar low-voltage zone and unipolar amplitude <5.5 mV as the low unipolar voltage. After the acquisition of endocardial and/or epicardial geometries, 3D-EAM geometry is registered with the imported MDCT model. Identifiable anatomic reference points (such as coronary sinus, RV apex, and tricuspid annulus [3, 6, 9, and 12 o'clock] or mitral annulus [3, 6, 9, and 12 o'clock]) is used as landmarks for alignment and orientation of the 3D-EAM and imaging models. For NavX system, to keep the coronary sinus catheter stable is very important, as the body of the coronary sinus catheter is taped to provide a stable spatial reference, and a discreet anatomic boundary for guidance of the 3D-EAM/imaging model registration that could be monitored fluoroscopically throughout the procedure. When using Carto, after initial alignment using these fixed reference points as landmarks for registration, automatic surface registration using CartoMerge (Biosense Webster) was performed. The NavX Fusion registration algorithm allowed dynamic molding of the 3D-EAM geometry to the static MDCT surface (Fig. 13.4a, b). After primary registration, the registered model was refined using a second set of fiducial points, judiciously placed in a stepwise fashion to further align both surfaces at sites of local mismatch [16].

While there are clear data that demonstrate 3-D mapping systems can decrease fluoroscopy use and minimize radiation exposure to patients undergoing ablation. Cardiac imaging merging with 3-D mapping systems process could provide valuable information to recognize the extent and specific distribution of VT substrate (such as local abnormal ventricular activities, LAVA), and guide the manipulation of ablation catheter without fluoroscopy. Integration of MDCT-imaged myocardial fat into 3D-EAM is feasible in patients with ARVC. Its segmentation superimposed on 3D-EAM provides valuable information to recognize the extent and specific distribution of VT substrate and demonstrates ablation targets clustering in its border zone.

Induction and Mapping of Ventricular Tachycardia with Structural Heart Disease

Induction of VT with Structural Heart Disease

In patients with SMVT, reproducible initiation by programmed stimulation is the rule. Reproducible initiation excludes both normal and abnormal automaticity. The common protocol of programmed stimulation includes up to four extra stimuli from two ventricular locations with coupling intervals down to 200 ms or refractoriness, whichever occurred first. The same induction protocol is used to reinduce the VT after catheter ablation.

For patients with ARVC, one study demonstrated that fast rate (≥250 beats/min) right ventricular burst stimulation might provide a useful supplemental method for VT induction in ARVC patients. The author concluded that localized mechanism including micro-reentry and triggered activity might be the main mechanism of VT in ARVC [17].

Mapping of VT with Structural Heart Disease

The mapping technique used to identify potential sites for ablation depends on the mechanism of the VT. Activation mapping and pace mapping are most useful for focal mechanisms, whereas substrate mapping (with or without associated pace mapping) and entrainment mapping are used for reentrant mechanisms. For patients with

SHD, the majority of VTs are not hemodynamically tolerated and therefore do not permit either activation or entrainment mapping. Substrate mapping has evolved over the past decade and a half as an alternative to activation and/or entrainment mapping to deal with hemodynamically untolerated VTs. This methodology reduces or eliminates that need for mapping during prolonged periods of tachycardia.

Substrate mapping is the characterization of areas likely to support reentry based on anatomy and electrophysiological characteristics that can be determined during stable sinus or paced rhythm. Current criteria to define the abnormal substrate rely on a combination of abnormal electrogram characteristics (such as wide, split, and late electrograms) with lower amplitude. Substrate mapping generally begins with identification of the region of ventricular scar, based on electrogram characteristics (usually voltage) in an electroanatomic map of the ventricle of interest. **Scar tissue** can be identified based on bipolar electrogram amplitude. Bipolar electrograms recorded from regions of infarction have a peak-to-peak amplitude <1.5 mV (1 mm interelectrode spacing with a 4-mm distal electrode and filtered at 10–400 Hz) [18]. Areas of extremely low voltage (<0.5 mV or even less) have been designated as ***dense scar***, but it is important to recognize that these regions can still contain viable myocytes and reentry circuit isthmuses. Other study suggested that a bipolar voltage of <0.1 mV could be used to define electrical inexcitability [19]. Changing the bipolar viability voltage range to 0.1–0.5 mV increased the heterogeneity within the area of previously defined "dense scar." Of note, use of different mapping catheters with different electrode sizes and interelectrode distances may have an impact on voltage and abnormal electrogram recording. For instance, catheters with large-tip electrodes (3.5–4.0 mm) often record low-amplitude signals in areas of heterogeneous scar, while catheters with smaller electrodes (0.4–1.0 mm) record high-voltage signals at similar scar sites, thus identifying surviving myocardial bundles. Similarly, decreasing the interelectrode distance may decrease the voltage amplitude and duration, but may better identify near-field obscure activity, increasing the resolution of mapping.

In patients with VT, these infarct regions are typically large, with a circumference exceeding 20 cm [20]. In order to limit the area of ablation within the scar, a region of the scar is targeted for ablation based on pace mapping or additional electrogram characteristics. ***Exits*** can be identified based on pace mapping along the border of the scar. Radiofrequency lesions can then be placed in the infarct border zone (where bipolar electrogram amplitude is typically between 0.5 and 1.0 mV) roughly parallel to the infarct border. ***Late potentials*** during sinus rhythm and **isolated potentials** during VT are usually present within these low-amplitude regions and are often produced by conduction through potential conduction channels in the infarct areas [21, 22]. A number of ablation approaches have been described with the aim of targeting the abnormal substrate defined with mapping in sinus or paced rhythm. Some of these strategies (such as late potential and local abnormal ventricular activity ablation or scar homogenization) target the entire abnormal substrate harboring abnormal electrograms, defined with a variety of different criteria [23]. Scar dechanneling, linear ablation through sites matching VT with pacing, and the core isolation approach focus on more discrete regions with in the abnormal substrate that have been proven relevant to the clinical and/or inducible arrhythmias by means of physiologic maneuvers.

Some randomized trials examined the effect of substrate-based ablation on the long-term success rate of VT ablation. The VISTA trial demonstrated that an extensive substrate-based approach was superior to a more focused activation mapping strategy [24]. The randomized, primary-prevention trial, SMASH VT, showed a reduction in VT events using a substrate-based approach [25]. However, the positive results of this trial, which achieved a 70% reduction in arrhythmic events at 2 years, have not been replicated.

Ablation of Common Ventricular Tachycardia with Structural Heart Disease

Ventricular Tachycardia in Patients with Ischemic Heart Disease

Ventricular tachycardia occurs in 1–2% of patients late after myocardial infarction (MI), often after an interval of several years. The mechanism of VT is usually macroreentry [26]; focal non-reentrant mechanisms are responsible for fewer than 5–10% of VTs [27]. Patients with scar-related VTs often have multiple potential reentry circuits, giving rise to more than one morphology of inducible monomorphic VT. VTs may be hemodynamically well tolerated and inducible, but the majority of patients have one or more VTs that are unstable and not amenable to extensive mapping, due to poor hemodynamic tolerance, or inconsistent inducibility. Substrate mapping approaches that identify target regions for ablation during stable sinus rhythm often allow ablation of these tachycardias.

Several large multicenter series have reported outcomes following combined entrainment and substrate mapping approaches (Table 13.1). The **SMASH-VT** (Substrate Mapping and Ablation in Sinus Rhythm to Halt Ventricular Tachycardia) trial compared ICD implantation along with VT substrate ablation to ICD implantation alone in patients with recent VT [25]. In this trial, ablation of the VT substrate reduced ICD shocks from 31 to 9% over a mean follow-up of 22.5 ± 5 months ($p = 0.003$) and reduced VT from 33 to 12% ($p = 0.007$) in comparison to a control group that did not use antiarrhythmic drug therapy. The **VTACH** (Ventricular Tachycardia Ablation in Coronary Heart Disease) **trial** [28] studied the effect of catheter ablation in patients with ischemic cardiomyopathy, who experienced hemodynamically tolerated SMVT without specific antiarrhythmic drug therapy in the control arm (approximately one-third of patients in both arms were treated with amiodarone). Over a mean follow-up of 22.5 months, ablation prolonged the time to recurrent VT significantly (HR = 0.61), with a relative risk reduction of 25% and an absolute risk reduction of 18% at 2 years. In the **SMS** (Substrate Modification Study) [29], catheter ablation failed to decrease the primary endpoint of time to first VT/VF recurrence in post-MI patients with LVEF ≤40% and hemodynamically unstable VT. However, ablation did result in a >50% reduction in total ICD interventions. The **VANISH** (Ventricular Tachycardia Ablation versus Escalated Antiarrhythmic Drug Therapy in Ischemic Heart Disease) trial randomly allocated patients with ICD, prior infarction, and SMVT despite first-line antiarrhythmic drug therapy to catheter ablation or more aggressive antiarrhythmic drug therapy [30]. During 28 months of follow-up, catheter ablation resulted in a 28% relative risk reduction in the composite endpoint of death, VT storm, and appropriate ICD shock ($p = 0.04$).

Ventricular Tachycardia in Patients with Dilated Cardiomyopathy

The ventricular myocardium of individuals with dilated cardiomyopathy (DCM) is histologically characterized by multiple regions of patchy interstitial and replacement fibrosis, myofiber disarray, and variable degrees of myocyte hypertrophy and atrophy. Sustained monomorphic ventricular tachycardia is not common in nonischemic dilated cardiomyopathies, but 80% of those that occur are due to scar-related reentry, with the remainder due to bundle branch reentry or a focal origin. Unlike post-MI scar that has a predilection for the subendocardium, scar in DCM may be mid-myocardial or epicardial and most often occurs in the basal anteroseptal and inferolateral LV regions [11, 31, 32]. The results of catheter ablation in dilated cardiomyopathy are generally worse than in ischemic cardiomyopathy, due to a higher preponderance of intramural substrate and infrequent substrate ablation targets (i.e., fractionated and late potentials) [33–35].

Table 13.1 Clinical trials of catheter ablation in patients with ischemic heart disease

Trial	Control therapy	No. of patients	Population	Mean follow-up (Mo)	Endpoint	Outcomes (%)		
						Ablation	ICD	*P*
SMASH-VT	ICD	128	OMI underwent ICD for VT or VF	22.5 ± 5.5	Appropriate ICD therapy	12	33	0.007
VTACH	ICD	107	OMI, LVEF ≤50%, stable VT	22.5	Survival free from VT or VF	47	29	0.045
SMS	ICD	111	Post-MI patients with LVEF ≤40%	27.6 ± 13.2	Event- free survival	49	52.4	0.84
VANISH	Escalated antiarrhythmic drug therapy	259	Prior infarction, ICD and SMVT	27.9 ± 17.1	Composite endpoint of death, VT storm, and appropriate ICD shock	59.1	68.5	0.04

SMASH-VT substrate mapping and ablation in sinus rhythm to halt ventricular tachycardia, *VTACH* ventricular tachycardia ablation in coronary heart disease, *SMS* substrate modification study, *VANISH* ventricular tachycardia ablation versus escalated antiarrhythmic drug therapy in ischemic heart disease, *Mo* month, *ICD* implantable cardioverter defibrillator, *MI* myocardial infarction, *LVEF* left ventricular ejection fraction, *SMVT* sustained monomorphic ventricular tachycardia, *VT* ventricular tachycardia, *VF* ventricular fibrillation

Ventricular Tachycardia in Patients with Arrhythmogenic Right Ventricular Cardiomyopathy/Dysplasia

Arrhythmogenic right ventricular dysplasia/cardiomyopathy (ARVC/D) is characterized by fibrofatty replacement of myocardium within the so-called triangle of dysplasia which encompasses the RV inflow, outflow, and apex. Scar-related reentry is the most common cause of VTs, focal VTs in ARVD/C have also been described, although some of these cases may represent epicardial reentry with a focal endocardial breakthrough [36].

Conventional VT induction protocols including extra-stimuli and incremental stimulation had been found to increase the yield of inducible VT; some study also found that fast rate (≥250 beats/min) right ventricular burst stimulation provides a useful supplemental method for VT induction in ARVC patients, which might indicate that localized mechanism including micro-reentry and triggered activity might be one of the mechanisms of VT in ARVC [17]. The methods for mapping and ablation are as for scar-related VTs; activation mapping, entrainment mapping, substrate mapping, and combined approaches have been used. Our previous study demonstrated the efficacy of endocardial regional RF catheter ablation under the guidance of noncontact mapping (Fig. 13.5) [37]. Endocardial VT ablation in this setting can produce acute success,

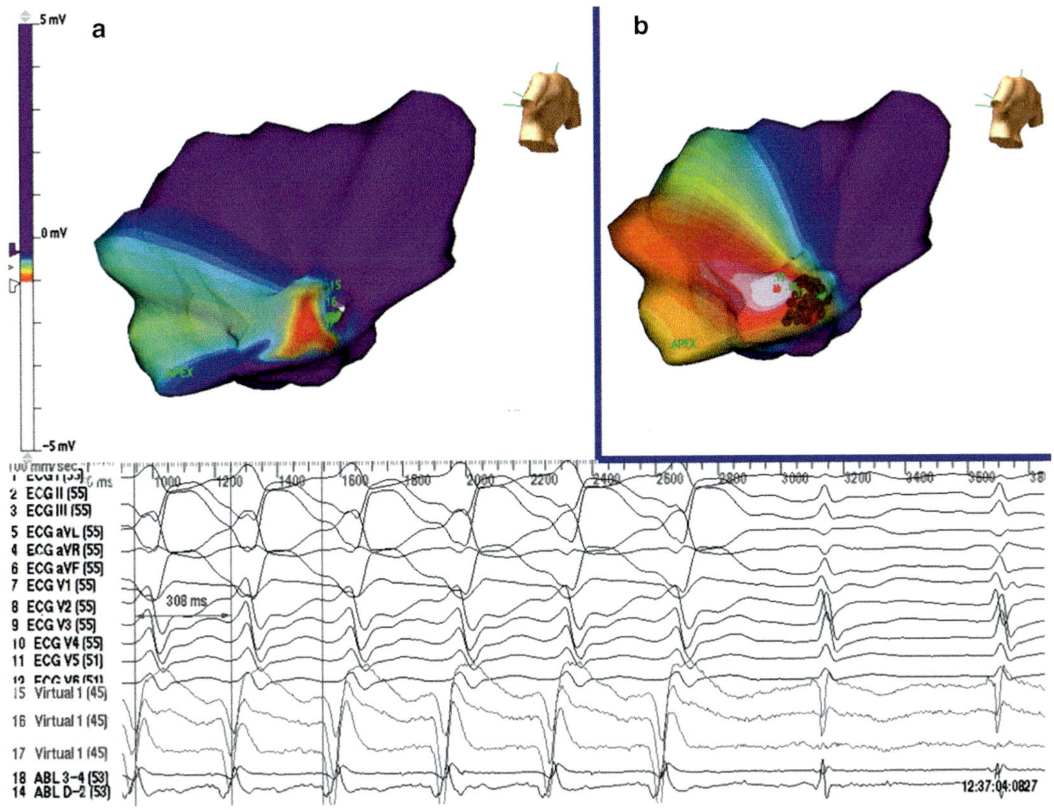

Fig. 13.5 Regional ablation under the guidance of isopotential mapping in a 36-year-old female with a 4-year history of palpitation and pre-syncope. The VT origin was at the basal septum. Panel **a** indicates that the VT with cycle length of 308 ms was terminated by RF ablation but was induced again. The ablation region was expanded stepwise according to the mapping results. Panel **b** indicates that VT was still inducible after 23 RF applications. The morphology of the VT is similar and was finally terminated after further attempts at adjacent sites. *HIS* His bundle, *Apex* apex of the right ventricle

though recurrence rate is quite high, which may be explained by the more epicardial and patchy nature of the disease. Combined endocardial-epicardial ablation has since been shown to be feasible, safe, and with significantly better acute and long-term success, particularly when combined with scar dechanneling or homogenization of the scar (Fig. 13.6a–c) [38].

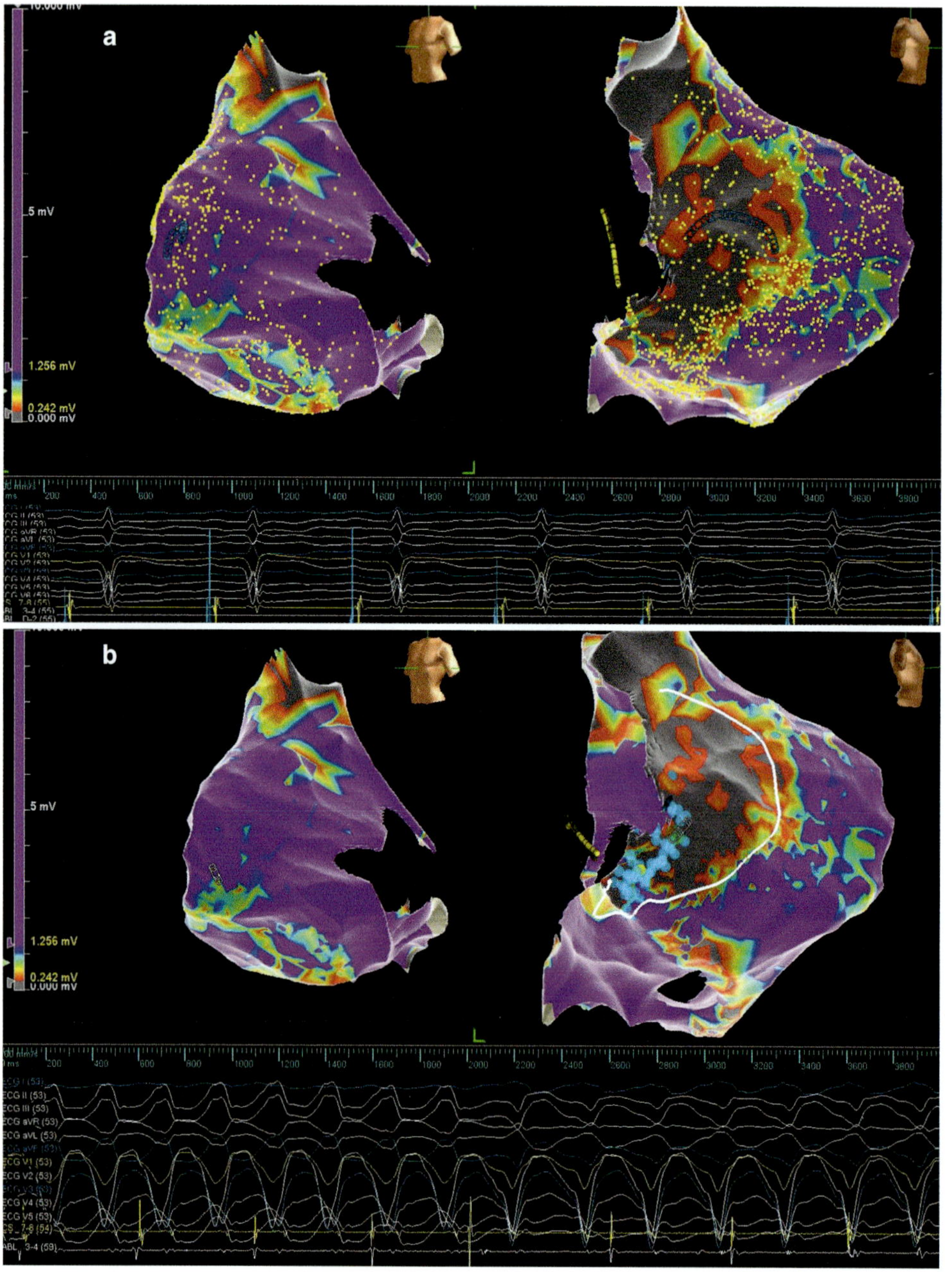

Fig. 13.6 (**a**) Epicardial mapping and ablation in patients with ARVC. Substrate mapping shows huge low-voltage area and scar at RVOT and basal-lateral wall of RV. (**b**) The morphology of VT changed after ablation at the basal-lateral wall of RV. (**c**) Extensive and regional ablation at the Basal-lateral wall of RV terminated the VT finally

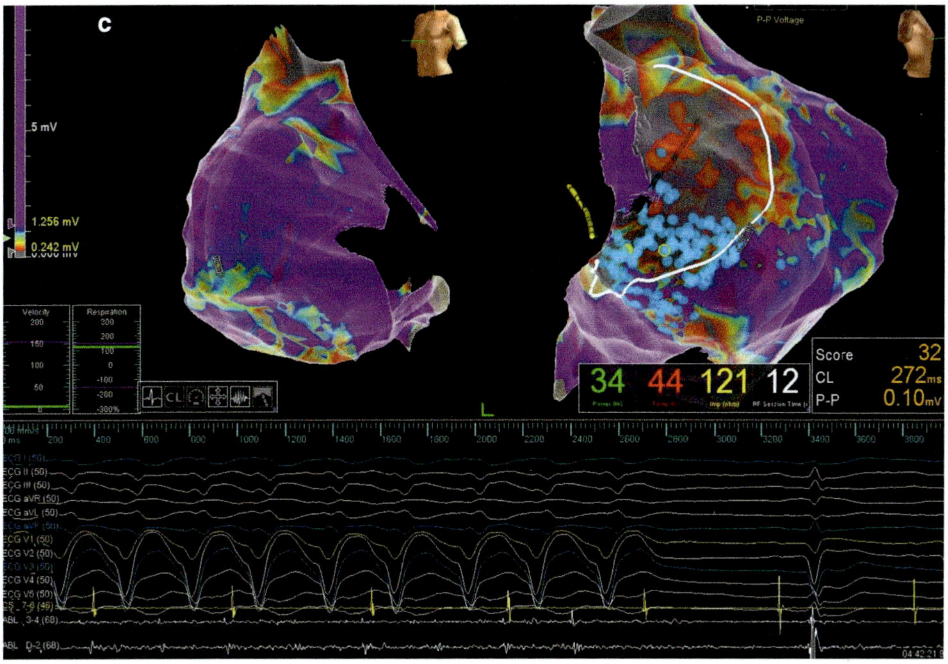

Fig. 13.6 (continued)

Ventricular Tachycardia in Patients with Hypertrophic Cardiomyopathy

In high-risk individuals with hypertrophic cardiomyopathy (HCM), monomorphic VT accounts for 38% of episodes [39]. HCM patients with LV aneurysms are at higher risk for the occurrence of monomorphic VT. Ventricular arrhythmias occur more frequently (4.7% vs. 0.9%/year; $p < 0.001$) in HCM patients with and without LV aneurysms [40]. The mechanism of monomorphic VT in these patients is also scar-related reentry and is amenable to catheter ablation [41]. Standard endocardial mapping and ablation alone are likely insufficient to target the relevant VT circuits. In this highly selected population, a combined epicardial and endocardial approach to catheter ablation is feasible and of reasonable efficacy to consider if aggressive trials of antiarrhythmic medications and trials of antitachycardia pacing fail to control VT [42].

Ventricular tachycardia could also occur in other diseases including valvular heart disease, sarcoidosis, Chagas disease, and in repaired congenital heart disease (Fig. 13.1). In patients with sarcoidosis, due to progressive inflammation and a complex underlying substrate, ventricular arrhythmias may have several mechanisms, including abnormal automaticity, triggered activity, or scar-related reentry [43]. When inflammation is present, the combination of immunosuppressive therapy and antiarrhythmic drugs may decrease VT recurrence. However, when these treatments fail, catheter ablation is feasible [44]. Chagas disease is caused by the flagellate protozoan parasite Trypanosoma cruzi and is transmitted by hematophagous triatomine insect vectors. It is endemic to Latin American countries, but is also prevalent in non-endemic areas due to population migration. Monomorphic VT due to scar-related reentry can arise from any scar location, but the inferolateral segment is the most common source, accounting for ~80% of VTs [45]. Combination of endocardial and epicardial mapping and ablation in Chagas patients markedly improved the long-term success rate [46].

Minimization of Fluoroscopy During Mapping and Ablation of VAs

Traditionally, mapping and catheter ablation of VAs in patients with structural heart disease is complex and guided by three-dimensional mapping system and fluoroscopy. Actually, it is quite difficult to perform the process with zero fluoroscopy, but minimization of the fluoroscopy is reasonable with the accumulation of more experiences.

The Placement of Diagnostic and Ablation Catheter

We can position the diagnostic (such as the His bundle, right ventricular, and coronary sinus catheter), mapping, and ablation catheter into the exact sites guided by the 3D mapping system with zero fluoroscopy (Fig. 13.7a, b). The trajectory of the catheter could be clearly monitored and observed under the guidance of the 3D mapping system. In addition, operators could continuously observe two projections at the same time through 3D mapping system—such as the position of CS catheter, firstly, the CS catheter is bent at 90° and direct to the lateral wall of right atrium in the left anterior oblique (LAO) 30° view, then rotate it clockwise and direct to the inferior septal wall of right atrium; it is generally easy to enter the ostium of coronary sinus. For the manipulation of retroaortic approach, we can bent the catheter as inverted U shape at ascend aorta, the tip of catheter direct to the anterior aorta, then push it and pass through the aortic valve in the right anterior oblique (RAO) 30° view. All the manipulation of catheter could be performed under the guidance of 3D mapping system without fluoroscopy.

Of note, retract the catheter and advance it again when we feel resistance during the procedure of placing catheter. However, it is necessary to replace the catheter under the X-ray guidance for the safety consideration, if persistent resistance encountered in the process of pushing the catheter, which may indicate the stenosis, distortion, or occlusion of vascular access. In this circumstance, angiography could be used to evaluate the vascular condition. Schwartz sheath can be applied by pushing long wire across narrow or twisted vessels if encounting the vascular stenosis or distortion. Otherwise, we need to choose other vascular accesses, such as the internal jugular vein, subclavian vein, contralateral femoral vein, or artery.

The Substrate Mapping and Ablation During Sinus Rhythm

The main challenges for catheter ablation of ventricular tachycardia are the complex arrhythmogenicity of the myocardial scar and hemodynamically unstable state during onset of VT. Substrate mapping in sinus rhythm could allow hemodynamically unstable VAs to be successfully mapping and ablation, and consequently minimizing the fluoroscopic dose [47]. This approach uses a non-fluoroscopic three-dimensional mapping system that produces an electroanatomical reconstruction of the heart.

The substrate mapping of RV/LV endocardium and epicardium could be performed using ablation or high-density mapping catheter (typically Pentaray® catheter, Biosense Webster, Diamond Bar, CA, USA). High-density EAM of RV/LV was obtained during stable sinus rhythm using the CARTO system (Biosense Webster, Diamond Bar, CA) or Ensite Navx (St Jude Medical, St Paul, MN). Endocardial access to the LV was obtained by single transseptal puncture or retroaortic approach. Transseptal LV access was achieved, and manipulation of the ablation catheter was assisted by a steerable sheath (Agilis St Jude Medical, St Paul, MN). Epicardial mapping and ablation are performed when preprocedural ce-CMR showed epicardial scar, endocardial mapping do not identify subendocardial scars, ECG of clinical or induced VT suggested epicardial origin, or endocardial ablation is unsuccessful.

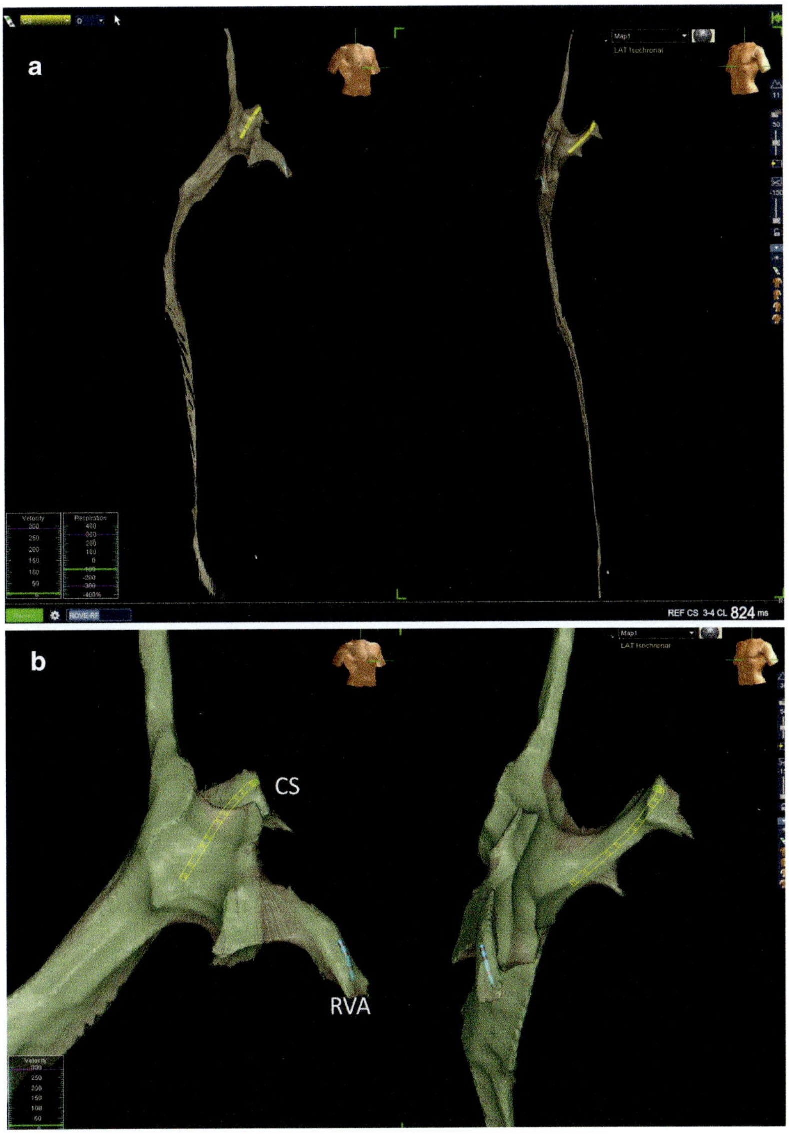

Fig. 13.7 (**a**) The trajectory of the catheter could be clearly monitored and observed under the guidance of the 3D mapping system. (**b**) The position of CS and RVA catheter under the guidance of Ensite system

All the mapping procedure could be performed under the guidance of EAM system during sinus rhythm, which minimizes the radiation dose. With regard to our previous procedural data with guidance of fluroscopy, we found that our total procedural times are comparable to previous data despite longer geometry times. We believe this highlights the importance of accurate geometry reconstruction, as it suggests that spending more time obtaining an accurate geometry reconstruction with voltage and abnormal electrograms may speed up subsequent phases of the procedure. Indeed, basing ablation on an accurate 3D model of cardiac anatomy provides certain remarkable technical advantages, which both save time and make the procedure easier. Electroanatomical mapping confers a deeper insight into the patient's individual cardiac anatomy, as geometry reconstruction will already have compelled the operator to exercise the movements necessary to reach the various intracardiac sites relevant to the subsequent ablation procedure. The latter is also speed up by the fact that the 3D model enables the operator to continuously observe two projections at the same time.

The Scar Homogenization and/or Dechanneling During Sinus Rhythm

The scar homogenization approach targets all the abnormal electrograms within the scar defined with conventional bipolar voltage criteria when mapping in sinus or paced rhythm (Fig. 13.8a–c). The acute ablation endpoint is either elimination of abnormal electrograms or loss of local capture at high-output pacing (20-mA output at 10 ms pulse width). One large multicenter randomized study comparing scar homogenization with stan-

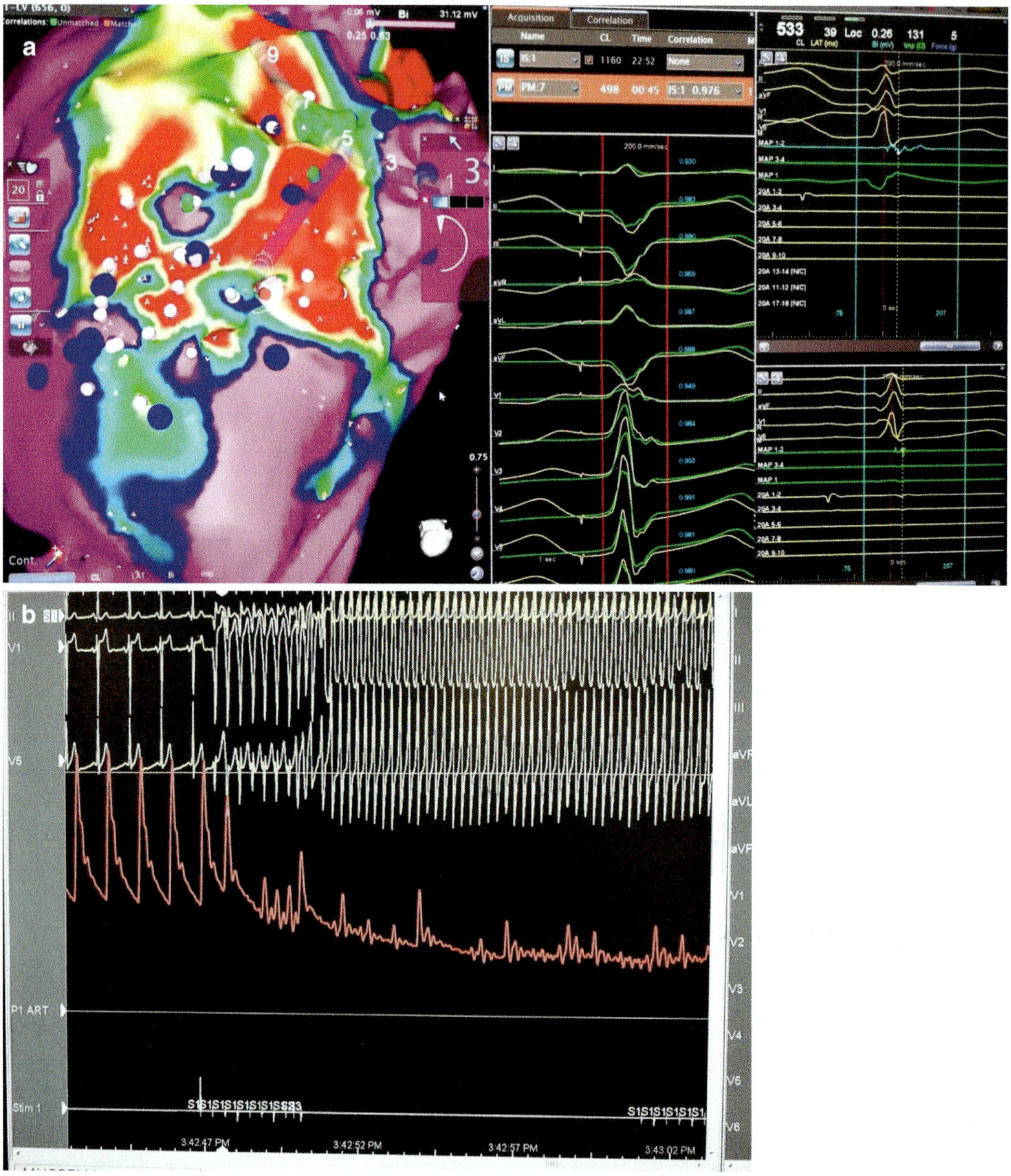

Fig. 13.8 (**a**) One VT patient with OMI (inferior wall). Late potential was recorded in the border zone of inferior wall during sinus rhythm, pace mapping at this site produce morphology was similar to the VT morphology. (**b**) Non-tolerable VT was induced using programmed stimulation. (**c**) The scar homogenization approach targets all the abnormal electrograms within the scar was performed (Thanks Dr. Ivan Ho of Cedars-Sinai Medical Center who performed the radiofrequency ablation for this patient)

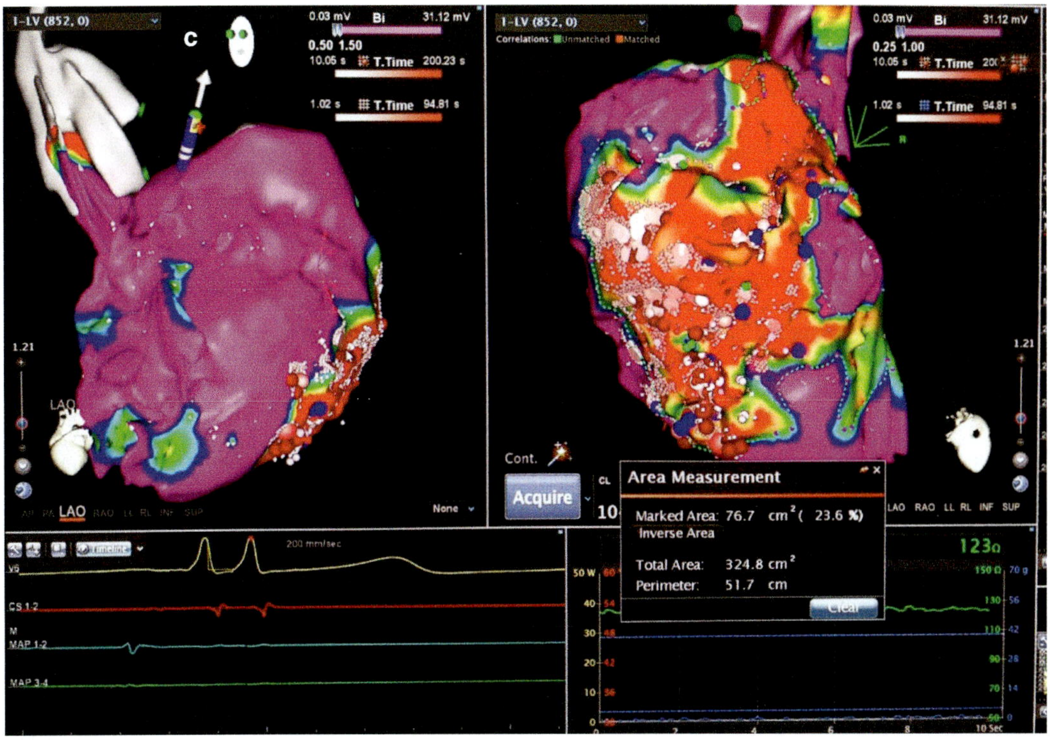

Fig. 13.8 (continued)

dard limited substrate ablation in 118 patients with ischemic cardiomyopathy presenting with stable VT demonstrated the efficacy of scar homogenization strategy. At 1 year post ablation, freedom from VT recurrence was achieved in 52% of patients who underwent clinical VT ablation only vs. 85% of patients who underwent scar homogenization.

The substrate ablation approach that targets channels within the abnormal substrate was described as scar dechanneling. After identified the conduction channel (CC), radiofrequency (RF) elimination of all identified CCs by RF ablation is performed at the CC entrance during sinus rhythm. In our center, substrate mapping routinely be performed as first step before VT induction and ablation in patients with hemodynamically stable or unstable VT. The acute and long-term outcomes of ablation are not inferior to the strategy of VT induction and mapping before substrate mapping. Our results are consistent with the findings reported by other centers [9, 47, 48]. As the accumulation of experience of VT ablation, the manipulation of mapping and/or ablation catheters could be done guided not by fluoroscopy but under three-dimensional mapping system. Therefore, minimization of radiation dose could be achieved during the whole procedure of mapping and ablation.

Conclusions

In general, catheter ablation of ventricular tachycardia in patients with structural heart disease can significantly reduce the incidence of recurrent ventricular arrhythmias. It is best used as an adjunct to ICDs, and as an alternative or adjunct to antiarrhythmic drugs. Nowadays, 3D mapping system provides an accurate geometry reconstruction with voltage information and abnormal electrograms, which is used to guide the subsequent mapping and ablation procedure without fluoroscopy. Technological advancements in substrate imaging, mapping, and ablation to improve outcomes and minimization of radiation dose are in the process of development.

Acknowledgments We are indebted to Dr. Zhenhui Zhu from Fuwai Hospital for his echo data, Dr. Ivan Ho from Cedars-Sinai Medical Center for the VT data, and Miss Xiaodan Yang for the drafting of schematic diagram.

References

1. Priori SG, Blomstrom-Lundqvist C, Mazzanti A, et al. 2015 ESC Guidelines for the management of patients with ventricular arrhythmias and the prevention of sudden cardiac death: the Task Force for the Management of Patients with Ventricular Arrhythmias and the Prevention of Sudden Cardiac Death of the European Society of Cardiology (ESC). Endorsed by: Association for European Paediatric and Congenital Cardiology (AEPC). Eur Heart J. 2015;36:2793–867.
2. Perisinakis K, Damilakis J, Theocharopoulos N, et al. Accurate assessment of patient effective radiation dose and associated detriment risk from radiofrequency catheter ablation procedures. Circulation. 2001;104:58–62.
3. Packer DL. Three-dimensional mapping in interventional electrophysiology: techniques and technology. J Cardiovasc Electrophysiol. 2005;16:1110–6.
4. Casella M, Pelargonio G, Dello RA, et al. "Near-zero" fluoroscopic exposure in supraventricular arrhythmia ablation using the EnSite NavX mapping system: personal experience and review of the literature. J Interv Card Electrophysiol. 2011;31:109–18.
5. Cherry EM, Fenton FH, Gilmour RJ. Mechanisms of ventricular arrhythmias: a dynamical systems-based perspective. Am J Physiol Heart Circ Physiol. 2012;302:H2451–63.
6. Pandit SV, Jalife J. Rotors and the dynamics of cardiac fibrillation. Circ Res. 2013;112:849–62.
7. Lerman BB. Mechanism, diagnosis, and treatment of outflow tract tachycardia. Nat Rev Cardiol. 2015;12:597–608.
8. Zhang J, Cooper DH, Desouza KA, et al. Electrophysiologic scar substrate in relation to VT: noninvasive high-resolution mapping and risk assessment with ECGI. Pacing Clin Electrophysiol. 2016;39:781–91.
9. Fernandez-Armenta J, Penela D, Acosta J, et al. Substrate modification or ventricular tachycardia induction, mapping, and ablation as the first step? A randomized study. Heart Rhythm. 2016;13:1589–95.
10. Tsuji Y, Heijman J, Nattel S, et al. Electrical storm: recent pathophysiological insights and therapeutic consequences. Basic Res Cardiol. 2013;108:336.
11. Bogun FM, Desjardins B, Good E, et al. Delayed-enhanced magnetic resonance imaging in nonischemic cardiomyopathy: utility for identifying the ventricular arrhythmia substrate. J Am Coll Cardiol. 2009;53:1138–45.
12. Andreu D, Ortiz-Perez JT, Boussy T, et al. Usefulness of contrast-enhanced cardiac magnetic resonance in identifying the ventricular arrhythmia substrate and the approach needed for ablation. Eur Heart J. 2014;35:1316–26.
13. Dickfeld T, Tian J, Ahmad G, et al. MRI-guided ventricular tachycardia ablation: integration of late gadolinium-enhanced 3D scar in patients with implantable cardioverter-defibrillators. Circ Arrhythm Electrophysiol. 2011;4:172–84.
14. Yamashita S, Sacher F, Mahida S, et al. Image integration to guide catheter ablation in scar-related ventricular tachycardia. J Cardiovasc Electrophysiol. 2016;27:699–708.
15. Soto-Iglesias D, Acosta J, Penela D, et al. Image-based criteria to identify the presence of epicardial arrhythmogenic substrate in patients with transmural myocardial infarction. Heart Rhythm. 2018;15(6):814–21.
16. Komatsu Y, Cochet H, Jadidi A, et al. Regional myocardial wall thinning at multidetector computed tomography correlates to arrhythmogenic substrate in postinfarction ventricular tachycardia: assessment of structural and electrical substrate. Circ Arrhythm Electrophysiol. 2013;6:342–50.
17. Wu LM, Bao JR, Yao Y, et al. Fast rate (≥250 beats/min) right ventricular burst stimulation is useful for ventricular tachycardia induction in arrhythmogenic right ventricular cardiomyopathy. J Geriatr Cardiol. 2016;13:70–4.
18. Stevenson WG, Friedman PL, Kocovic D, et al. Radiofrequency catheter ablation of ventricular tachycardia after myocardial infarction. Circulation. 1998;98:308–14.
19. Josephson ME, Anter E. Substrate mapping for ventricular tachycardia: assumptions and misconceptions. JACC Clin Electrophysiol. 2015;1:341–52.
20. Soejima K, Suzuki M, Maisel WH, et al. Catheter ablation in patients with multiple and unstable ventricular tachycardias after myocardial infarction: short ablation lines guided by reentry circuit isthmuses and sinus rhythm mapping. Circulation. 2001;104:664–9.
21. Harada T, Stevenson WG, Kocovic DZ, et al. Catheter ablation of ventricular tachycardia after myocardial infarction: relation of endocardial sinus rhythm late potentials to the reentry circuit. J Am Coll Cardiol. 1997;30:1015–23.
22. Arenal A, Glez-Torrecilla E, Ortiz M, et al. Ablation of electrograms with an isolated, delayed component as treatment of unmappable monomorphic ventricular tachycardias in patients with structural heart disease. J Am Coll Cardiol. 2003;41:81–92.
23. Di Biase L, Santangeli P, Burkhardt DJ, et al. Endo-epicardial homogenization of the scar versus limited substrate ablation for the treatment of electrical storms in patients with ischemic cardiomyopathy. J Am Coll Cardiol. 2012;60:132–41.
24. Di Biase L, Burkhardt JD, Lakkireddy D, et al. Ablation of stable VTs versus substrate ablation in ischemic cardiomyopathy: the VISTA randomized multicenter trial. J Am Coll Cardiol. 2015;66:2872–82.
25. Reddy VY, Reynolds MR, Neuzil P, et al. Prophylactic catheter ablation for the prevention of defibrillator therapy. N Engl J Med. 2007;357:2657–65.

26. de Chillou C, Lacroix D, Klug D, et al. Isthmus characteristics of reentrant ventricular tachycardia after myocardial infarction. Circulation. 2002;105:726–31.
27. Pogwizd SM, Hoyt RH, Saffitz JE, et al. Reentrant and focal mechanisms underlying ventricular tachycardia in the human heart. Circulation. 1992;86:1872–87.
28. Kuck KH, Schaumann A, Eckardt L, et al. Catheter ablation of stable ventricular tachycardia before defibrillator implantation in patients with coronary heart disease (VTACH): a multicentre randomised controlled trial. Lancet. 2010;375:31–40.
29. Kuck KH, Tilz RR, Deneke T, et al. Impact of substrate modification by catheter ablation on implantable cardioverter-defibrillator interventions in patients with unstable ventricular arrhythmias and coronary artery disease: results from the multicenter randomized controlled SMS (substrate modification study). Circ Arrhythm Electrophysiol. 2017;10:e004422.
30. Sapp JL, Wells GA, Parkash R, et al. Ventricular tachycardia ablation versus escalation of antiarrhythmic drugs. N Engl J Med. 2016;375:111–21.
31. Jackson JA, Leake DR, Schneiders NJ, et al. Magnetic resonance imaging in multiple sclerosis: results in 32 cases. AJNR Am J Neuroradiol. 1985;6:171–6.
32. Delacretaz E, Stevenson WG, Ellison KE, et al. Mapping and radiofrequency catheter ablation of the three types of sustained monomorphic ventricular tachycardia in nonischemic heart disease. J Cardiovasc Electrophysiol. 2000;11:11–7.
33. Oloriz T, Silberbauer J, Maccabelli G, et al. Catheter ablation of ventricular arrhythmia in nonischemic cardiomyopathy: anteroseptal versus inferolateral scar sub-types. Circ Arrhythm Electrophysiol. 2014;7:414–23.
34. Muser D, Santangeli P, Castro SA, et al. Long-term outcome after catheter ablation of ventricular tachycardia in patients with nonischemic dilated cardiomyopathy. Circ Arrhythm Electrophysiol. 2016;9:e004328.
35. Gokoglan Y, Mohanty S, Gianni C, et al. Scar homogenization versus limited-substrate ablation in patients with nonischemic cardiomyopathy and ventricular tachycardia. J Am Coll Cardiol. 2016;68:1990–8.
36. Miljoen H, State S, de Chillou C, et al. Electroanatomic mapping characteristics of ventricular tachycardia in patients with arrhythmogenic right ventricular cardiomyopathy/dysplasia. Europace. 2005;7:516–24.
37. Yao Y, Zhang S, He DS, et al. Radiofrequency ablation of the ventricular tachycardia with arrhythmogenic right ventricular cardiomyopathy using non-contact mapping. Pacing Clin Electrophysiol. 2007;30:526–33.
38. Garcia FC, Bazan V, Zado ES, et al. Epicardial substrate and outcome with epicardial ablation of ventricular tachycardia in arrhythmogenic right ventricular cardiomyopathy/dysplasia. Circulation. 2009;120:366–75.
39. Link MS, Bockstall K, Weinstock J, et al. Ventricular tachyarrhythmias in patients with hypertrophic cardiomyopathy and defibrillators: triggers, treatment, and implications. J Cardiovasc Electrophysiol. 2017;28:531–7.
40. Furushima H, Chinushi M, Iijima K, et al. Ventricular tachyarrhythmia associated with hypertrophic cardiomyopathy: incidence, prognosis, and relation to type of hypertrophy. J Cardiovasc Electrophysiol. 2010;21:991–9.
41. Dukkipati SR, D'Avila A, Soejima K, et al. Long-term outcomes of combined epicardial and endocardial ablation of monomorphic ventricular tachycardia related to hypertrophic cardiomyopathy. Circ Arrhythm Electrophysiol. 2011;4:185–94.
42. Santangeli P, Di Biase L, Lakkireddy D, et al. Radiofrequency catheter ablation of ventricular arrhythmias in patients with hypertrophic cardiomyopathy: safety and feasibility. Heart Rhythm. 2010;7:1036–42.
43. Furushima H, Chinushi M, Sugiura H, et al. Ventricular tachyarrhythmia associated with cardiac sarcoidosis: its mechanisms and outcome. Clin Cardiol. 2004;27:217–22.
44. Kumar S, Barbhaiya C, Nagashima K, et al. Ventricular tachycardia in cardiac sarcoidosis: characterization of ventricular substrate and outcomes of catheter ablation. Circ Arrhythm Electrophysiol. 2015;8:87–93.
45. Sarabanda AV, Sosa E, Simoes MV, et al. Ventricular tachycardia in Chagas' disease: a comparison of clinical, angiographic, electrophysiologic and myocardial perfusion disturbances between patients presenting with either sustained or nonsustained forms. Int J Cardiol. 2005;102:9–19.
46. Scanavacca M, Sosa E. Epicardial ablation of ventricular tachycardia in Chagas heart disease. Card Electrophysiol Clin. 2010;2:55–67.
47. Proietti R, Roux JF, Essebag V. Recent advances in ablation of ventricular tachycardia associated with structural heart disease: overcoming the challenges of functional and fixed barriers. Curr Opin Cardiol. 2016;31:64–71.
48. Proietti R, Essebag V, Beardsall J, et al. Substrate-guided ablation of haemodynamically tolerated and untolerated ventricular tachycardia in patients with structural heart disease: effect of cardiomyopathy type and acute success on long-term outcome. Europace. 2015;17:461–7.

The Demise of Fluoroscopy in Pediatric Electrophysiology

14

Amee M. Bigelow and John M. Clark

Introduction

> Given the known risks of ionizing radiation, particularly relevant in the pediatric population, there has been an increasing effort to limit its use. Indeed, the era of low and even fluoroscopy-free electrophysiology study and ablation procedures has arrived [1]—D. Bradley

The above statement highlights the change currently in progress in the profession of pediatric electrophysiology. In little more than one decade, there has been a revolution in the treatment of arrhythmias in children. This revolution has been facilitated entirely by the development and refinement of three-dimensional mapping systems, which allow for the nonfluoroscopic visualization of catheter electrodes. The current millennium began with catheter ablation being the treatment of choice for arrhythmia management in children. Catheter guidance at that time was entirely dependent upon fluoroscopy. Today, three-dimensional mapping tools have allowed dramatic decreases in radiation exposure in nearly all-pediatric electrophysiology (EP) labs. This "fluoroless" movement, away from radiologic guidance, has been spurred by reports revealing the significant increase in medical radiation exposure, as well as the potential associated health risks [2–4]. Between 1987 and 2009 there was a 730% increase in medical radiation exposure in the United States. As a result, patient tracking of lifetime radiation dosing is becoming prevalent.

Ten years ago, fluoroscopy was the sole means of catheter guidance in the vast majority of pediatric electrophysiology labs. Today, virtually all EP labs use some form of three-dimensional guidance. Ten years from now, fluoroscopic guidance for routine pediatric ablation procedures will be rare.

Pediatric electrophysiologists have been the leaders in this revolution. As the fluoroless procedure becomes more common in the pediatric world, the techniques will spill over into the adult arena. The purpose of this chapter is to discuss the role of no-fluoro ablation techniques in the treatment of pediatric arrhythmias. Data relating to the performance and outcomes of this new approach are presented to help the practitioner incorporate the techniques into his or her daily practice. For many of the studies cited, we will also quote the rationale given for the importance of the particular study.

A. M. Bigelow
Division of Cardiology, Department of Pediatrics, Heart Institute, Cincinnati Children's Hospital Medical Center, Cincinnati, OH, USA
e-mail: amee.bigelow@cchmc.org

J. M. Clark (✉)
Division of Cardiology, Department of Pediatrics, Heart Center, Akron Children's Hospital, Akron, OH, USA
e-mail: jclark@akronchildrens.org

R. Proietti et al. (eds.), *Cardiac Electrophysiology Without Fluoroscopy*,
https://doi.org/10.1007/978-3-030-16992-3_14

There has been a steady improvement in fluoroscopy times since the start of catheter ablation. Data from the pediatric registry (1998) showed the mean fluoroscopy time to be 47.6 min. Data from the earliest years of that registry (1991–1992) showed a mean of 60 min [5]. The next large study was the PAPCA registry. It was published in 2004, and showed a mean fluoro time of 38.3 min for supraventricular tachycardia (SVT) ablation in children [6].

The interest in minimizing radiation dose is due to the associated risks. Clay et al. using radiation dosimeters during EP procedures estimated that a single 15 min biplane fluoroscopy exposure during pediatric ablation conferred a lifetime risk to the patient of about 1:5000 for development of a fatal malignancy [7]. Extrapolating that to the early registry data would suggest that those patients could carry a risk as high as 1:1000 per procedure, for lifetime cancer. For a single procedure, the risk is greater for the patient than for the physician. However, over an entire career, the risk of radiation exposure for the staff can also be significant. The Expert Consensus Document on Radiation Safety in the Practice of Cardiology estimates that a busy interventional cardiologist, working an entire career, has about a 4% risk of fatal malignancy due to occupational radiation exposure [3]. That document recommends radiation doses, "As Low As Reasonably Achievable" (ALARA).

For these reasons, broad interest remains in lowering radiation dose. Some of these efforts have gone toward optimizing fluoroscopy use. Gellis et al. developed an "ALARA" protocol to help minimize radiation dose when fluoro was being used [8]. But the greatest benefit would come from nonfluoroscopic guidance systems.

Three-Dimensional Mapping: What Does It Involve?

Broadly, nonfluoroscopic mapping, or electroanatomic mapping systems (EAM), use computers to localize electrodes in three-dimensional space. The location is then displayed on a screen. Relevant blood vessels and cardiac chambers can be drawn, creating a three-dimensional shell within which the catheter can be manipulated.

There have been two mapping systems which have impacted the direction of patient care: the CARTO® system (Biosense-Webster) and the EnSite system (Abbott, Abbott Park, Ill, USA). The CARTO system was the first system clinically available. The first report of its use was by Worley in 1998 [8]. That system works on magnetic detection. The patient is positioned on the cath table, lying on an array of magnets. A proprietary catheter contains a magnetic detector in its tip. By detection of the magnetic field strength at the tip, a computer can triangulate the position of the tip in three-dimensional space. The EnSite system functions by electrical impedance measurement. The patient has three sets of patches positioned on the torso to create three orthogonal electrical fields, anterior-posterior, superior-inferior, and right-left. Any electrode from any catheter can detect the three fields, and the computer can then triangulate the location of that electrode relative to a reference electrode, usually on the patient's abdomen.

Each system has its own strengths. The CARTO system does not need a reference electrode, and shows good geometry stability provided the patient remains stationary on the magnet pad. However, geometry creation in the early versions was a slow, tedious process, with little resemblance to anatomic structures (Fig. 14.1). It requires a proprietary ablation catheter with a

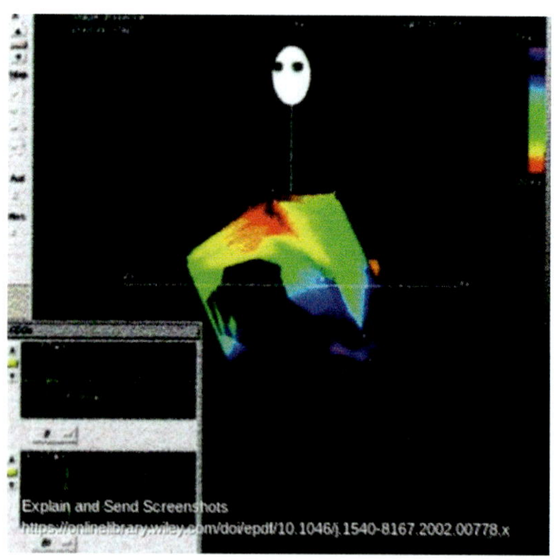

Fig. 14.1 Geometry as drawn for early CARTO procedures

magnetic detector, which makes it poorly functional with cryoablation catheters. The EnSite system can create anatomically detailed geometry in a very short period of time (Fig. 14.2). However, being impedance based, anything that changes electrical impedance can cause the geometry to shift. These include air volume within the lung, and fluid volume and distribution within the body. It can function with any brand or type of catheter, and therefore makes cryoablation a readily available option.

In 2002, using the CARTO system, Drago et al. were the first to report catheter ablation without fluoroscopy [9]. In their report, they performed ablations on 21 children with right-sided manifest accessory pathways. In nine of the patients no fluoroscopy was used. While this marked a milestone in catheter ablation technique, it was never duplicated by another laboratory. The reason why is that the original CARTO system was only compatible with one catheter, a radiofrequency ablation catheter. To perform an ablation without fluoroscopy meant completing the procedure using just one catheter. The only patients who were potentially eligible would be patients with right-sided manifest accessory pathways. All other arrhythmias would require more than one catheter, and therefore were not candidates for a fluoroless procedure. It would be five more years before any other groups would report fluoroless procedures, and those would all utilize EnSite.

The CARTO system, in its early versions, had many weaknesses which prohibited it from functioning as a viable tool for fluoroless procedures. With the release of CARTO 3, those handicaps had mostly been resolved. As the second decade of the new millennium unfolded, some labs were beginning to assess CARTO 3's utility for decreasing fluoroscopy.

As noted by Pass, "Efforts to reduce fluoroscopic dose are of great potential benefit to both patients and staff to reduce both deterministic and stochastic risk" [10].

As previously stated, Gellis reported the experience in Dr. Pass' lab of an "ALARA" protocol, which attempted to decrease radiation exposure using only fluoroscopic guidance of catheters. They reported less total radiation dose, with fluoroscopy alone, than another published study, which utilized CARTO 3 in addition to fluoroscopy [11]. It is important to note that, while the study clearly demonstrates radiation reduction through manipulation of fluoro equipment, it also demonstrates the importance of experience with EAM systems. Just 1 year after publishing his data demonstrating lower radiation exposure than a current EAM system, Pass reported his labs experience with that same EAM system (CARTO 3), while

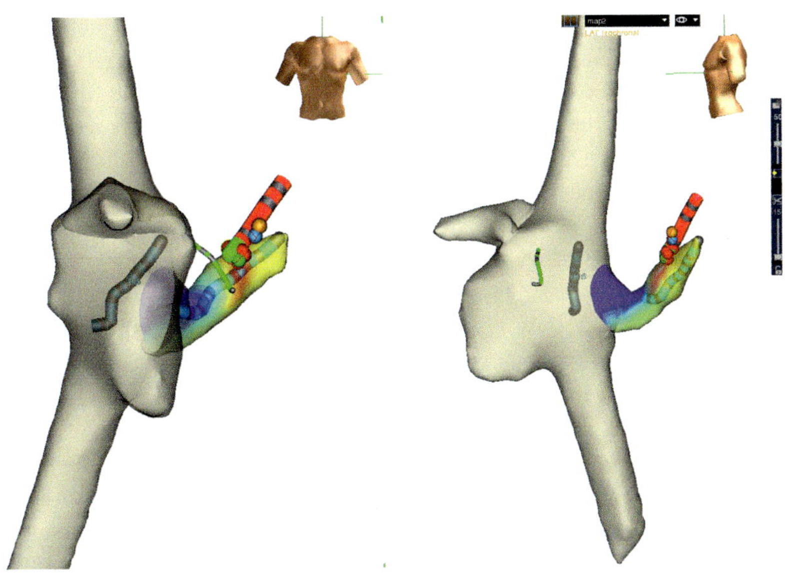

Fig. 14.2 Typical geometry as drawn for early EnSite procedures

still following their own ALARA protocol. In his own words: "When CARTO 3 was added… we observed a nearly sevenfold drop in average dose from 93 to 13 mGy/case" [10]. Others reporting a benefit from the newer CARTO system included Dr. Berul, who noted "The use of high levels of radiation is potentially dangerous, especially in a pediatric population undergoing rapid somatic growth and cellular maturation." They report a 60–70% decrease in all measures of radiation exposure after introduction of CARTO 3 [12].

The competitor of CARTO was EnSite. EnSite was the mapping system that triggered the revolution. Being a nonproprietary, "open" system, it allowed the use of all available mapping and ablation catheters. It also localized transseptal needle tips, and certain guidewires. All of those characteristics made it the leading system for broad application of fluoroless interventions. Tuzcu was the first to begin that process. He reported his early experience in 2007, taking note of the fact that, "Patients and staff can be exposed to a significant amount of fluoroscopy during these (fluoroscopic) procedures." His study involved 28 children with right-sided SVT mechanisms undergoing ablation. Of the 28 procedures, 24 were completed without the use of fluoroscopy. He had acute success in 22 of the 24. There were no complications [13].

That same year, our group reported our experience using EnSite in a pediatric lab. Of 30 patients undergoing SVT ablation, 80% required no fluoroscopy. Five of the six patients requiring fluoro needed it only for transseptal puncture. There was 100% acute success and no complications [14]. For the next 5 years, all publications describing fluoroless procedures utilized the Ensite system. With the release of CARTO 3, reports began to be published around 2013 of its utility to eliminate fluoro. Today, both systems are viable for fluoroless procedures in the majority of instances. One of the benefits of both systems is the continuous localization of electrodes throughout the entire procedure. One does not need to activate fluoroscopy to determine if the catheter has moved. However, both systems can still be improved.

Arrhythmias Amenable to Fluoroless Ablation in Pediatric Labs

Right-Sided Accessory Pathways

While all arrhythmias are approachable without fluoroscopy, there are differing levels of difficulty. Right-sided accessory pathways are the obvious first choice for a fluoroless intervention in children. As a catheter leaves the femoral sheath and enters the femoral vein, it is visible on the EAM. Its movement and direction can be followed as it ascends the IVC. If the catheter redirects into a renal or hepatic vein, that is easily seen. When the catheter enters the liver, it takes a slight leftward direction. With a couple more inches of travel, the catheter enters the right atrium and atrial electrograms will be visible from the electrodes. After optimizing the system, and collecting respiratory compensation, the relevant geometry can then be drawn, using a steerable catheter. The usual procedure for SVT ablation is to draw Superior Vena Cava (SVC), Inferior Vena Cava (IVC), right atrium, coronary sinus (cs), and tricuspid valve. The location of the *His* electrogram is identified and marked. In our early experience, we drew the tricuspid valve by taking points with good atrial and ventricular electrograms. However, with time, one usually finds that, by letting the catheter advance across the tricuspid valve into the ventricle and moving it within the ventricle, the tricuspid valve draws itself. Into this geometry, one can place as many catheters as is deemed appropriate for the procedure. Pacing, EP study, mapping, and ablation can all proceed normally. Since all structures can be directly accessed from the femoral vein, the only reason for the use of fluoroscopy with right-sided accessory pathways is inexperience with the equipment. Fluoroscopy does not localize the *His* bundle better than EAM. Ergul published Tuzcu's results using EnSite for fluoroless ablation of anteroseptal accessory pathways. In 24 patients, they reported a 96% acute success, an 8% recurrence, and no complications [15].

Gaita noted, in explaining their use of CARTO 3 for right-sided accessory pathways, that, "The use of fluoroscopy exposes children to the potential harmful effects of radiation due to the longer life expectancy of this subset of patients." His work, reported by Scaglione, describes 47 accessory pathways in 44 children. They had 100% acute success, 15% recurrence, and no complications [16].

Atrioventricular Nodal Reentrant Tachycardia

AV nodal reentrant tachycardia (AVNRT) is the next simplest arrhythmia to approach without fluoroscopy. Catheter introduction and geometry creation are the same as described, but more attention is paid to Koch's triangle. The *His* bundle is identified and either marked, or a catheter is left in place for continuous recording of the *His* electrogram. The coronary sinus is drawn, and usually a catheter is left in place. This, then, gives an excellent real-time orientation of Koch's triangle. If the EnSite system is used, then either radiofrequency (RF) or cryoenergy can be employed, at the physician's discretion. If CARTO 3 is used, the system will make RF the preferred energy, due to relative incompatibility of cryo with CARTO, as Dr. Ceresnak notes in 2016: "The CARTO 3 system requires the use of specific, proprietary Biosense-Webster ablation catheters. This can be particularly problematic when using the CARTO 3 system if cryoenergy is needed for ablation." Fortunately, his group has been able to outline a workaround for the problem. By employing a "jumper cable," they were able to "trick" CARTO into visualizing the cryocath during ablation [17]. As an alternative to jumper cables, Scaglione used CARTO 3 to position the cryocatheter in the slow pathway location, and then disconnected it from CARTO and plugged into the cryo console for immediate lesion delivery. This approach results in loss of visualization of the catheter during the lesion. Given the high safety factor of cryo, the authors felt this was an acceptable solution. They report 21 ablation procedures of AVNRT. Nineteen were completed without fluoro. Two patients required fluoro to navigate the catheters from the femoral vein to the heart, which is a potential remaining handicap of the CARTO system. They had 100% acute success, with 5 recurrences at 2 years, and no complications [18]. Alvarez reported their experience comparing a traditional fluoro approach to EnSite for ablation of AVNRT. With 25 patients in each group, they achieved zero fluoroscopy in 24/25 with EnSite. All other outcomes, including success, complications, procedure time, and recurrence, were the same between the two groups [19]. Gist reported our group's learning curve for fluoroless ablation of AVNRT using EnSite (Table 14.1). Comparing our first 2 years experience to the most recent 2 years, we noted a 20% improvement in procedure time. No patient required fluoro in either the early or late era. The success, complication, and recurrence rates were equal [20].

Table 14.1 Comparison of early versus recent era for ablation of AVNRT

Results of study versus control			
Variable	Early ($N = 27$)	Recent ($N = 35$)	P-value
Female	17 (63%)	23 (66%)	0.8
Mean age (years)	14 ± 5	14 + 7	0.8
Mean height (cm)	160 ± 21	156 + 21	0.4
Mean weight (kg)	55 ± 16	56 ± 22	0.8
Mean lesion no.	6 + 3	6 ± 3	1
Mean lesion time	25 ± 14	25 + 12	0.9
Cath tip size (4 mm)	26 (96%)	32 (91%)	0.4
Transient AV block	12 (44%)	13 (38%)	0.6
Procedure time	202 ± 76	160 ± 61	0.014
Room time	265 ± 72	221 ± 63	0.01
Setup time	63 + 15	61 ± 17	0.63
Procedural success	27 (100%)	34 (97%)	1
Recurrences	4 (15%)	3 (9%)	0.69

Learning curve for AVNRT ablation. All parameters are similar between the early and late groups except procedure time, which is shorter in the later group

Other Right-Sided Mechanisms of Tachycardia

Less common mechanisms of tachycardia can also be approached without fluoroscopy. These include atrial flutter, ectopic tachycardia, and intra-atrial reentry. Typical atrial flutter is uncommon in children, but easily managed. The tricuspid annulus and isthmus are readily defined. Creating a line of block is documented by standard EP protocols.

Ectopic atrial tachycardia (EAT) may be better treated with EAM than with standard fluoroscopy. This is because EAM systems have the added benefit of being able to create an activation map, which can graphically show the wavefront of depolarization within the atrium (Figs. 14.3 and 14.4) demonstrates this in a patient with an ectopic tachycardia from the left atrial appendage. Dieks reported her group's experience of the Ensite system for guiding ablation of focal atrial tachycardia. Over a 10-year period, they

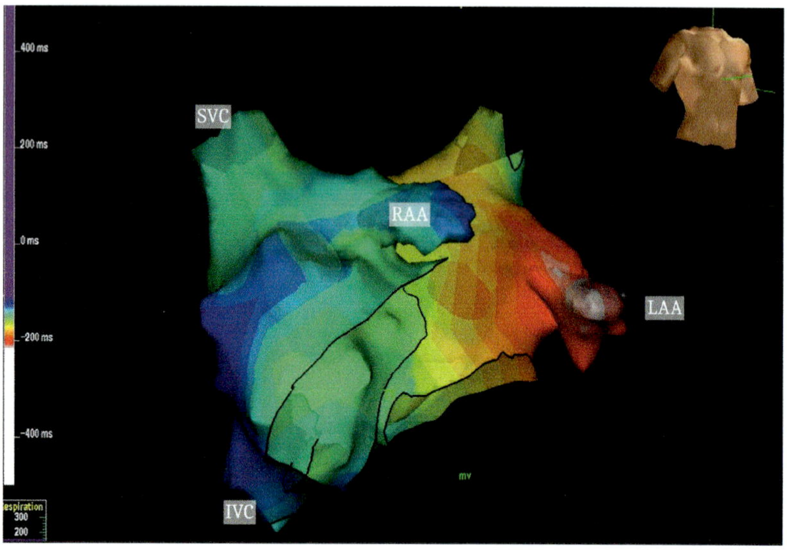

Fig. 14.3 Activation map in a patient with ectopic tachycardia from the left atrial appendage. White and red color represents area of earliest atrial activation. *SVC* superior vena cava, *IVC* inferior vena cava, *RAA* right atrial appendage, *LAA* left atrial appendage

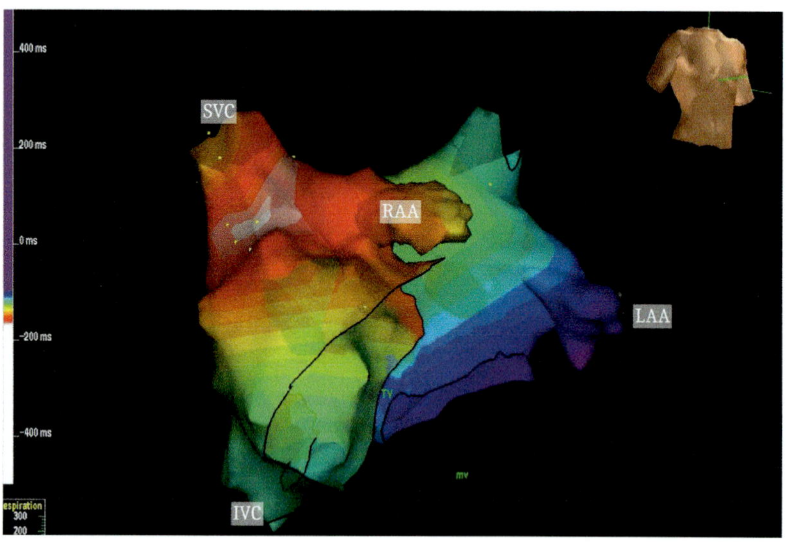

Fig. 14.4 Same patient as Fig. 14.3, after ablation. Notice earliest activation now maps to area near sinus node

attempted 16 ablations, with acute success in 14/16. Compared to other published series', they found higher success rate and lower fluoroscopy times [21]. Intra-atrial reentrant tachycardia (IART) is a troublesome rhythm to deal with regardless of approach. It is most often seen in complex congenital heart disease. Because of this, it is more likely to require fluoroscopy. However, because these patients are exposed to multiple procedures over their lifetime, it is also the reason to attempt to minimize radiation exposure.

Three-dimensional mapping tools can increase the success of the procedure due to their ability to provide both activation maps and voltage maps. Voltage maps can help in defining areas of scar that might be serving to support the reentrant circuit. There is not a set approach to ablation in this population, and each patient needs to be assessed and treated individually. However, there are reports of fluoroless ablations being performed for this arrhythmia in complex congenital heart disease (CHD) [22].

Left-Sided Mechanisms

Left-sided arrhythmias have all the same treatment issues that right-sided mechanisms do, plus the added factor of access. To access left-sided tachycardias, there are three options available in the usual EP lab: patent foramen ovale, transseptal puncture, or retrograde arterial. These will be discussed individually.

The patent foramen ovale (PFO) is somewhat of a buried treasure to the electrophysiologist. Few things bring the sense of good personal fortune like discovering ready-made access to a left-sided accessory pathway. When present, a PFO is easily identified on EAM. When drawing geometry, the catheter will take an unmistakable course. With the catheter facing the atrial septum, as it is advanced superiorly, it will take a course aiming leftward and posteriorly. There will generally still be excellent atrial electrograms noted, unless the catheter is advanced into a pulmonary vein. When a PFO is discovered during geometry creation, the operating physician should pause and say a short prayer that the patient's tachycardia mechanism is a left-sided concealed pathway. The remainder of the procedure can then continue according to standard protocol.

In the absence of a PFO, the options become transseptal or retrograde. If patient size allows a retrograde approach, then the ablation can proceed without fluoro. Advancing the ablation catheter into the left ventricle (LV) is not technically different with EAM guidance than with fluoroscopy. Positioning of the catheter tip on the mitral annulus is aided by electrograms, and the presence of a coronary sinus catheter. It will not take long to develop a comfort level with the 3D images, which replace the fluoro images to which we are accustomed. Gaita has embraced this approach, noting that, "the use of fluoroscopy exposes children to the potential harmful effects of radiation due to the longer life expectancy of this subset of patients." His lab has reported fluoroless ablation in 21 children with left-sided accessory pathways. Two patients had PFO, and the remainder a retrograde approach. None of the cases required fluoroscopy. They had 100% acute success and no complications [16].

If a transseptal approach is needed, then the current options are transesophageal (TEE) or intracardiac echo (ICE). We prefer TEE because it is not restricted by venous access issues, and can be performed on any size patient. However, the downsides of TEE are that it is more time consuming, and requires the assistance of a second physician. For those individuals wishing to learn the TEE approach, it is relatively simple. A guidewire is advanced from the femoral vein to the SVC. A bicaval TEE view confirms the position of the guidewire. The transseptal sheath and dilator are advanced to the SVC, with visualization by TEE. The guidewire is then removed and replaced with the transseptal needle. Continuing with a bicaval view, the sheath and dilator are pulled down to engage the atrial septum. The view is then changed to an aortic valve en-face view. From this angle, the thin membranous septum is well visualized. The dilator is manipulated

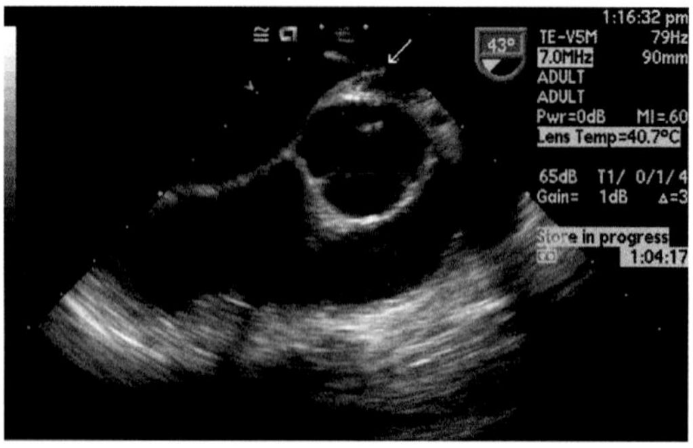

Fig. 14.5 Typical transesophageal image guiding transseptal puncture. Arrow identifies tip of dilator as it "tents" the atrial septum prior to advancing the transseptal needle

to demonstrate tenting of the membranous atrial septum, with care being taken to visualize the tip of the dilator (Fig. 14.5). The needle is then advanced into the left atrium. Saline is injected to confirm left atrial position of the needle, and then the sheath is advanced over the needle. Ablation then continues per standard protocols. We began this approach in 2006, and published our data in 2008 [23]. Since that time, it has remained our standard approach. Others have reported use of ICE to accomplish the same goal [24].

Many labs are now approaching all arrhythmias with a zero-fluoroscopy intention. In Gersak's lab, they performed 43 consecutive ablations for SVT in children, with an intention of zero fluoroscopy. Utilizing EAM and ICE, they achieved 100% success with 0 fluoro and no complications. They concluded that stochastic and deterministic effects potentially express a greater risk in this population. Therefore, there seems to be some rationale to go even beyond the utilization of the ALARA principle in pediatric catheter ablation procedures [25].

In Aziz's lab, they report an 88% decrease in fluoro time, and 54% of cases achieving zero fluoroscopy for SVT ablation in children. These numbers are what they achieved when first attempting fluoroless procedures, having not yet gone through a learning curve [26]. Wan reported very similar results as they went through their learning curve [27].

Ventricular Arrhythmias

Ventricular arrhythmia ablation presents additional challenges if the intention is to reach zero fluoroscopy. These procedures often require special catheters and sheaths to successfully ablate the substrate. It takes a little more practice to reach zero fluoroscopy in this setting. A common situation for ventricular arrhythmia ablation is to place a spiral catheter in the right ventricular outflow tract (RVOT). This requires a long sheath. But, sheaths are not visible on EAM systems. To deal with this issue, one must take note of the fact that the sheath insulates the electrodes from the electrical fields generated by the surface patches. Translated, that means that whenever an electrode is pulled back into a sheath, the catheter is distorted on the EAM. It is, therefore, possible to identify when the tip of the sheath is right at the proximal electrode of a catheter. With that fact understood, it becomes possible to place a spiral catheter into the RVOT. Start by inserting the particular sheath needed. Through this sheath, advance a steerable catheter into the main pulmonary artery (MPA). Next, advance the sheath over the catheter until you see the distortion of the proximal electrode. This will inform you that the tip of the sheath is now positioned in the MPA. Remove the steerable catheter and advance the spiral catheter through the sheath. As the distal electrode emerges from the sheath, hold the catheter steady and pull the sheath back. This will allow the catheter to coil in the MPA. It can then be pulled back and positioned in the RVOT. This technique can allow a zero fluoroscopy procedure for those wishing to pursue it. Utilizing this technique, Von Bergen et al. were able to achieve zero fluoroscopy in three out of five ventricular arrhythmia ablations [28]. In Tuzcu's lab, they achieved 6/17 fluoroless ablations of ventricular tachycardia in their early results, and 19/35 in their later report [29, 30]. Figure 14.6 demonstrates the three-dimensional anatomy of a patient with left ventricular outflow tract (LVOT) tachycardia, mapped from both the RV and the LV.

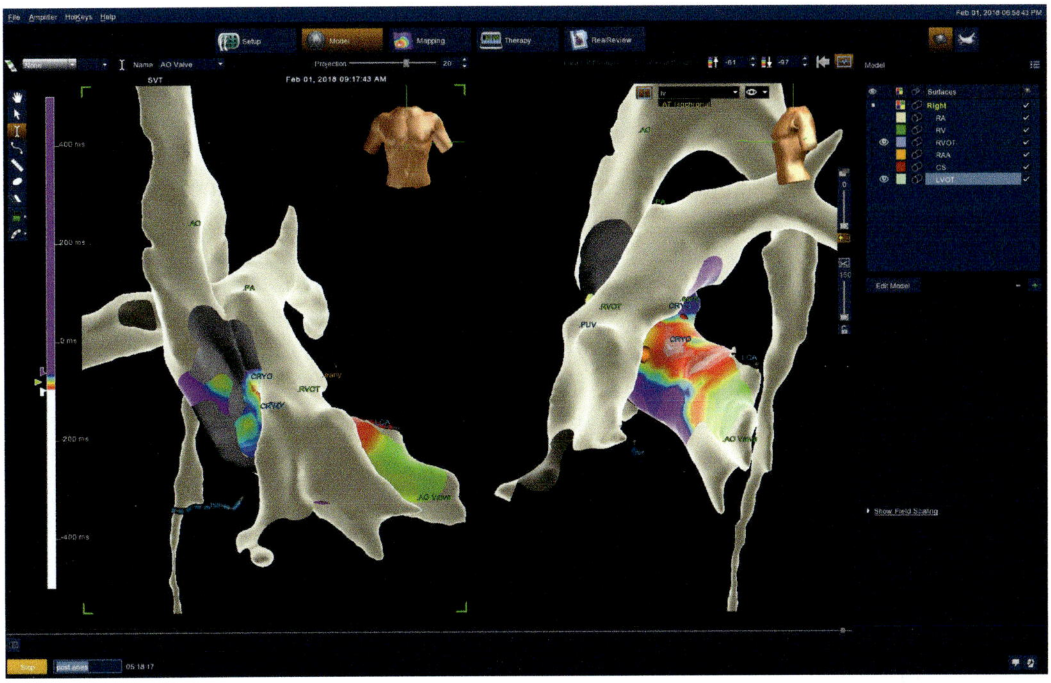

Fig. 14.6 AP and lateral view in patient with left ventricular outflow tract (LVOT) tachycardia. Geometry drawn shows 3-D relationship of LVOT and RVOT

Special Considerations

Other issues of particular import to the pediatric electrophysiologist are congenital heart disease and small patient size. As previously noted, patients with significant CHD require more radiologic procedures over their lifetime, and require more fluoroscopy per procedure. They may be the group of patients who will benefit the most from EAM systems. Most reports of fluoroless ablation in patients with CHD are isolated case reports [22, 31]. We have reported on two neonates with WPW and CHD undergoing fluoroless ablation [32]. One patient had Ebstein's anomaly, and the other had pulmonary atresia. Both procedures were accomplished without fluoroscopy, and neither patient has had recurrence at 3 years follow-up.

Small size is a known risk for complication in catheter ablation, with patients <15 kg at greater risk [5]. Mapping and ablation catheters are developed for adult-sized patients. At the lower limits of our patient size, the curves and stiffness of the available catheters become a detriment to patient care. This is true regardless of the method of catheter guidance. The EnSite system suffers from similar technical difficulties. The total surface area of all patches and electrodes for an EnSite procedure is 1380 cm^2, while the typical torso surface area of a newborn is 900 cm^2. However, since most of the navigation patches are gel, with only a small portion of it being the wire mesh, it is possible to remove up to 90% of the gel pad without interfering with the wiring of the patch. Viewing the patches under fluoroscopy can identify the extent of the wire mesh antenna. This has allowed us to create a template for removing excess gel pad from the patch as a less than ideal, but systematic work-around.

Benefits

The benefits of a no-fluoro approach in pediatric electrophysiology include avoidance of lead protective equipment, elimination of stochastic complication risk, allowing safer performance of procedures during pregnancy, improved outcomes, and potential portability of the procedure.

Wearing lead aprons, thyroid shields, and goggles is held to be an absolute requirement within the profession of electrophysiology. But the utility of EAM systems raises the possibility of removing those cumbersome defenses. Stec et al. report their experience from 188 consecutive SVT ablations performed with an intention of zero fluoroscopy [33]. Of the 188, 179 were completed without fluoro. Based on this data, and noting that the "need for lead aprons and eye protection to protect medical staff increases workplace discomfort and the risk of neck, back and joint complications," they have recommended a "no lead" approach. We have followed this approach for over 10 years, and the increased comfort associated with it will very likely be the impetus that ultimately drives most labs to adopt a no-fluoro technique.

Long-term stochastic complication risks are low enough that electrophysiologists are habituated to ignore them. However, a recent publication makes a sobering point. Roguin et al. reported on 31 physicians with head and neck tumors [34]. The physicians were interventional cardiologists, radiologists, and electrophysiologists. Of the 31 tumors, the sidedness of the tumor could be defined in 26. Of the 26 in which the sidedness of the tumor was identified in the chart, 22 of them were left sided, one was midline, and only three were right sided. Given that the X-ray source is always to the physician's left, it is unsettling to find that 85% of head and neck tumors in this population were on the left side.

Arrhythmias during pregnancy are another uncommon but troublesome scenario. There are a number of case reports now demonstrating the utility of EAM to perform fluoroless procedures during pregnancy [35–44]. Given the risks of fluoroscopy, and the risks of antiarrhythmic medications during pregnancy, fluoroless ablation may eventually become the treatment of choice for arrhythmia management in pregnancy. In addition to benefits to the pregnant patient, there are also potential benefits to staff. In the last 12 years in our lab, we have had multiple staff members who were able to maintain their jobs in the EP lab throughout pregnancy because we were not using fluoroscopy.

Portability of electrophysiology procedures remains just over the horizon. Routine fluoroless procedures will first need to become commonplace before the profession will be ready to accept routine portability. However, the reason to consider it is due to the rare but difficult scenario of tachycardia-induced cardiomyopathy in the patient who requires ECMO support. In that setting, ablation is the treatment of choice, and can be life saving. But, transporting an ECMO patient to the EP lab is fraught with risk. Eliminating the need for fluoroscopy has the potential to eliminate the need for the stationary EP lab. It is technically feasible to perform an ablation in the intensive care unit (ICU). While we have not yet performed an ablation on an ECMO patient in an ICU, we have developed our service in a way that will easily allow it when needed. Our system is maintained on a portable cart, which can be transported to any room where a procedure is necessary. Thus far, we have performed ablations in various operating rooms within the hospital. We have performed more than 100 ablations outside of the cath lab. Our early data was recently published [45]. While this is unique at the moment, it will become more common as greater worldwide experience is obtained.

In addition to minimizing radiation exposure, there may also be other benefits to 3D mapping. Ceresnak et al. reported improved acute success when EAM was used for catheter guidance in ablation of WPW, as opposed to fluoroscopy alone [46]. This was a multicenter, retrospective review. Tuzcu reported similar findings from a single institution [47].

The Future

The future of pediatric electrophysiology is fascinating to consider from this moment in time. Unquestionably, fluoroscopy will be eliminated from all but the most difficult or complex cases. As Giuseppe Stabile notes, "Once the decision has been made to use a navigation system to reduce fluoroscopy time, the next step is just a question of learning and confidence" [48]. What is not clear about the future is, what will be the changes in the tools and technology that will expedite the transformation, and who will lead the revolution. Immediate needs include sheaths, dilators, guidewires, and needles that are visible on EAM systems. Those simple tools would markedly increase the acceptance of fluoroless procedures. Once the elimination of fluoroscopy has become commonplace, it is only a little further down the road before we reach the point of elimination of the traditional EP lab. As L Szydlowski notes, "Growing experience with this radiation-free approach should lead to the complete elimination of fluoroscopy during SVT ablations, and in the training of a new generation of invasive electrophysiologists" [33].

Indeed, the era of fluoroscopy-free ablation procedures has arrived.

References

1. Kean AC, LaPage MJ, Yu S, Dick M 2nd, Bradley DJ. Patient and procedural correlates of fluoroscopy use during catheter ablation in the pediatric and congenital electrophysiology lab. Congenit Heart Dis. 2015;10(3):281–7.
2. Beels L, Bacher K, De Wolf D, Werbrouck J, Thierens H. Gamma-H2AX foci as a biomarker for patient X-ray exposure in pediatric cardiac catheterization: are we underestimating radiation risks? Circulation. 2009;120(19):1903–9.
3. Limacher MC, Douglas PS, Germano G, et al. ACC expert consensus document. Radiation safety in the practice of cardiology. American college of cardiology. J Am Coll Cardiol. 1998;31(4):892–913.
4. Broga D. Ionizing radiation exposure of the population of the united states. National Council on Radiation. 1st edn. Wiley: Hoboken, NJ: 2009. https://doi.org/10.1118/1.3245881.
5. Kugler JD, Danford DA, Houston K, Felix G. Radiofrequency catheter ablation for paroxysmal supraventricular tachycardia in children and adolescents without structural heart disease. Pediatric EP society, radiofrequency catheter ablation registry. Am J Cardiol. 1997;80(11):1438–43.
6. Van Hare GF, Javitz H, Carmelli D, et al. Prospective assessment after pediatric cardiac ablation: demographics, medical profiles, and initial outcomes. J Cardiovasc Electrophysiol. 2004;15(7):759–70.
7. Clay MA, Campbell RM, Strieper M, Frias PA, Stevens M, Mahle WT. Long-term risk of fatal malignancy following pediatric radiofrequency ablation. Am J Cardiol. 2008;102(7):913–5.
8. Gellis LA, Ceresnak SR, Gates GJ, Nappo L, Pass RH. Reducing patient radiation dosage during pediatric SVT ablations using an "ALARA" radiation reduction protocol in the modern fluoroscopic era. Pacing Clin Electrophysiol. 2013;36(6):688–94.
9. Drago F, Silvetti MS, Di Pino A, Grutter G, Bevilacqua M, Leibovich S. Exclusion of fluoroscopy during ablation treatment of right accessory pathway in children. J Cardiovasc Electrophysiol. 2002;13(8):778–82.
10. Pass RH, Gates GG, Gellis LA, Nappo L, Ceresnak SR. Reducing patient radiation exposure during paediatric SVT ablations: use of CARTO(R) 3 in concert with "ALARA" principles profoundly lowers total dose. Cardiol Young. 2015;25(5):963–8.
11. Miyake CY, Mah DY, Atallah J, et al. Nonfluoroscopic imaging systems reduce radiation exposure in children undergoing ablation of supraventricular tachycardia. Heart Rhythm. 2011;8(4):519–25.
12. Clark BC, Sumihara K, McCarter R, Berul CI, Moak JP. Getting to zero: impact of electroanatomical mapping on fluoroscopy use in pediatric catheter ablation. J Interv Card Electrophysiol. 2016;46(2):183–9.
13. Tuzcu V. A nonfluoroscopic approach for electrophysiology and catheter ablation procedures using a three-dimensional navigation system. Pacing Clin Electrophysiol. 2007;30(4):519–25.
14. Smith G, Clark JM. Elimination of fluoroscopy use in a pediatric electrophysiology laboratory utilizing three-dimensional mapping. Pacing Clin Electrophysiol. 2007;30(4):510–8.
15. Ergul Y, Tola HT, Kiplapinar N, Akdeniz C, Saygi M, Tuzcu V. Cryoablation of anteroseptal accessory pathways in children with limited fluoroscopy exposure. Pediatr Cardiol. 2013;34(4):802–8.
16. Scaglione M, Ebrille E, Caponi D, et al. Zero-fluoroscopy ablation of accessory pathways in children and adolescents: CARTO3 electroanatomic mapping combined with RF and cryoenergy. Pacing Clin Electrophysiol. 2015;38(6):675–81.
17. Ceresnak SR, Nappo L, Janson CM, Pass RH. Tricking CARTO: cryoablation of supraventricular tachycardia in children with minimal radiation exposure using the CARTO3 system. Pacing Clin Electrophysiol. 2016;39(1):36–41.
18. Scaglione M, Ebrille E, Caponi D, et al. Single center experience of fluoroless AVNRT ablation guided by electroanatomic reconstruction in children and adolescents. Pacing Clin Electrophysiol. 2013;36(12):1460–7.
19. Alvarez M, Tercedor L, Almansa I, et al. Safety and feasibility of catheter ablation for atrioventricular

nodal re-entrant tachycardia without fluoroscopic guidance. Heart Rhythm. 2009;6(12):1714–20.
20. Gist K, Tigges C, Smith G, Clark J. Learning curve for zero-fluoroscopy catheter ablation of AVNRT: early versus late experience. Pacing Clin Electrophysiol. 2011;34(3):264–8.
21. Dieks JK, Muller MJ, Schneider HE, et al. Catheter ablation of pediatric focal atrial tachycardia: ten-year experience using modern mapping systems. Pediatr Cardiol. 2016;37(3):459–64.
22. Zambito MP, Samuel BP, Vettukattil JJ, Ratnasamy C. Fluoroless catheter ablation of intraatrial reentrant tachycardia status post fontan procedure: fluoroless catheter ablation in fontan patient. Int J Cardiol. 2015;201:126–8.
23. Clark J, Bockoven JR, Lane J, Patel CR, Smith G. Use of three-dimensional catheter guidance and trans-esophageal echocardiography to eliminate fluoroscopy in catheter ablation of left-sided accessory pathways. Pacing Clin Electrophysiol. 2008;31(3):283–9.
24. Mah DY, Miyake CY, Sherwin ED, et al. The use of an integrated electroanatomic mapping system and intracardiac echocardiography to reduce radiation exposure in children and young adults undergoing ablation of supraventricular tachycardia. Europace. 2014;16(2):277–83.
25. Jan M, Zizek D, Rupar K, et al. Fluoroless catheter ablation of various right and left sided supraventricular tachycardias in children and adolescents. Int J Cardiovasc Imaging. 2016;32(11):1609–16.
26. Nagaraju L, Menon D, Aziz PF. Use of 3D electroanatomical navigation (CARTO-3) to minimize or eliminate fluoroscopy use in the ablation of pediatric supraventricular tachyarrhythmias. Pacing Clin Electrophysiol. 2016;39(6):574–80.
27. Wan G, Shannon KM, Moore JP. Factors associated with fluoroscopy exposure during pediatric catheter ablation utilizing electroanatomical mapping. J Interv Card Electrophysiol. 2012;35(2):235–42.
28. Von Bergen NH, Bansal S, Gingerich J, Law IH. Nonfluoroscopic and radiation-limited ablation of ventricular arrhythmias in children and young adults: a case series. Pediatr Cardiol. 2011;32(6):743–7.
29. Ozyilmaz I, Ergul Y, Akdeniz C, Ozturk E, Tanidir IC, Tuzcu V. Catheter ablation of idiopathic ventricular tachycardia in children using the EnSite NavX system with/without fluoroscopy. Cardiol Young. 2014;24(5):886–92.
30. Akdeniz C, Gul EE, Celik N, Karacan M, Tuzcu V. Catheter ablation of idiopathic right ventricular arrhythmias in children with limited fluoroscopy. J Interv Card Electrophysiol. 2016;46(3):355–60.
31. Giaccardi M, Chiodi L, Del Rosso A, Colella A. 'Zero' fluoroscopic exposure for ventricular tachycardia ablation in a patient with situs viscerum inversus totalis. Europace. 2012;14(3):449–50.
32. Bigelow AM, Arnold BS, Padrutt GC, Clark JM. Nonfluoroscopic cardiac ablation of neonates with CHD. Cardiol Young. 2017;27(3):592–6.
33. Stec S, Sledz J, Mazij M, et al. Feasibility of implementation of a "simplified, no-X-ray, no-lead apron, two-catheter approach" for ablation of supraventricular arrhythmias in children and adults. J Cardiovasc Electrophysiol. 2014;25(8):866–74.
34. Roguin A, Goldstein J, Bar O, Goldstein JA. Brain and neck tumors among physicians performing interventional procedures. Am J Cardiol. 2013;111(9):1368–72.
35. Szumowski L, Szufladowicz E, Orczykowski M, et al. Ablation of severe drug-resistant tachyarrhythmia during pregnancy. J Cardiovasc Electrophysiol. 2010;21(8):877–82.
36. Wu H, Ling LH, Lee G, Kistler PM. Successful catheter ablation of incessant atrial tachycardia in pregnancy using three-dimensional electroanatomical mapping with minimal radiation. Intern Med J. 2012;42(6):709–12.
37. Hogarth AJ, Graham LN. Normal heart ventricular tachycardia associated with pregnancy: successful treatment with catheter ablation. Indian Pacing Electrophysiol J. 2014;14(2):79–82.
38. Raman AS, Sharma S, Hariharan R. Minimal use of fluoroscopy to reduce fetal radiation exposure during radiofrequency catheter ablation of maternal supraventricular tachycardia. Tex Heart Inst J. 2015;42(2):152–4.
39. Bigelow AM, Crane SS, Khoury FR, Clark JM. Catheter ablation of supraventricular tachycardia without fluoroscopy during pregnancy. Obstet Gynecol. 2015;125(6):1338–41.
40. Chen G, Sun G, Xu R, et al. Zero-fluoroscopy catheter ablation of severe drug-resistant arrhythmia guided by ensite NavX system during pregnancy: two case reports and literature review. Medicine (Baltimore). 2016;95(32):e4487.
41. Prolic Kalinsek T, Jan M, Rupar K, Razen L, Antolic B, Zizek D. Zero-fluoroscopy catheter ablation of concealed left accessory pathway in a pregnant woman. Europace. 2017;19(8):1384.
42. Kozluk E, Piatkowska A, Kiliszek M, et al. Catheter ablation of cardiac arrhythmias in pregnancy without fluoroscopy: a case control retrospective study. Adv Clin Exp Med. 2017;26(1):129–34.
43. Rossi L, Penela D, Villani GQ. Intracardiac echocardiography catheter-guided zero fluoroscopy transeptal puncture technique for ablation of left-sided accessory pathway in a pregnant woman. Europace. 2017;19(11):1825.
44. Lahiri A, Srinath SC, Chase D, Roshan J. Zero fluoroscopy radiofrequency ablation for typical atrioventricular nodal reentrant tachycardia (AVNRT). Indian Pacing Electrophysiol J. 2017;17(6):180–2.
45. Bigelow AM, Smith PC, Timberlake DT, et al. Procedural outcomes of fluoroless catheter ablation outside the traditional catheterization lab. Europace. 2017;19(8):1378–84.
46. Ceresnak SR, Dubin AM, Kim JJ, et al. Success rates in pediatric WPW ablation are improved with

3-dimensional mapping systems compared with fluoroscopy alone: a multicenter study. J Cardiovasc Electrophysiol. 2015;26(4):412–6.
47. Tuzcu V. Significant reduction of fluoroscopy in pediatric catheter ablation procedures: long-term experience from a single center. Pacing Clin Electrophysiol. 2012;35(9):1067–73.
48. Solimene F, Donnici G, Shopova G, et al. Trends in fluoroscopy time during radiofrequency catheter ablation of supraventricular tachycardias. Int J Cardiol. 2016;202:124–5.

Complications of Radiofrequency Catheter Ablation and Prevention Methods

15

Andres C. Klein, Riccardo Proietti, and Félix Ayala-Paredes

Introduction

It is a global trending in EP labs all around the world to try to reduce fluoroscopy; to reduce impact on patients, but also in personnel working at those labs, much more exposed to radiation everyday. As with any new approach, safety should be a main topic to consider. X-rays have been so much time in use that despite the low resolution we have all learnt to work with, but the use of radiation has never prevented the complications related to RFCA.

With the development of new technologies such as very precise 3D mapping systems, contact force catheters, intravascular ultrasound and other technologies adding more and useful information about the position of the catheters and its interaction with the cardiac structures fluoroscopy became a dispensable tool.

In the next paragraphs, we describe how to change the paradigm using as close to zero radiation as possible, for most ablation procedures, and to prevent and manage related complications.

The more radiofrequency (RF) applied, the more the chances to have complications. RFCA of atrial fibrillation is by far the procedure that needs more RF, and it is even worse when non PVI foci are target (substrate modification); in a recent series with 10,795 patients from Japan, the total rate of complications occurred in 3% of patients; with pericardial effusion in 1%, massive bleeding in 1%, stroke 0.05% and atrial-oesophageal fistula in 0.02% of patients [1].

The next substrate that requires considerable amounts of RFCA is ventricular arrhythmias; a multicentre report on idiopathic PVC ablation, with 1185 patients, showed fluoroscopy times of 30 ± 24 min, RF time of 12 ± 11 min, with a total of 5.5% of complications (2.4% of major complications, including 0.8% of cardiac tamponades, 1.3% of major groin complications, and one complete AV block; no strokes and no deaths were reported) [2]. A Chinese series of 1231 patients, single centre, on the same substrate reported 2.7% of complications, mostly pericardial effusion and tamponade, but also with stroke reported and two deaths [3]. Finally, a retrospective analysis of RFCA of ventricular arrhythmias in 34,907 patients (51.6% with

A. C. Klein
Division of Cardiology (Arrhythmia Service), University of Ottawa Heart Institute, Ottawa, ON, Canada

Canadian Working Group on Radiation Reduction in Arrhythmia Management, Toronto, ON, Canada
e-mail: aklein@ottawaheart.ca

R. Proietti
University of Padua, Padua, Italy

F. Ayala-Paredes (✉)
Canadian Working Group on Radiation Reduction in Arrhythmia Management, Toronto, ON, Canada

Division of Cardiology, Centre Hospitalier Universitaire de Sherbrooke, Sherbrooke, QC, Canada
e-mail: felix.ayala-paredes@usherbrooke.ca

R. Proietti et al. (eds.), *Cardiac Electrophysiology Without Fluoroscopy*,
https://doi.org/10.1007/978-3-030-16992-3_15

structural heart disease, SHD); major complications occurred in 6.3% of SHD patients compared to 2.1% of patients without SHD; death rate was also superior in patients with SHD 2.5% versus 0.12% in patients without SHD [4].

In supraventricular RFCA a paediatric report of more than 20 years and three different registries shows a complication rate varying between 3.2% before 1996 (n = 3653), 4% between 1999 and 2001 (n = 2761), and 3.6% between 2014 and 2015 (n = 1417); cryoablation was used in 53% of AVNRT resulting in a 0.1% of complete AV block; the use of 3-D mapping systems reduced fluoroscopy times from 47.6 ± 40 min in the previous registries to 7 ± 12 min in the latter registry [5].

A report on 519951 adult patients in the USA ablated from 2000 to 2013 showed that 5.46% of patients had at least one complication (rates increased from 3.07% in 2000 to 7.04% in 2013) (mostly bleeding or hematoma at access sites in 2.57% followed by pericardial complications in 1.3% of patients); ventricular tachycardia ablation had the highest rate of complications 9.9%, followed by atrial fibrillation ablation 7.21%, and supraventricular ablations with only 3.29% of reported complications [6].

In the NO-PARTY trial, a prospective, multicentre, randomized controlled trial in six electrophysiology laboratories in Italy, comparing a minimally fluoroscopic radiofrequency catheter ablation (MFA) with conventional fluoroscopy-guided ablation for supraventricular tachycardia, 231 patients underwent an ablation following the EP study with a complications rate of 1.1% (P = ns). The procedural complications were as follows: one arteriovenous fistula solved by compression in MFA group and two first-degree atrioventricular node blocks spontaneously solved in 48 h in ConvA group. The mean follow-up time was 12 + 4 months, during which no procedure-related complication occurred [7]. Sommer et al. showed in a cohort of 1000 patients who underwent AF ablation using near-zero fluoroscopy approach an overall complication rate of 2.0% including femoral pseudoaneurysm (n = 10, 1%), arteriovenous fistula (n = 1, 0.1%), pericardial effusion (n = 7, 0.7%), phrenic nerve palsy (n = 1, 0.1%), and stroke (n = 1, 0.1%). The median procedure time was 120 min, median fluoroscopy time was 0.90 min, and the median fluoroscopy dose was 345.1 cGy/cm^2 [8].

There are mainly three types of complications we want to prevent: perforation of vascular structures and bleeding, thromboembolic complications, and damage of the normal conduction system. We are going to discuss how to avoid and manage each one of these complications.

Bleeding

1. Vascular access: Venous and arterial punctures carry the inherent risk of bleeding. The need of fluoroscopy in this seeting is, in some labs, the visualization of the femoral head, to guide a high arterial puncture, and the potential use of an arterial closing device at the end of the procedure without the risk of blocking the femoral bifurcation, which also needs an arteriography at the end. If it is the case, a way to reduce fluoroscopy utilization could be an arterial puncture guided by vascular ultrasound, but at the end the arteriography will would be still necessary, before the deployment of the vascular closing device; if the puncture was done too close to the bifurcation, manual compression is needed. For most of EP procedures however, venous punctures are needed, they do not need any special equipment or fluoroscopy, but vascular ultrasound is also gaining acceptability to reduce the risks of inadvertent arterial puncture. Some labs use the left antecubital venous access to place a non-deflectable coronary sinus 6F catheter from above, it is an area easier to compress and with less bleeding risk than the usual groin access. Even in left-sided procedures with retrograde access we routinely use 7F introducers, and manual compression is the default, applied by trained nurses in an adjacent compression room, to speed workflow at our busy lab. Arterial closure devices and "figure-of-eight" suture [9, 10] have dramatically reduced bleeding after introducer retrieval, even if full anticoagulation is used. Finally, the use of 3-D mapping

systems helps to reduce the number of catheters needed, in our lab the two-catheter technique is the default setting for the clear majority of substrates, and less punctures mean also less risk of complications.

2. Catheter placement: Once the vascular access is achieved, catheters need to follow the vessel chosen to arrive to the heart chambers; unless extreme force is applied, it is very unlikely to cause any bleeding while advancing the catheters; radiofrequency is never used while the ablation catheter progresses (and once the ablation catheter is in the vasculature, we keep power in zero values until it is time to ablate, to prevent inadvertent activation of the RF pedal). If there is abnormal resistance to catheter advancement, we should try first to introduce a softer and smaller catheter; we can try to advance a long guide wire and then connect it to the 3-D mapping system (please refer to Chap. 5) to confirm the position and use it as a rail for a longer introducer (especially for arterial retrograde access in patients with vascular peripheral disease), or if a guidewire does not progress easily, sometimes fluoroscopy and arteriography is needed to exclude dissection. One helpful manoeuvre using deflectable catheters is to full bend the catheter just after it went through the sheath for preventing it to go into smaller collateral branches of the vessel. Arriving to the right atrium through the inferior vena cava has no major challenges, other than catheters sometimes directing to hepatic or diaphragmatic veins; all systems allow visualization of the catheters at this level and even further, gentle retrieval, torque and advancement allow the catheter to arrive to the atrium and record atrial EGMs. Arriving to the aorta possess a different challenge; the catheter should start acquiring the virtual anatomy at the arch level, and movements of advancement, rotation and retrieval should be done smoothly; while working with fluoroscopy most centres would perform a selective angiography to guide then the procedure; in a non-fluoroscopic environment, the coronary arteries are not visualized and their ostia cannot be estimated unless the aortic valve cusps are depicted; once the ascending aorta shell has been created, we can flex the ablation catheter and use both RAO and LAO incidences to protrude into the ventricle. Intracardiac echocardiography (ICE) is very useful in aortic cusp assessment and is also capable of showing the ostium of the coronary arteries. Transeptal puncture is extensively discussed in the atrial fibrillation chapter. It is impossible to achieve without the use of ICE or TEE, to prevent perforation and bleeding.

3. Ablation: The higher the force applied and the higher the power delivered at any location, the higher the chances to cause perforation and bleeding. The contact force and power setting applied are independent of the fluoroscopy utilization, but it is a common knowledge the usefulness of fluoroscopy to assess the heart silhouette and the heart moving to rule out perforation and tamponade. To prevent perforation there are different options available: we can use proprietary catheters displaying the force applied (Carto and Abbot have catheters available); but, as it would be too expensive to use these catheters in a daily basis for all substrates, we should also carefully titrate the power delivered based on the location targeted. Most of the sensible locations as the junction of the inferior vena to the cavotricuspid isthmus, the coronary sinus, the right atrial appendage, the superior vena cava, the right ventricular outflow tract, and the aortic cusps rarely need more than 20–30 W to achieve ablation with non-irrigated catheters and 20 W when an irrigated catheter is used. Ablation in the left atrium also needs titration between 30 and 40 W (exception to high power short application time emerging as a new modality of atrial fibrillation ablation). If despite our efforts perforation occurs, to wait until a "silent heart" is observed in fluoroscopy is usually too late, we should recognize faster the complication, to react in a timely manner: Hemodynamic monitoring (arterial line or beat-to-beat blood pressure if patient heavily sedated or general anaesthesia used)

and ultrasound readily available (most of EP labs have now ultrasound machines in the lab) are the best friends to easily recognize a perforation and impending tamponade. Every unexpected drop in blood pressure (even if associated to a vagal phenomenon) should be investigated. Sudden impedance rise and steam popping are ominous markers of charring and perforation if in sensitive areas, they should trigger a quick look ultrasound before continuing RF. Finally, if a pericardiocentesis is needed, ultrasound guided puncture is now the recommended mean to place the drain, making fluoroscopy rarely necessary, even if a complication arise.

Thromboembolic Complications

The more thrombogenic material we put into the vasculature, the higher the risk of thrombosis. There is also a relation between anticoagulation levels used and the risk of bleeding. It should be stated that any bleeding is easier to deal than a thromboembolic complication; if we need to balance bleeding risk versus thromboembolic risk, we should always prefer more bleeding and less thromboembolic events in any setting or ablation procedure.

We routinely administer empiric 5000 units IV of unfractionated heparine once the venous punctures are achieved for any procedure (even right sided), and switch to full anticoagulation (targeting with ACT monitoring depending on ablation type) if for any reason a left-sided access is needed. In atrial fibrillation ablation setting, most of the labs perform now the ablation on uninterrupted warfarine, and there is also evidence that uninterrupted dabigatran is as safe warfarin in this setting [11]. Flutter ablation is also performed with uninterrupted anticoagulation, there is few evidence available, but ablation with uninterrupted warfarine has been tested safer than bridge with heparine, in this setting [12].

The potential need of fewer catheters when a 3-D system is used could contribute to diminish also the risk of thromboembolic complications.

AV Block

In AVNRT, para-Hisian accessory pathways, or any other septal ablation—as some outflow tract ventricular arrhythmias—there is an associated risk of AV block. The goal to prevent AV nodal or His damage is to be able to visualize always catheter movement, a task rarely feasible with fluoroscopy, as it would mean the constant use of radiation; even most conservative labs would not use fluoroscopy every time the radiofrequency is on. 3-D mapping systems allows to visualize all catheters, always, and not only in standard simultaneous RAO and LAO views; but other, multiple and infinite angulations are also possible, depending on the area of interest.

Using 3-D mapping systems for all arrhythmia settings, we have developed the habit to annotate any His recording seen in the virtual anatomy (as only two catheter approach is used, we do not place an extra His catheter), to prevent the ablation catheter to move close.

As we describe in the AVNRT ablation chapter, tagging all His potentials found in the virtual anatomy, we recorded a mean His area of 1.44 cm^2; it is clearly not a fact that a His bundle occupies that big area, but the His displaces with every heart beat and respiratory movements, while our shell of virtual anatomy is a still structure. We judge than working in a non-fluoroscopy environment, no RF lesion should be applied closer than 10 mm far (caudal) from the lowest His found and tagged (Fig. 15.1a, b) [13]. Ablation of para-Hisian accessory pathways is also a challenge, but we should keep in mind that any accessory pathway has always a ventricular insertion (in this case, the para-Hisian one), but also an atrial insertion, with some anecdotic reports showing this insertion sometimes faraway (as aortic cusps) making it safe for RF to ablate [14].

If security versus cost is not a trade-off situation, cryoablation provides—at a higher cost—unsurpassed security while dealing with ablation in the septal area close to the His or AV node. Any cryocatheter can be used with Abbot Nav-X or Boston Rythmia systems; Carto needs a Navistar plugged in order to construct the virtual anatomy to navigate; some centres use a Navistar

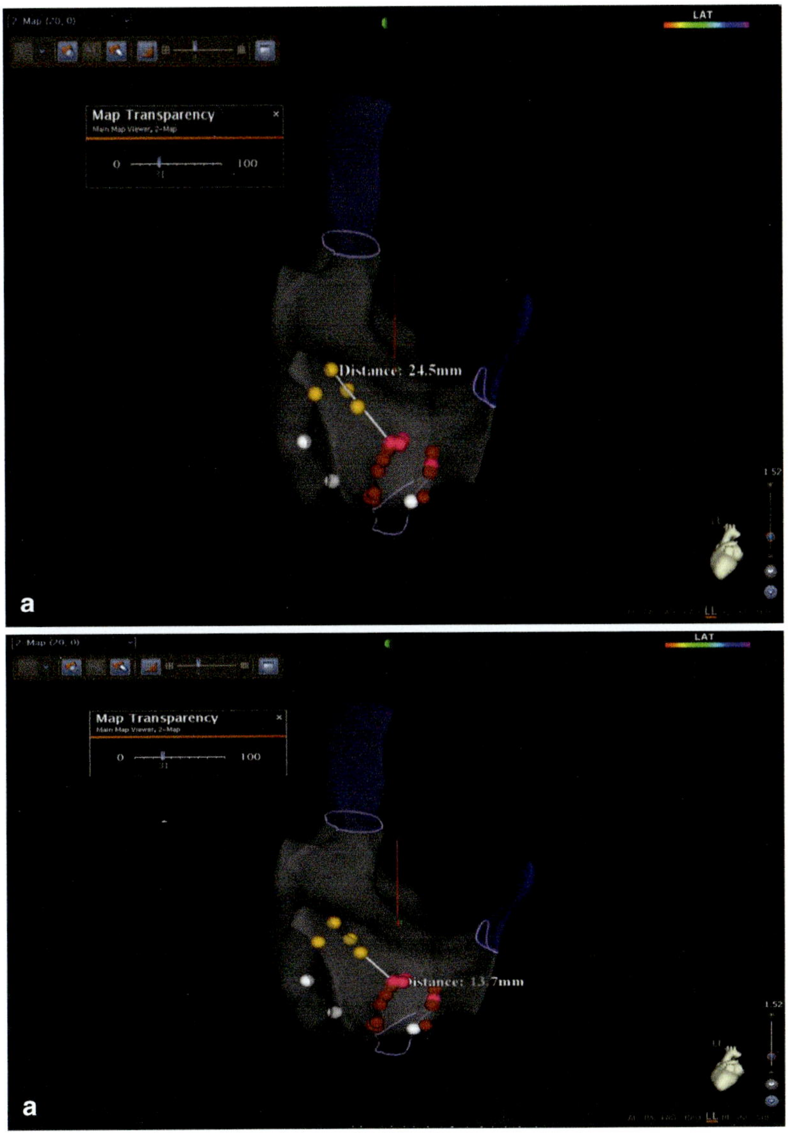

Fig. 15.1 (**a**, **b**) Carto 3 system. LAO for both figures. (**a**) Shows the distance between successful ablation sites and the highest His recorded (usually where a His catheter sits, a comfortable 24.5 mm); (**b**) shows that His signals can be recorded far down, and that the real distance was 13.7 mm from the successful RF site and lowest His recorded

and a cryoablation catheter, especially in young patients; as described in the AVNRT ablation chapter, we use a previous patient Navistar catheter placed in a bag beneath the thoracic region (usually under the mattress) of the new case, the virtual anatomy is then created with a decaNAV catheter, and finally the cryocatheter is now visualized as any other catheter and used for ablation. If there is no data showing when cryoablation is mandatory, when 1% of risk is deemed too high, the newer cryocatheters have shown a similar efficacy profile, with a lesser risk [15].

Catheter Entrapment

One mandatory need of fluoroscopy in a non-fluoroscopic ablation setting is to prevent catheter entrapment. To date we can visualize only the distal part of catheters, when a 3-D mapping system is used to reduce or eliminate fluoroscopy; there are some rare situations when a catheter "loops" while entering in the vasculature, we had in more than 700 procedures done without fluoroscopy, three cases when it occurred. Systematically, the first feature detected was that the catheter was not responding to torque applied in the usual way. While trying to remove the catheter it blocked with the loop entrapped outside the introducer, at the groin level; further effort to remove the catheter "shrinks" the introducer (always with the loop out of it) to a level that it was impossible to either advance neither retrieve the catheter. A vascular surgery was prevented, accessing the vessel from the contralateral groin with a "lasso" catching the tip of the catheter to undo the loop. It can occur either in the venous or in the arterial bed. The advice is, once a catheter is not answering in a standard fashion to torque applied, please use the fluoroscopy, advance the catheter forcing the loop to enter a heart chamber (it is almost impossible to unloop a catheter in the inferior vena cava or the aorta) and turn it to undo the loop; the procedure can be continued then without fluoroscopy (Fig. 15.2).

Finally, a very rare catheter entrapment case happened us also once, using the Rhythmia Orion basket catheter without fluoroscopy: when the case was finished we close the basket catheter and tried to retrieve it but even if it well advanced until the groin level, it was impossible to remove; the fluoroscopy showed the ablation catheter entrapped between the splines of the basket catheter; we advanced the Orion back to the atrium, we open the splines, remove the ablation catheter and then easily retrieve the basket catheter without

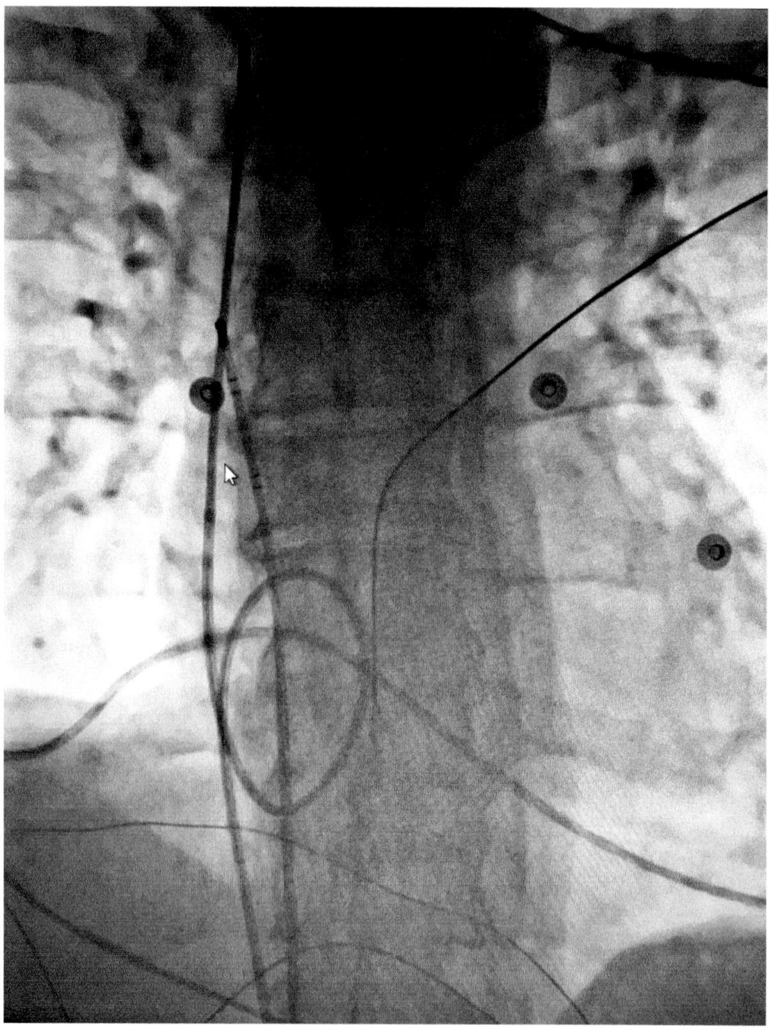

Fig. 15.2 A looped ablation catheter (at the inferior vena cava level) was advanced until the loop entered the right atrium. It was then easy to turn the catheter (the tip is located almost at the cervical level) to undo the loop. If we try to just retrieve the catheter, the loop becomes small and it can be entrapped "shrinking" the introducer at the groin level

further difficulty. We recommend so, to remove all catheters before the basket catheter, and while it is still at the heart level with the splines yet open.

Conclusion

The non-fluoroscopic approach is a feasible and safe alternative to fluoroscopy for any ablation procedure. We have described some methods to prevent and deal with complications that could arise when using this approach. Newer developments on catheter visualization would help to easy our journeys without fluoroscopy.

Finally, we should keep in mind that the main propose of the non-fluoroscopic ablation is to make the procedure safer (for the patient and for the operator). So, we should never have to hesitate in use a few seconds of fluoroscopy trying to avoid further complications if necessary.

References

1. Murakawa Y, Yamane T, Goya M, Inoue K, Naito S, Kumagai K, Miyauchi Y, Morita N, Nogami A, Shoda M, Okumura K, Hirao K, Japanese Heart Rhythm Society Members. Influence of substrate modification in catheter ablation of atrial fibrillation on the incidence of acute complications: analysis of 10 795 procedures in J-CARAF study 2011–2016. J Arrhythm. 2018;34(4):435–40.
2. Latchamsetty R, Yokokawa M, Morady F, Kim HM, Mathew S, Tilz R, Kuck KH, Nagashima K, Tedrow U, Stevenson WG, Yu R, Tung R, Shivkumar K, Sarrazin JF, Arya A, Hindricks G, Vunnam R, Dickfeld T, Daoud EG, Oza NM, Bogun F. Multicenter outcomes for catheter ablation of idiopathic premature ventricular complexes. JACC Clin Electrophysiol. 2015;1(3):116–23.
3. Wang JS, Shen YG, Yin RP, Thapa S, Peng YP, Ji KT, Liao LM, Lin JF, Xue YJ. The safety of catheter ablation for premature ventricular contractions in patients without structural heart disease. BMC Cardiovasc Disord. 2018;18(1):177.
4. Ogunbayo GO, Charnigo R, Darrat Y, Shah J, Patel R, Suffredini J, Wilson W, Parrott K, Kusterer N, Biase LD, Natale A, Morales G, Elayi CS. Comparison of complications of catheter ablation for ventricular arrhythmias in adults with versus without structural heart disease. Am J Cardiol. 2018;122(8):1345–51.
5. Dubin AM, Jorgensen NW, Radbill AE, Bradley DJ, Silva JN, Tsao S, Kanter RJ, Tanel RE, Trivedi B, Young ML, Pflaumer A, McCormack J, Seslar SP. What have we learned in the last 20 years? A comparison of a modern era pediatric and congenital catheter ablation registry to previous pediatric ablation registries. Heart Rhythm. 2019;16(1):57–63. https://doi.org/10.1016/j.hrthm.2018.08.013. pii: S1547-5271(18)30800-2
6. Hosseini SM, Rozen G, Saleh A, Vaid J, Biton Y, Moazzami K, Heist EK, Mansour MC, Kaadan MI, Vangel M, Ruskin JN. Catheter ablation for cardiac arrhythmias: utilization and in-hospital complications, 2000 to 2013. JACC Clin Electrophysiol. 2017;3(11):1240–8.
7. Casella M, Dello Russo A, Pelargonio G, Del Greco M, Zingarini G, Piacenti M, Di Cori A, Casula V, Marini M, Pizzamiglio F, Zucchetti M, Riva S, Russo E, Narducci ML, Soldati E, Panchetti L, Startari U, Bencardino G, Perna F, Santangeli P, Di Biase L, Cichocki F, Fattore G, Bongiorni M, Picano E, Natale A, Tondo C. Near zerO fluoroscopic exPosure during catheter ablAtion of supRavenTricular arrhYthmias: the NO-PARTY multicentre randomized trial. Europace. 2016;18(10):1565–72.
8. Sommer P, Bertagnolli L, Kircher S, Arya A, Bollmann A, Richter S, Rolf S, Hindricks G. Safety profile of near-zero fluoroscopy atrial fibrillation ablation with non-fluoroscopic catheter visualization: experience from 1000 consecutive procedures. Europace. 2018;20(12):1952–8.
9. Aytemir K, Canpolat U, Yorgun H, Evranos B, Kaya EB, Sahiner ML, Ozer N. Usefulness of 'figure-of-eight' suture to achieve haemostasis after removal of 15-French calibre femoral venous sheath in patients undergoing cryoablation. Europace. 2016;18:1545–50.
10. Kottmaier M, Bourier F, Reents T, Reiter A, Kornmayer M, Semmler V, Telishevska M, Koch-Büttner K, Deiss M, Brooks S, Grebmer C, Lennerz C, Kolb C, Hessling G, Deisenhofer I. Safety and feasibility of subcutaneous purse-string suture of the femoral vein after electrophysiological procedures on uninterrupted oral anticoagulation. Am J Cardiol. 2017;119(11):1781–4.
11. Calkins H, Willems S, Gerstenfeld EP, Verma A, Schilling R, Hohnloser SH, Okumura K, Serota H, Nordaby M, Guiver K, Biss B, Brouwer MA, Grimaldi M, RE-CIRCUIT Investigators. Uninterrupted dabigatran versus warfarin for ablation in atrial fibrillation. N Engl J Med. 2017;376(17):1627–36.
12. Finlay M, Sawhney V, Schilling R, Thomas G, Duncan E, Hunter R, Virdi G, Abrams D, Sporton S, Dhinoja M, Earley M. Uninterrupted warfarin for periprocedural anticoagulation in catheter ablation of typical atrial flutter: a safe and cost-effective strategy. J Cardiovasc Electrophysiol. 2010;21(2):150–4.
13. Chaumont J, Al Baridi E, Roux J-F, Badra M, Arseneau F, Ayala-Paredes F. His area is closer than expected to RF ablation lesions in AVNR Tachycardia. Abstract 612. CCS Congress. October 30, 2012. Toronto. Canada. Can J Cardiol. 2012;28(5):S327.

14. Liao Z, Zhan X, Wu S. Successful radiofrequency ablation of a parahisian accessory pathway from the right coronary cusp. Int J Cardiol. 2015;186:41–2.
15. Wells P, Dubuc M, Klein GJ, Dan D, Roux JF, et al. Intracardiac ablation for atrioventricular nodal re-entry tachycardia using a 6 mm distal electrode cryoablation catheter: prospective, multicenter, North American study (ICY-AVNRT). J Cardiovasc Electrophysiol. 2018;29(1):167–76.

Safety of Zero-Fluoroscopic Catheter Ablation During Pregnancy

16

Matevž Jan, David Žižek, Vesna Fabjan Vodušek, and Bor Antolič

Introduction

Incidence of all types of arrhythmias is higher during pregnancy. Li et al. reported an incidence of 166 per 100,000 unselected pregnancy-related hospital admissions [1]. The majority of symptomatic cardiac rhythm disturbances are benign with sinus tachycardia being the most common. Supra-ventricular tachycardia (SVT) is the most prevalent type of sustained tachycardia, followed by atrial fibrillation (AF) and flutter (AFL). Ventricular tachycardias (VTs) can occur but are infrequent. Furthermore, various tachycardia recurrences during pregnancy are frequent in women with previously documented tachycardias. Recurrences can be as high as 50%, 52%, and 27% for SVT, AF/AFL, and VTs, respectively [2]. Fortunately, clinically significant tachyarrhythmias are rare during normal pregnancy.

When maternal tachycardias cause hemodynamic compromise, they could account for adverse fetal complications. Thus, early recognition of the type of tachycardia, followed by timely and effective treatment are main goals of patient management. Arrhythmia management relies on anti-arrhythmic drugs (AADs) and catheter ablation (CA). As certain AADs may cross the placental barrier, careful consideration should be given in selecting the medication to prevent adverse effects on the fetus. Although catheter ablation for various arrhythmias is now widely regarded as the therapy of choice in the nonpregnant patients, there has been a hesitation to perform CA during pregnancy [3–5]. First, CA is an invasive procedure and procedure-related complications can cause harm to the gravid patient and the fetus. Second, CA is traditionally performed with the use of fluoroscopy that causes radiation exposure that can be potentially harmful to maternal health and fetal development.

This chapter will deal with fluoroless approach to catheter ablation and its safety during pregnancy.

Changes in Physiology During Pregnancy Relevant to Occurrence of Arrhythmias

During pregnancy there are some changes in cardiovascular physiology that result in two major hemodynamic changes: fall in systemic

M. Jan (✉)
Department of Cardiovascular Surgery, University Medical Centre Ljubljana, Ljubljana, Slovenia

D. Žižek · B. Antolič
Department of Cardiology, University Medical Centre Ljubljana, Ljubljana, Slovenia

V. Fabjan Vodušek
Department of Gynecology and Perinatology, University Medical Centre Ljubljana, Ljubljana, Slovenia
e-mail: vesna.fabjan@mf.uni-lj.si

R. Proietti et al. (eds.), *Cardiac Electrophysiology Without Fluoroscopy*,
https://doi.org/10.1007/978-3-030-16992-3_16

vascular resistance and increase in cardiac output. Cardiovascular and hemodynamic changes begin as early as in the fourth week of gestation and persist for several months postpartum. The largest change in the cardiac output starts at about 22–24 weeks. Systemic vascular resistance decreases, heart rate increases by 15–20 beats/min, and preload increases due to an increase in blood volume. These changes result in a 30–50% increase in cardiac output above baseline. Also occurring is a physiological dilution anemia due to a 50% increase in plasma volume accompanied by a 30% increase in red blood cell mass [6].

Pregnancy is associated with an increased thromboembolic risk due to lower extremity venous stasis resulting from inferior vena cava compression by the gravid uterus, and to a hyper-coagulable state due to an increase in vitamin K dependent clotting factors and a reduction in free protein S [7].

During labor, cardiac output progressively increases due to pain, anxiety, and auto-transfusion during contractions. Stroke volume and heart rate rise and fall with each contraction, with peaks as high as 50% above pre-labor values [8].

Immediately after either vaginal or cesarean delivery, cardiac output peaks as the evacuated uterus contracts and blood from myometrial veins is auto-transfused into the systemic venous system. Also, the contracted uterus lifts off the vena cava, resulting in greater venous blood return to the heart, which increases the stroke volume. In fact, within the first 10 min following a term vaginal delivery, cardiac output increases by about 59% and stroke volume by about 71% [9]. Due to the described hemodynamic changes acting as a "natural stress test" it seems obvious that various symptoms and conditions related to heart disease become evident during pregnancy and labor. Thus, arrhythmias are the most common cardiac complication encountered during pregnancy in women with and without structural heart disease [7].

Available Data on Catheter Ablation Without the Use of Fluoroscopy During Pregnancy

CA for treatment of various tachyarrhythmias is gaining widespread adoption, as recent studies show not only symptomatic but also mortality benefit [10, 11]. As more centers start performing CA procedures in a diverse population of patients, specific safety accommodations should be recognized to limit complications in specific subpopulation of patients.

Only few case reports and small series of patients are available on completely fluoroless CA in pregnant patients (Table 16.1). According to the data in the described publications CAs were performed for various SVTs and frequent PVCs. There are no reports on fluoroless CA for VTs related to structural heart disease and AF in pregnant patients. There is some data available in the literature regarding non-randomized comparison of fluoroless and fluoro-based CA in nonpregnant population for various SVTs, frequent PVCs, and other tachyarrhythmias which indicates that procedural time and success rates are similar regardless of fluoroscopy use [21–25]. In addition, complication rates are similar in both techniques.

Possible Complications of Catheter Ablation During Pregnancy

Complications related to CA procedure can result from radiation exposure, vascular access (access site related hemorrhage, hematoma and arteriovenous fistula, deep venous thrombosis, pneumothorax), catheter manipulation (valvular damage, myocardial wall/coronary sinus perforation with tamponade, coronary artery dissection), and delivery of RF energy (AV block, myocardial wall perforation with tamponade, coronary artery occlusion, thromboembolic stroke or TIA). The most common complications of CA according to the type of tachycardia are listed in Table 16.2. Very limited information is available on complication rates of CA in pregnancy. However, we can only assume that safety profile of ablation procedures for different tachycardia types in pregnancy is likely similar to the one reported in the nonpregnant population.

Hemodynamically important complications such as cardiac tamponade and complete AV block can cause hypoxemia in the fetus which can, in the worst-case scenario, end in fetal distress and even intrauterine death. The end result is dependent on

Table 16.1 Publications on fluoroless CA in pregnant patients

Author, year of publication	Number of cases	Tachycardia type	Indication for procedure	Outcome	Complications
Ferguson (2011) [12]	1	Focal AT	Incessant, drug-resistant tachycardia causing tachycardia-related cardiomyopathy	Successful	No
Leiria (2014) [13]	1	AVRT	Drug-resistant recurrent tachycardias with syncope	Successful	No
Bigelow (2015) [14]	1	AVNRT	Incessant, drug-resistant tachycardia	Successful	No
Chen (2016) [15]	2	PVC; AVRT	Drug-resistant frequent PVCs; frequent very symptomatic AVRTs	Both procedures successful	No
Kozluk (2017) [16]	11	3 WPWs; 2 AVNRTs, PJRT, 3 ATs, 2 PVCs	Not specified	1 recurrence	No
Karbarz (2017) [17]	1	WPW	Recurrent very symptomatic tachycardias	Successful	No
Prolič Kalinšek (2017) [18]	1	AVRT	Drug-resistant recurrent very symptomatic tachycardias	Successful	No
Rossi (2017) [19]	1	AVRT	Drug-resistant tachycardia	Successful	No
Jan (2018) [20]	1	Focal AT	Incessant, drug-resistant tachycardia causing tachycardia-related cardiomyopathy	Successful	No

AT atrial tachycardia, *AVRT* atrio-ventricular reentrant tachycardia, *AVNRT* atrio-ventricular nodal reentrant tachycardia, *WPW* Wolff-Parkinson-White syndrome, *PJRT* persistent junctional reciprocating tachycardia, *PVC* premature ventricular complex

the duration of the hypoxemia. A short-lasting hypoxemia with fast and effective resuscitation and reversal of the hemodynamic compromise in the mother usually do not have long-term effect on the development of the fetus. However, if the hypoxemia lasts more than 10 min it usually causes severe fetal distress and results in some degree of acute ischemic brain injury. This 10-min time interval of the effect of hypoxemia was deduced from several clinical cases using fetal surveillance with the cardio-tocogram (CTG) in various obstetrical complications that influence uterine perfusion (uterine rupture, hypertonus, placental abruption, etc.) [33].

Safety of Common Drugs Used During Catheter Ablation Procedures

Unfractionated heparin (UFH) is used as an anticoagulant during left-sided CA procedures, i.e., when ablation in the left atrium, left ventricle, or aortic root is needed. Serious side effects are bleeding and heparin-induced thrombocytopenia. Heparin appears to be relatively safe for use during pregnancy (FDA group C).

Protamine sulfate is a medication that is used to reverse the effects of heparin. It can be used during CA to reverse the effect of heparin at the end of the procedure or when bleeding occurs as a side effect of heparin use. Common side effects in pregnancy and also after birth include low blood pressure, slow heart rate, allergic reactions, dyspnea, and vomiting. While there is no evidence of harm from using it during pregnancy it has not been well studied in pregnant patients, so the FDA rules it in group C.

Isoprenaline is a medication used during CA for induction of tachycardia, often together with fast or programmed atrial or ventricular stimulation. It is a nonselective β adrenoreceptor agonist that is the isopropyl-amine analog of epinephrine (adrenaline). Common side effects include

Table 16.2 Publications on complications of CA according to the tachycardia type

Author, year of publication	Number of cases	Tachycardia type	Type of complication	Complication rate	Use of fluoroscopy	Inclusion of pregnant patients
Gupta (2013) [26]	Systematic review	AF	All Stroke/TIA Tamponade DVT/PE Pneumothorax Hemothorax Vascular complications	2.9% 0.6% 1% 0.15% 0.2% 0.2% 1.4%	Yes	No
Rodriguez-Entem (2013) [27]	119 (cryo + RF group)	AVNRT	Complete AV block in the RF group	1%	Yes	No
Estner (2005) [28]	506	AVNRT	Complete AV block (procedurally + follow-up)	1%	Yes	No
Ceresnak (2015) [29]	650 (cryo+RF)	AVRT	NS	0%	Yes	No
Busch (2018) [30]	413	AT	All Vascular complication Pericardial effusion Phrenic palsy Nonfatal atrio-esophageal fistula	2.4% 1% 1% 0.02% 0.02%	Yes	No
Latchamsetty (2015) [31]	1185	Idiopathic PVCs	All Tamponade Vascular complications Complete AV block	2.4% 0.8% 1.3% 0.1%	Yes	No
Peichl (2014) [32]	473	Structural heart disease-related VT	All Perforation of the heart Thromboembolism Complete AV block Vascular complications	8% 0.6% 0.8% 1% 4.7%	Yes	No

nervousness, headache, dizziness, nausea, visual blurring, palpitations, angina pectoris, hypotension, dyspnea, tremors, weakness, and pallor. Isoprenaline is ruled in group C according to the FDA.

Conclusion

Catheter ablation of various tachycardias without the use of fluoroscopy is becoming an established method with comparable success rates and safety profile compared to fluoro-based procedures. It seems that pregnant patients with tachycardias are the ideal target population for this new and emerging method. Limited evidence in the form of case reports or small retrospective case series has reported CA in pregnancy to be effective with no maternal and fetal complications. However, the evidence is scant and further research is needed in this area, particularly comparing the risks of therapy with anti-arrhythmic drugs and ablation therapy with no or minimal fluoroscopy. Drug therapy should be judiciously used, understanding physiological changes (increase of distribution volumes during pregnancy requires at least to double standard doses used in nonpregnant patients or to reduce the dosing interval to achieve effective plasma concentrations). Recent advances in nonfluoroscopic catheter navigation have helped minimize the radiation exposure during ablation. Such techniques could lower the threshold to perform ablation in pregnant women and thus avoid use of potentially harmful and less effective medications.

Thus, it seems prudent to still generally follow the recommendations of the ECS Guidelines on the management if cardiovascular disease during pregnancy to try ADD as the first-line treatment and proceed to CA (IIb indication) in case of drug-resistant tachycardia causing severe symptoms [6]. In case of development of tachycardia-induced cardiomyopathy or hemodynamic compromise causing fetal distress, the anti-arrhythmic drug trial should be short lived and possibility of urgent CA kept in mind. In the absence of clear guidelines and evidence, the decision on treatment management should be made by using a multidisciplinary approach with a careful and well-documented risk benefit discussion with the patient.

It is clear that invasive procedures are, to date, the last resort, when approaching a pregnant patient, nonetheless, we should be prepared to succeed in this setting, having acquired confidence and effectiveness in non-fluoro ablation in standard, nonpregnant patients; a pregnant patient should be never the first non-fluoro case to approach.

References

1. Li JM, Nguyen C, Joglar JA, Hamdan MH, Page RL. Frequency and outcome of arrhythmias complicating admission during pregnancy: experience from a high-volume and ethnically-diverse obstetric service. Clin Cardiol. 2008;31(11):538–41.
2. Silversides CK, Harris L, Haberer K, Sermer M, Colman JM, Siu SC. Recurrence rates of arrhythmias during pregnancy in women with previous tachyarrhythmia and impact on fetal and neonatal outcomes. Am J Cardiol. 2006;97(8):1206–12.
3. Blomström-Lundqvist C, Scheinman MM, Aliot EM, Alpert JS, Calkins H, Camm AJ, Campbell WB, Haines DE, Kuck KH, Lerman BB, Miller DD, Shaeffer CW Jr, Stevenson WG, Tomaselli GF, Antman EM, Smith SC Jr, Alpert JS, Faxon DP, Fuster V, Gibbons RJ, Gregoratos G, Hiratzka LF, Hunt SA, Jacobs AK, Russell RO Jr, Priori SG, Blanc JJ, Budaj A, Burgos EF, Cowie M, Deckers JW, Garcia MA, Klein WW, Lekakis J, Lindahl B, Mazzotta G, Morais JC, Oto A, Smiseth O, Trappe HJ, American College of Cardiology; American Heart Association Task Force on Practice Guidelines; European Society of Cardiology Committee for Practice Guidelines. Writing Committee to Develop Guidelines for the Management of Patients with Supraventricular Arrhythmias. ACC/AHA/ESC guidelines for the management of patients with supraventricular arrhythmias—executive summary: a report of the American College of Cardiology/American Heart Association Task Force on Practice Guidelines and the European Society of Cardiology Committee for Practice Guidelines (Writing Committee to Develop Guidelines for the Management of Patients With Supraventricular Arrhythmias). Circulation. 2003;108(15):1871–909.
4. Priori SG, Blomström-Lundqvist C, Mazzanti A, Blom N, Borggrefe M, Camm J, Elliott PM, Fitzsimons D, Hatala R, Hindricks G, Kirchhof P, Kjeldsen K, Kuck KH, Hernandez-Madrid A, Nikolaou N, Norekvål TM, Spaulding C, Van Veldhuisen DJ, Task Force for the Management of Patients with Ventricular Arrhythmias and the Prevention of Sudden Cardiac Death of the European Society of Cardiology (ESC). 2015 ESC Guidelines for the management of patients with ventricular arrhythmias and the prevention of sudden cardiac death: The Task Force for the management of patients with Ventricular Arrhythmias and the Prevention of Sudden Cardiac Death of the European Society of Cardiology (ESC)Endorsed by: Association for European Paediatric and Congenital Cardiology (AEPC). Europace. 2015;17(11):1601–87.
5. Kirchhof P, Benussi S, Kotecha D, Ahlsson A, Atar D, Casadei B, Castella M, Diener HC, Heidbuchel H, Hendriks J, Hindricks G, Manolis AS, Oldgren J, Popescu BA, Schotten U, Van Putte B, Vardas P, ESC Scientific Document Group. 2016 ESC Guidelines for the management of atrial fibrillation developed in collaboration with EACTS. Eur Heart J. 2016;37(38):2893–962.
6. European Society of Gynecology (ESG); Association for European Paediatric Cardiology (AEPC); German Society for Gender Medicine (DGesGM), Regitz-Zagrosek V, Blomstrom Lundqvist C, Borghi C, Cifkova R, Ferreira R, Foidart JM, Gibbs JS, Gohlke-Baerwolf C, Gorenek B, Iung B, Kirby M, Maas AH, Morais J, Nihoyannopoulos P, Pieper PG, Presbitero P, Roos-Hesselink JW, Schaufelberger M, Seeland U, Torracca L, ESC Committee for Practice Guidelines. ESC Guidelines on the management of cardiovascular diseases during pregnancy: the Task Force on the Management of Cardiovascular Diseases during Pregnancy of the European Society of Cardiology (ESC). Eur Heart J. 2011;32(24):3147–9.
7. Drenthen W, Pieper PG, Roos-Hesselink JW, van Lottum WA, Voors AA, Mulder BJ, van Dijk AP, Vliegen HW, Yap SC, Moons P, Ebels T, Van Veldhuisen DJ, ZAHARA Investigators. Outcome of pregnancy in women with congenital heart disease: a literature review. J Am Coll Cardiol. 2007;49(24):2303–11.
8. Ueland K, Hansen JM. Maternal cardiovascular dynamics. II. Posture and uterine contractions. Am J Obstet Gynecol. 1969;103(1):1–7.

9. Kjeldsen J. Hemodynamic investigations during labour and delivery. Acta Obstet Gynecol Scand Suppl. 1979;89:1.
10. Marrouche NF, Brachmann J, Andresen D, Siebels J, Boersma L, Jordaens L, Merkely B, Pokushalov E, Sanders P, Proff J, Schunkert H, Christ H, Vogt J, Bänsch D, CASTLE-AF Investigators. Catheter ablation for atrial fibrillation with heart failure. N Engl J Med. 2018;378(5):417–27.
11. Tung R, Vaseghi M, Frankel DS, Vergara P, Di Biase L, Nagashima K, Yu R, Vangala S, Tseng CH, Choi EK, Khurshid S, Patel M, Mathuria N, Nakahara S, Tzou WS, Sauer WH, Vakil K, Tedrow U, Burkhardt JD, Tholakanahalli VN, Saliaris A, Dickfeld T, Weiss JP, Bunch TJ, Reddy M, Kanmanthareddy A, Callans DJ, Lakkireddy D, Natale A, Marchlinski F, Stevenson WG, Della Bella P, Shivkumar K. Freedom from recurrent ventricular tachycardia after catheter ablation is associated with improved survival in patients with structural heart disease: an International VT Ablation Center Collaborative Group study. Heart Rhythm. 2015;12(9):1997–2007.
12. Ferguson JD, Helms A, Mangrum JM, DiMarco JP. Ablation of incessant left atrial tachycardia without fluoroscopy in a pregnant woman. J Cardiovasc Electrophysiol. 2011;22(3):346–9.
13. Leiria TL, Martins Pires L, Lapa Kruse M, Glotz de Lima G. Supraventricular tachycardia and syncope during pregnancy: a case for catheter ablation without fluoroscopy. Rev Port Cardiol. 2014;33(12):805.e1–5.
14. Bigelow AM, Crane SS, Khoury FR, Clark JM. Catheter ablation of supraventricular tachycardia without fluoroscopy during pregnancy. Obstet Gynecol. 2015;125(6):1338–41.
15. Chen G, Sun G, Xu R, Chen X, Yang L, Bai Y, Yang S, Guo P, Zhang Y, Zhao C, Wang DW, Wang Y. Zero-fluoroscopy catheter ablation of severe drug-resistant arrhythmia guided by Ensite NavX system during pregnancy: two case reports and literature review. Medicine (Baltimore). 2016;95(32):e4487.
16. Koźluk E, Piątkowska A, Kiliszek M, Lodziński P, Małkowska S, Balsam P, Rodkiewicz D, Piątkowski R, Zyśko D, Opolski G. Catheter ablation of cardiac arrhythmias in pregnancy without fluoroscopy: a case control retrospective study. Adv Clin Exp Med. 2017;26(1):129–34.
17. Karbarz D, Stec PJ, Deutsch K, Śledź J, Stec S. Zero-fluoroscopy catheter ablation of symptomatic pre-excitation from non-coronary cusp during pregnancy. Kardiol Pol. 2017;75(12):1351.
18. Prolič Kalinšek T, Jan M, Rupar K, Ražen L, Antolič B, Žižek D. Zero-fluoroscopy catheter ablation of concealed left accessory pathway in a pregnant woman. Europace. 2017;19(8):1384.
19. Rossi L, Penela D, Villani GQ. Intracardiac echocardiography catheter-guided zero fluoroscopy transseptal puncture technique for ablation of left-sided accessory pathway in a pregnant woman. Europace. 2017;19(11):1825.
20. Jan M, Ružič Medvešček N, Fabjan VV. Zero-fluoroscopy catheter ablation of focal atrial tachycardia in a pregnant woman with tachycardia induced cardiomyopathy. Zdrav Vestn. 2018;87(3–4):163–6.
21. Jan M, Žižek D, Rupar K, Mazić U, Kuhelj D, Lakič N, Geršak B. Fluoroless catheter ablation of various right and left sided supra-ventricular tachycardias in children and adolescents. Int J Cardiovasc Imaging. 2016;32(11):1609–16.
22. Stec S, Śledź J, Mazij M, Raś M, Ludwik B, Chrabąszcz M, Śledź A, Banasik M, Bzymek M, Młynarczyk K, Deutsch K, Labus M, Śpikowski J, Szydłowski L. "Feasibility of implementation of a simplified, No-X-Ray, no-lead apron, two-catheter approach" for ablation of supraventricular arrhythmias in children and adults. J Cardiovasc Electrophysiol. 2014;25(8):866–74.
23. Fernández-Gómez JM, Moriña-Vázquez P, Morales Edel R, Venegas-Gamero J, Barba-Pichardo R, Carranza MH. Exclusion of fluoroscopy use in catheter ablation procedures: six years of experience at a single center. J Cardiovasc Electrophysiol. 2014;25(6):638–44.
24. Wang Y, Chen GZ, Yao Y, Bai Y, Chu HM, Ma KZ, Liew R, Liu H, Zhong GQ, Xue YM, Wu SL, Li YF, Zhao CX, Liu QG, Lin L, Wang L, Wang DW. Ablation of idiopathic ventricular arrhythmia using zero-fluoroscopy approach with equivalent efficacy and less fatigue: a multicenter comparative study. Medicine (Baltimore). 2017;96(6):e6080.
25. Razminia M, Willoughby MC, Demo H, Keshmiri H, Wang T, D'Silva OJ, Zheutlin TA, Jibawi H, Okhumale P, Kehoe RF. Fluoroless catheter ablation of cardiac arrhythmias: a 5-year experience. Pacing Clin Electrophysiol. 2017;40(4):425–33.
26. Gupta A, Perera T, Ganesan A, Sullivan T, Lau DH, Roberts-Thomson KC, Brooks AG, Sanders P. Complications of catheter ablation of atrial fibrillation: a systematic review. Circ Arrhythm Electrophysiol. 2013;6(6):1082–8.
27. Rodriguez-Entem FJ, Expósito V, Gonzalez-Enriquez S, Olalla-Antolin JJ. Cryoablation versus radiofrequency ablation for the treatment of atrioventricular nodal reentrant tachycardia: results of a prospective randomized study. J Interv Card Electrophysiol. 2013;36(1):41–5.
28. Estner HL, Ndrepepa G, Dong J, Deisenhofer I, Schreieck J, Schneider M, Plewan A, Karch M, Weyerbrock S, Wade D, Zrenner B, Schmitt C. Acute and long-term results of slow pathway ablation in patients with atrioventricular nodal reentrant tachycardia--an analysis of the predictive factors for arrhythmia recurrence. Pacing Clin Electrophysiol. 2005;28(2):102–10.
29. Ceresnak SR, Dubin AM, Kim JJ, Valdes SO, Fishberger SB, Shetty I, Zimmerman F, Tanel RE, Epstein MR, Motonaga KS, Capone CA, Nappo L, Gates GJ, Pass RH. Success rates in pediatric WPW ablation are improved with 3-dimensional mapping systems compared with fluoroscopy alone:

a multicenter study. J Cardiovasc Electrophysiol. 2015;26(4):412–6.

30. Busch S, Forkmann M, Kuck KH, Lewalter T, Ince H, Straube F, Wieneke H, Julian Chun KR, Eckardt L, Schmitt C, Hochadel M, Senges J, Brachmann J. Acute and long-term outcome of focal atrial tachycardia ablation in the real world: results of the german ablation registry. Clin Res Cardiol. 2018;107(5):430–6.
31. Latchamsetty R, Yokokawa M, Morady F, Kim HM, Mathew S, Tilz R, Kuck KH, Nagashima K, Tedrow U, Stevenson WG, Yu R, Tung R, Shivkumar K, Sarrazin JF, Arya A, Hindricks G, Vunnam R, Dickfeld T, Daoud EG, Oza NM, Bogun F. Multicenter outcomes for catheter ablation of idiopathic premature ventricular complexes. JACC Clin Electrophysiol. 2015;1(3):116–23.
32. Peichl P, Wichterle D, Pavlu L, Cihak R, Aldhoon B, Kautzner J. Complications of catheter ablation of ventricular tachycardia: a single-center experience. Circ Arrhythm Electrophysiol. 2014;7(4):684–90.
33. Rennie J, Rosenbloom L. How long have we got to get the baby out? A review of the effects of acute and profound intrapartum hypoxia and ischaemia. Obstet Gynaecol. 2011;13:169–74.

17 Cost Optimization When Using 3-D Mapping Systems for a Non-fluoroscopic EP Lab

Pablo Moriña Vazquez and Félix Ayala-Paredes

Introduction

The days of radiation and fluoroscopy as a mean to guide catheters inside the heart in the EP lab are counted. Awareness from EP physicians and health personnel trends to reduce fluoroscopy utilization, not only to reduce impact of radiation on patients, but also to reduce the higher impact on the EP personnel exposed to radiation in an everyday basis (Chap. 2 is dedicated to this matter); in the next paragraphs we describe how to expand 3-D mapping system utilization and how to justify the increment in cost expected.

Components of Cost at the EP Lab

It would be too simple to ascribe cost only to the material used for each procedure, of course there is cost related to the consumable or expandable material, but even this cost varies widely around the world, as many countries accept the reutilization of single-use catheters for EP procedures. We will analyze all components of cost at the EP lab, and how 3-D mapping systems could actually help in cost content, using different strategies.

- **EP lab construction:** The highest piece of cost at any EP lab is actually the fluoroscopy equipment; it requires the construction of a special room, with radiation blinding, and with a structure to support the heavy weight of single or biplane systems. The cost to set up a new EP lab counts for 4–5 times the marketed price of any 3-D mapping system. We can argue that we do need anyway the lab to perform EP procedures, but, what if 90% of EP procedures could be done outside the EP lab? This is the case now. Most of single centers reporting their experience on non-fluoroscopic procedures (all substrates: left sided and atrial fibrillation included) achieve in 90–100% of cases a total fluoroscopy-free procedure [1–4]. When less experienced or all comer operators report their results, there is also a 80–90% of chances that a case finishes without the need of any fluoroscopy [5, 6]. It is then tempting to perform procedures outside the EP lab, so we can eliminate the cost of an EP lab; this approach has been already tested by a pediatric center, left-sided ablations included, with same results, same complication rate, and no need of fluoroscopy in either environment (neither at the cath lab nor at the operating room used for this experience) [7]. We can affirm that ablation of most substrates, with a

P. Moriña Vazquez
Arrhythmia and Pacing Unit,
Hospital Juan Ramon Jiménez, Huelva, Spain

F. Ayala-Paredes (✉)
Division of Cardiology, Centre Hospitalier
Universitaire de Sherbrooke, Sherbrooke, Canada
e-mail: felix.ayala-paredes@usherbrooke.ca

R. Proietti et al. (eds.), *Cardiac Electrophysiology Without Fluoroscopy*,
https://doi.org/10.1007/978-3-030-16992-3_17

3-D mapping system only use, outside the traditional EP or cath lab will be the norm in following years, thus reducing the cost of building new and expensive cath or EP labs. In the rare case the fluorsocopy is needed, to use a mobile digital X-ray equipment (widely available in all institutions) is a cost-conscious option, providing enough detail with a fraction of the cost of the standard EP lab.

- **Consumables, catheters, and patches**: As many places in the world reuse catheters intended to single use (a survey published in 2001 showed that in the USA, 49% of EP labs reprocess and reuse catheter to a some extent [8]), most of 3-D mapping system providers have developed different strategies to force to adhere to a single-use policy of at least some part of their system components. EnSite NavX™, one of the systems mostly utilized, is an open platform; any catheter can be used, so they base their business model selling the patches needed at around twice the price of any standard ablation catheter; they have evolved now to the EnSite Precision™ (latest version) that better perform with the use of proprietary sensor-enabled diagnostic and ablation catheters. Carto™ uses since the beginning proprietary sensor ablation catheters with cost escalating at least at four times the cost of a standard ablation catheters, the patches needed are marketed at very low price, encouraging users to start a case always with the patches on board in case Carto™ is needed later during the case because of a clinical reason. Rhythmia™ started with a proprietary unsurpassed diagnostic ultra density mapping basket catheter, marketed around ten times the cost of any standard ablation catheter, and there are also now available sensor-enabled proprietary catheters, matching Carto™ features. Cost of consumables is, however, a business moving target; the less units a company sell, the higher the price that consumable needs to be marketed; in other words: we can deal the price on volume: if a 3-D mapping system is used 3–5 times a day instead of only once or twice a week, prices could go down. In our lab where strict single-catheter use policy is in place, we started with one of the three providers, we calculate the cost of a standard procedure using 4–5 catheters, we agreed on how much more we could bear as an extra cost for a bundled non-fluoro kit (patches, ablation catheter and coronary sinus catheter, as we judged that for most of standard cases a two catheter approach would be enough) and we now use that kit for every patient. Once the first agreement was achieved, we approached the other two providers, and we informed them that if they wanted to do business with us, they should match the non-fluoro kit bundled price; and they did. As a beneficial side effects (for both sides) we never cancel now a difficult arrhythmia substrate (in the past as the provider representative technician needed to be scheduled, we ended some times in EP study only and scheduling the case for a later date with a 3-D mapping system), and even if this cost has not been calculated yet, it cuts hospital and consumables costs; companies can also save as their technicians are not longer always needed, and they can even train their technicians at our lab (ours have become independent and due to our high volume). Another way to save money is to rely on most company policies where always a new—and expensive—catheter is developed with time. Most of simple substrate arrhythmias need also a standard catheter, and as for complex ablation targets sensor-based, irrigated, and force-measuring catheters are now the norm, there is less need and a surplus of standard noncontact force, nonirrigated catheters still produced and less and less utilized other than for non-fluoroscopic approaches. Every country and every institution has its own policy when acquiring 3-D mapping systems (purchasing with lower consumable costs versus leasing and higher consumable cost); in all cases an agreement can be obtained with one or more providers, based on volume to deal a win-win scenario.
- **Patients and health personnel work force**: There should be no cost trading to prevent a cancer at a later stage in life (either for a patient or health provider), or to prevent

lumbar (four times higher in EP physicians than non-interventional cardiologists in Canada [9]) or cervical spondylosis. There is no safe radiation exposure for pregnant patients needing an invasive EP procedure (a need appearing four times in our first 300 patients), and policies in most labs prevent further work in a standard EP lab for any member of the personnel once pregnancy has been confirmed due to radiation exposure risk. A small but increasing trend in most EP labs is also the choice of this field for more and more female physicians, nurses, and technicians: in 2003 only 8% of all cardiologist were female in the USA [10], but a more recent German survey showed an increase of female cardiologist training in EP from 26% in 2010 to 38% in 2015 [11]. There are some economic models derived from a randomized Italian study (NO-PARTY trial, assigning patients to conventional fluoroscopy or minimally fluoroscopic approach—MFA—for supraventricular arrhythmias with EnSite NavX™); the study showed a complete elimination of fluoroscopy in 72% of patients assigned to MFA; however this was enough to model a reduction of 96% of the risk of cancer incidence and mortality in the MFA group, and to consider the cost increment due to 3-D mapping system utilization, affordable for most European countries [6]. Another study on cost-effectiveness on a pediatric population stated that modeling for an effective dose reduction of 2.8 mSv per procedure, the additional cost incurred was not cost-effective for most countries, but when a children correction factor was added, the use of 3-D mapping systems is cost-effective [12]. If these models using modest exposure reductions, work for patients, imagine how much more they should work for physicians (the ones closer to the X-ray source) and health care personal, exposed in busy labs to constant radiation; there are no models yet on this matter as all interventional cardiologists we have grown with fluoroscopy as a friend; newer generations would see the benefits of working in a fluoroscopy-free EP lab. Once more, we prone that cost-effectiveness is a moving target, only incremental cost of 3-D mappings is calculated in most models; once this technique becomes widely adopted, cost of hardware will decrease; and once we use less and less fluoroscopy effective dose reductions will be even greater. In the mean time we cannot wait and we should be prepared when a pregnant patient needs our expertise, or the more frequent scenario: when a female health care provider wants to continue her professional career while pregnant.

Cost Containment When Using 3-D Mapping Systems for All Cases at the EP Lab

As we mention before, using a 3-D mapping system for everyday cases, prepares for success: there is no arrhythmia substrate that cannot be addressed, and if a complex arrhythmia appears, masked as an easy target, we have all the hardware needed to finish the case without the need to reschedule. It saves costs for the patient and the system.

An approach with lesser catheters (due to the other features available with any 3-D mapping system) makes it easier to discharge the patient the same day; two punctures only at the same groin side would eventually reduce vascular complications and helps to earlier mobilization and discharge. It saves costs for the patient and the system.

Pregnancy in a female health provider working in a fluoroscopy-free EP lab is no longer a problem. If she decides to continue working, it allows to smoothly prepare replacement personnel or to work as long as decided with no harm for the baby. It saves costs for the system, but specially welcomes female colleagues to EP labs.

I briefly mention—as there is no cost analysis yet done—the benefits for primary operators: once we have adopted this technique, there is no way to come back and to bear the weight of lead aprons; cancer and spine problems prevented would never been counted, as we would be retired at that time, only newer generations of EP will see the benefits of a fluoroscopy-free EP lab.

Catheter reutilization is another way to save money, but as previously described, most of 3-D providers have hardware or software in place to force physicians to single use, please see next section for details. If a single-use policy applies to your center, the only way to decrease costs is to deal on volume, as described before. If reuse of catheters is available, either ethylene oxide [13] or hydrogen peroxide plasma [14] sterilization is an accepted option, with a 15 h of detoxification period suggested before another use when ethylene oxide is utilized [13].

We will discuss now less orthodox methods to cut on costs when using specific 3-D mapping systems. We should disclose that these methods could not be approved or not be feasible in different jurisdictions, and for sure the specific providers do not promote these inventive utilization of their systems; however, as they cannot harm, we let the reader to decide if they are applicable at each individual institution.

- **EnSite NavX™**: The cost comes not from catheters but from patches that are labeled as single use. If in most countries reuse of a patch is not acceptable because of hygiene and contamination reasons, however, the patch can be actually used in more than one patient, provided that the session is still open for the same patient: the day starts with a case that ends just at the end of that day or when a new set of patches is used. For uninsured populations or low-income countries, it can decrease at least in three or four times the cost of a 3-D procedure without fluoroscopy (the anecdotic reuse of patches in a single day), a luxury not otherwise affordable in these settings.
- **Carto™**: Cost is attached to the ablation catheter. If reuse is allowed in your lab, the company states that internal software prevent all Navistar catheter utilization after 24 h of first use. Anecdotic reports showed the use of a catheter as the last case of a day on the lab, to send it to sterilization at night, and to still be able to reuse as the first case in the next morning, before the 24 h expiration period. In centers when a single-use policy is the norm, we decrease the costs of an EP study only (when no arrhythmia target is found) or when cryoablation is needed, in the following way: we start the day with a case where ablation is always needed (usually flutter ablation); if the next case has no arrhythmia documentation or cryoablation is the source of energy chosen, after brief decontamination, we keep the first Navistar catheter of the day and we place it on a plastic bag beneath the next patient mattress or under the table linen, still connected to the system. A decaNav catheter (marketed usually at the same price of a standard decapolar catheter) or any other sensor-enabled catheter needed is then used to create a virtual anatomy. An extra quadripolar catheter is used to complete the set up, and if the case ended up as an EP study, only two cheap diagnostic catheters have been used, without fluoroscopy and without compromising the single-use policy as the reused catheter is at the exterior of the patient. When a cryoablation catheter is needed, once the virtual anatomy has been created, it can be used and visualized as other any non-sensor-enabled catheter.
- **Rhythmia™**: We have not developed yet any trick for Orion reuse, it is supposed to have the same constraints as any sensor-based catheters, same tricks as Carto™ mentioned applies for sensor-based catheters (but there is no sensor-enabled decapolar catheter as the decaNav from Carto™ to acquire virtual anatomy).

Conclusion

The non-fluoroscopic approach for a daily life EP lab has grown as a feasible and safe alternative to fluoroscopy for any ablation procedure. With actual parameters on reduction to radiation exposure, for patients it is either cost-effective (pediatric populations) or borderline cost-effective (adult only population). There is no data on cost-related issues related to the operator and health allied professional exposure. Further developments should decrease costs. In the meantime, greater volume utilization allows to better deal when 3-D mapping systems are widely applied to all arrhythmia substrates. We have also described some methods to cost containment (applicable only if local regulation allows), to help to easy our journeys without fluoroscopy.

References

1. Ayala Valani L, Al Baridi E, Rivera S, Brambilla C, Brahim Y, Klein A, Coluccini P, Compagno P, Fortes Etchepare R, Badra M, Dusault C, Roux JF, Ayala Paredes F. Real life EP lab without fluoroscopy. Eur Heart J. 2018;39(Suppl 1):P6646.
2. Fernández-Gómez JM, Moriña-Vázquez P, Morales Edel R, Venegas-Gamero J, Barba-Pichardo R, Carranza MH. Exclusion of fluoroscopy use in catheter ablation procedures: six years of experience at a single center. J Cardiovasc Electrophysiol. 2014;25(6):638–44.
3. Razminia M, Willoughby MC, Demo H, Keshmiri H, Wang T, D'Silva OJ, Zheutlin TA, Jibawi H, Okhumale P, Kehoe RF. Fluoroless catheter ablation of cardiac arrhythmias: a 5-year experience. Pacing Clin Electrophysiol. 2017;40(4):425–33.
4. Sánchez JM, Yanics MA, Wilson P, Doshi A, Kurian T, Pieper S. Fluoroless catheter ablation in adults: a single center experience. J Interv Card Electrophysiol. 2016;45(2):199–207.
5. Álvarez M, Bertomeu-González V, Arcocha MF, Moriña P, Tercedor L, Ferrero de Loma Á, Pachón M, García A, Pardo M, Datino T, Alonso C, Osca J, Investigators of the Spanish Multicenter registry of Fluoroscopy-free Ablation. Nonfluoroscopic catheter ablation. Results from a prospective multicenter registry. Rev Esp Cardiol. 2017;70:699–705.
6. Casella M, Dello Russo A, Pelargonio G, et al. Near zerO fluoroscopic exPosure during catheter ablAtion of supRavenTricular arrhYthmias: the NO-PARTY multi-center randomized trial. Europace. 2016;18:1565–72.. https://www.ncbi.nlm.nih.gov/pmc/articles/PMC5072134/#sup1.
7. Bigelow AM, Smith PC, Timberlake DT, et al. Procedural outcomes of fluoroless catheter ablation outside the traditional catheterization lab. Europace. 2017;19(8):1378–84.
8. Mickelsen S, Mickelsen C, MacIndoe C, Jaramillo J, Bass S, West G, Kusumoto FM. Trends and patterns in electrophysiologic and ablation catheter reuse in the United States. Am J Cardiol. 2001;87(3):351–3.. A9
9. Birnie D, Healey JS, Krahn AD, Ahmad K, Crystal E, Khaykin Y, Chauhan V, Philippon F, Exner D, Thibault B, Hruczkowski T, Nery P, Keren A, Redfearn D. Prevalence and risk factors for cervical and lumbar spondylosis in interventional electrophysiologists. J Cardiovasc Electrophysiol. 2011;22(9):957–60.
10. Wenger NK. Women in cardiology : the US experience. Heart. 2005;91(3):277–9.
11. Eckardt L, Frommeyer G, Sommer P, Steven D, Deneke T, Estner HL, Kriatselis C, Kuniss M, Busch S, Tilz RR, Bonnemeier H, von Bary C, Voss F, Meyer C, Thomas D, Neuberger HR. Updated survey on interventional electrophysiology: 5-year follow-up of infrastructure, procedures, and training positions in Germany. JACC Clin Electrophysiol. 2018;4(6):820–7.
12. Marini M, Ravanelli D, Guarracini F, Del Greco M, Quintarelli S, Cima A, Coser A, Martin M, Valentini A, Bonmassari RA. Cost-effective analysis of systematically using mapping systems during catheter ablation procedures in children and teenagers. Pediatr Cardiol. 2018;39:1581–9. https://doi.org/10.1007/s00246-018-1933-5.
13. Ferrell M, Wolf CE 2nd, Ellenbogen KA, Wood MA, Clemo HF, Gilligan DM. Ethylene oxide on electrophysiology catheters following resterilization: implications for catheter reuse. Am J Cardiol. 1997;80(12):1558–61.
14. Bathina MN, Mickelsen S, Brooks C, Jaramillo J, Hepton T, Kusumoto FM. Safety and efficacy of hydrogen peroxide plasma sterilization for repeated use of electrophysiology catheters. J Am Coll Cardiol. 1998;32(5):1384–8.

18 Zero-Fluoroscopic Implantation of Cardiac Electronic Device

Yan Wang

Abbreviations

CRT	Cardiac resynchronization therapy
ICD	Implantable cardioverter
LAO	Left anterior oblique
RAO	Right anterior oblique

In the past decade, three-dimensional navigation systems, such as Ensite NavX (St. Jude Medical, St. Paul, MN, USA), CARTO (Biosense Webster, Diamond Bar, CA, USA), and LocaLisa (Medtronic, Minneapolis, MN, USA), have been developed and implemented in electrophysiological procedures; those systems are used to guide catheters inside the heart and can significantly reduce radiation exposure to patients and medical staffs [1–7].

In this chapter, we introduce the techniques to perform zero- or near zero-fluoroscopic implantation of cardiac electronic device. As for the first implantation of single-chamber pacemaker, dual-chamber pacemaker, or implantable cardioverter defibrillator (ICD), almost all of the procedures can be performed without fluoroscopy, whereas a few cases may need very low dose of fluoroscopy, especially during the implantation of cardiac resynchronization therapy (CRT) [8–12].

Y. Wang (✉)
Cardiovascular Division, Tongji Hospital, Tongji Medical College, Huazhong University of Science and Technology, Wuhan, China
e-mail: newswangyan@tjh.tjmu.edu.cn

Candidate

Generally, a zero- or near zero-fluoroscopic implantation of cardiac electronic device may be considered in the following situations: (1) it is the first time to implant a cardiac electronic device; (2) there is no evidence of abnormality in implantation-related vessels; (3) the patient is sensitive to radiation exposure or unwilling to be exposed to fluoroscopy; (4) an emergent implantation is required while the X-ray machine is not available.

Preparation

Confirmation of Venous Access Without Fluoroscopic Guidance

1. Extension tube with stopcock: It is a tube routinely used for pump injection; it comprises a male luer slip connector plus a female luer slip connector, which is applied here for confirming a real venous access; the male connector is used for collecting a needle and the female connector is for collecting a three-way stopcock or a syringe (Fig. 18.1).

R. Proietti et al. (eds.), *Cardiac Electrophysiology Without Fluoroscopy*,
https://doi.org/10.1007/978-3-030-16992-3_18

2. Clip-clip cable: a cable is routinely used for testing pacing parameters; usually two to three cables are required (Fig. 18.2).
3. Clip-pin cable (Optional): the alligator style clip can be attached to the conductive tail of a monopolar guide wire; the pin can be attached to a three-dimensional system for navigation (Fig. 18.3).
4. Monopolar guide wire (Optional): the tip of monopolar guide wire is conductive and extends to a conductive metal tail whereas the rest is insulated; it can be used for verifying a venous access (Figs. 18.4 and 18.5).

As for other apparatus or facilities for confirming a venous access, refer the chapter concerning catheter placement without fluoroscopic guidance.

Navigation System

All the navigation systems can be used for this purpose. Generally Ensite NavX™ system is preferred for guiding a zero-fluoroscopic implantation; it needs at least the patches and a diagnostic—ideally—steerable catheter to reconstruct

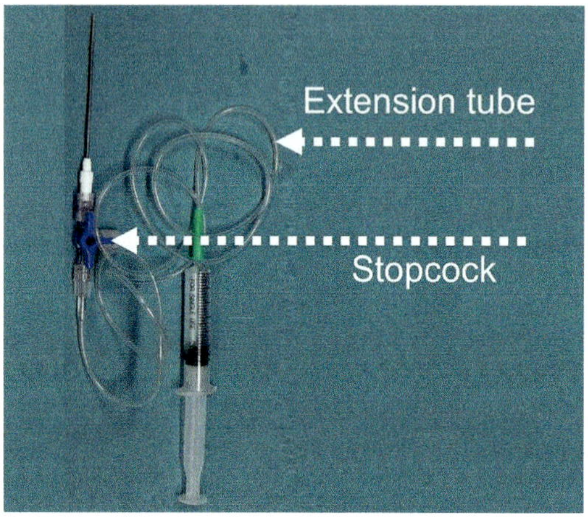

Fig. 18.1 Extension tube with stopcock

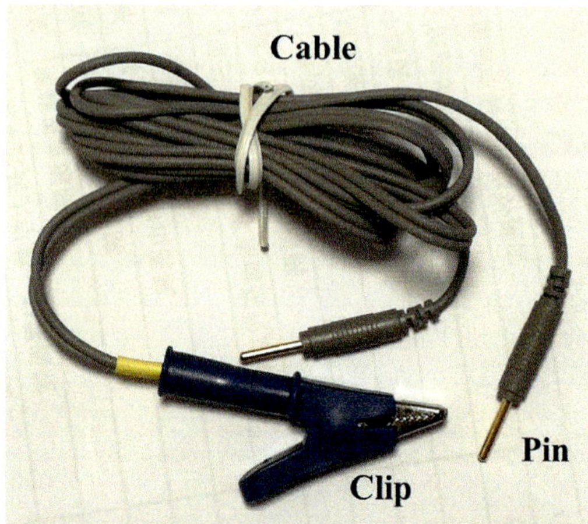

Fig. 18.3 Clip-pin cable

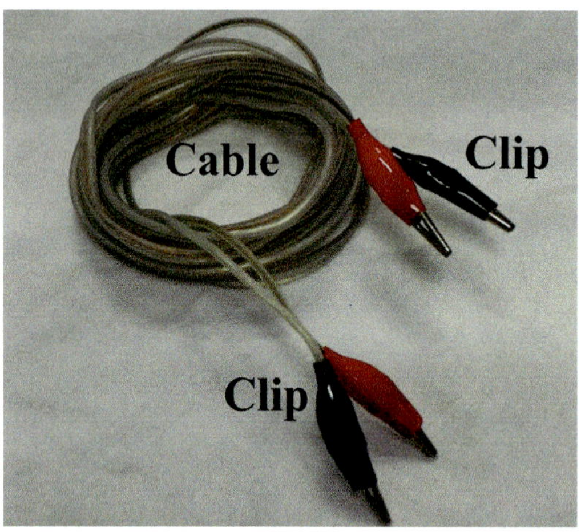

Fig. 18.2 Clip-clip cable

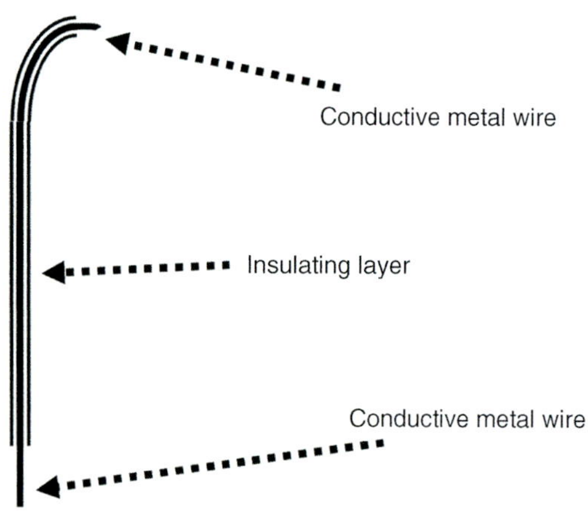

Fig. 18.4 Monopolar guide wire

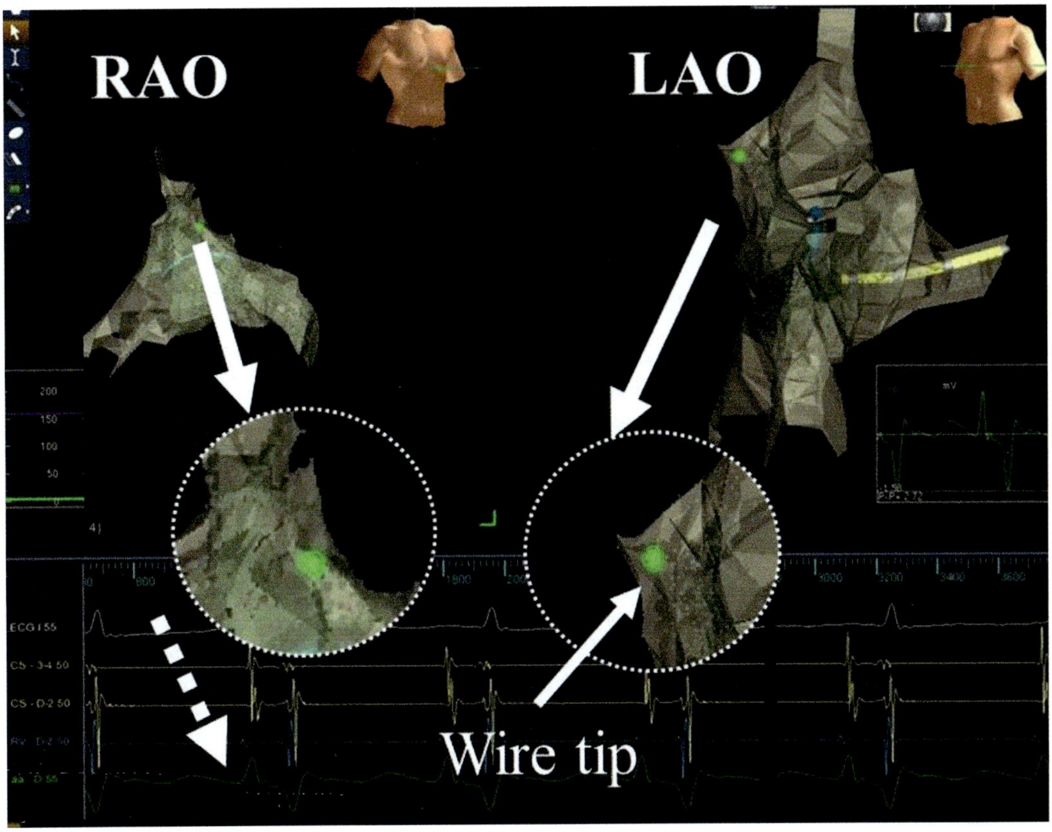

Fig. 18.5 Monopolar guide-wire placed in right atrium. *Green* dot shows the wire tip and the dashed arrow shows the intracardiac electrogram recorded by the wire tip

the heart anatomy of the chambers of interest. As described in other chapters, the Carto system can also be used: a Navistar magnetic-enabled catheter needs to be placed outside the patient at the thorax level—connected to the system—, and a decaNav diagnostic catheter can be used to reconstruct the heart anatomy.

Other Materials for Navigation

- One set of surface electrode patches (Ensite NavX, St Jude Medical, MN, USA)
- A diagnostic catheter plus a connecting cable
- Long sheath (SR0)
- Short sheaths (6F)

A steerable catheter is usually preferred for model reconstruction.

Echocardiography

Other imaging modalities, such as transthoracic echocardiography or transesophageal echocardiography, can be helpful for visualizing the catheter in the heart chamber; however we will not introduce them here due to the consideration of additional manipulation and adjunctive staffs, increased discomfort, or increased risk of infection.

Anyway, a standby transthoracic echocardiography is recommended for each patient.

Implantation-Related Articles

- Cardiac electronic device
- Pacing Leads (active or passive)
- Introducer sheaths

Implantation

Place a set of surface electrode patches on the patient's skin; sterilize and drape the planned operative region; use surface patches as system reference and positional reference.

Pacemaker

Lead Insertion

Under anesthesia, left or right subclavian or axillary vein can be used for lead implantation according to the clinical status. If needed, a puncture of the right femoral vein is obtained for temporary pacing.

As for a single-chamber pacemaker, only a puncture of the subclavian vein or axillary vein is needed unless temporary pacing is required.

Puncture the subclavian vein or axillary vein with the Seldinger technique and insert J-shaped wires. In some centers vascular ultrasound could guide to safely obtain a venous puncture. Once blood is obtained, verify a venipuncture by the following manifestations:

(a) The characteristic dark color of venous blood
(b) Pressure measurement or blood return test
(c) The movement of a catheter placed via femoral vein entangled by pushing-pulling the J-shaped wire placed via subclavian vein, which can be displayed on the monitor
(d) The presence of interference signal on intracardiac electrogram resulted from entanglement of the wire by rotating the catheter place at the middle of right atrium via femoral vein [6].

Blood return test is recommended for verifying venipuncture because of its simplicity. The test can be performed with a fluid-filled extension tube with stopcock. Collect the male luer slip connector with the needle and then put down and lift the extension tube. The blood will flow through to-and-fro the needle. More details for confirming a venipuncture have been discussed in previous chapter concerning catheter placement.

Tractive movement or interference signal can be observed on the monitor screen after the following preparation: insert a monopolar or a routinely used guide wire into the needle and connect the tail of the wire using a clip-pin cable, to obtain the intracardiac electrogram into the three-dimensional system (wire pacing test).

Advance an introducer sheath after the verification and withdraw the wire. Insert a pacing lead and remove the sheath.

Lead Connection

Connect the cables searching for one to two sites to obtain an ideal pacing site (Fig. 18.6). Connect one cable with the three-dimensional mapping system and another cable with a pacemaker test instrument.

(a) Use a clip-pin cable; connect the pacing lead with the clip and insert the pin into the pin-box linking with the three-dimensional navigation system.
(b) Utilize a clip-clip cable if clip-pin cable is not available; thus the operator need to peel the plastic shroud of the pins of a cable designed for linking diagnostic electrophysiological catheter; link one clip to the pacing lead and another clip to the peeled pin; finally insert the peeled pin into the pin-box.

Model Reconstruction

Right atrium and ventricle, as the coronary sinus shells could be constructed as in any standard EP procedure; then the leads can be placed using

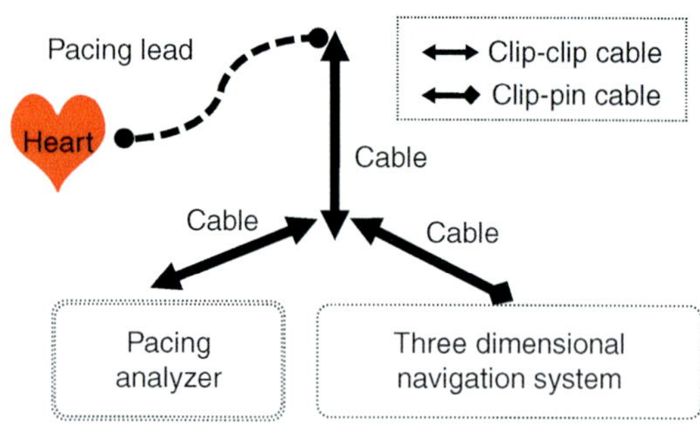

Fig. 18.6 One to two collection pattern with three cables

this reconstructed virtual anatomy to choose the desired pacing site. We are going to describe in the following paragraphs how to use directly the pacing leads to construct the desired anatomy with the NavX system.

Once the lead is connected to the system, the tip appears already in our screens, we can use them to acquire anatomy. Mainly focus on the target area (e.g., right atrial appendage) and construct the model as the following steps:

(a) Set the electrode spacing according the type of pacing lead used.
(b) Ask the patient to avoid body movement and avoid deep breathing.
(c) Perform an optimization and a respiratory compensation.
(d) Move the lead, record the track of the lead tip, and reconstruct an essential model, mainly focusing on the target area.
(e) Choose a soft steerable diagnostic catheter or even a mapping catheter if a more detailed high-density model is required.
(f) Generally, two guide wires are placed before lead insertion for the implantation of dual chamber pacemaker.
(g) Do remember to remove any guide wire during model reconstruction since a guide wire in the heart chamber may lead to obvious deformity of the model. We recommend to replace other guide wires with six French sheaths before model reconstruction.
(h) Be cautious to avoid any unexpected and deep insertion into the coronary sinus; it is helpful to observe the lead tip's track both in right anterior oblique (RAO) view and in left anterior oblique (LAO) view.
(i) The presence of typical atrial, ventricular, or coronary sinus electrogram is helpful to identify the site where the lead tip is located.
(j) Roughly create the geometry of the superior vena cava, right atrium, and right ventricular apex by wagging the pacing lead inside the target cavity (pre-shaped stylets would help to arrive to the chamber or site of interest).

Ventricular Lead Implantation

(a) Pacing 10–20 beats per minute faster than the patient's basic heart rate and set the pacing voltage at 1.0 V for seeking and screening an ideal site.
(b) Manipulate the tip of the ventricular lead to an ideal site in right ventricle in right anterior oblique plus left anterior oblique views.
(c) Observe and mark the inserted length when the lead just touch the target site and achieve a stable pacing capture; a maker can be made using a sterile suture or elastic at about three fingers away from where the lead enter into the tissue in the vasculature; label the position of the lead tip with a point on the three-dimensional model and continuously monitor the spatial stability of the lead tip.
(d) Further advance the ventricular lead 2–5 cm, usually varying from 2 to 3 cm.
(e) Check the stability of the lead tip as the following: (1) repeatedly advance and tract the lead about one to two centimeters; (2) ask the patient to breathe and cough deeply; (3) observe if the lead tip has a fixed position both in RAO plus LAO views; (4) has stable capture even pacing at a low voltage (Fig. 18.7).
(f) Evaluate the parameters including pacing thresholds, lead impedance, and sensitivity, and exclude the existence of diaphragmatic stimulation.
(g) Once acceptable parameters are obtained, the lead is fixed to the pectoral muscle with a suture.
(h) Sometimes, point-labels can be made to identify those sites reached easily and repetitively by the lead's tip, but with unsatisfactory pacing parameters, so as to improve procedural efficiency.
(i) The labeled positions can be monitored continuously and checked at any time during the procedure.
(j) As to zero-fluoroscopic implantation, an active fixation lead is relatively easier for determining the proper length for insertion than a passive fixation lead.

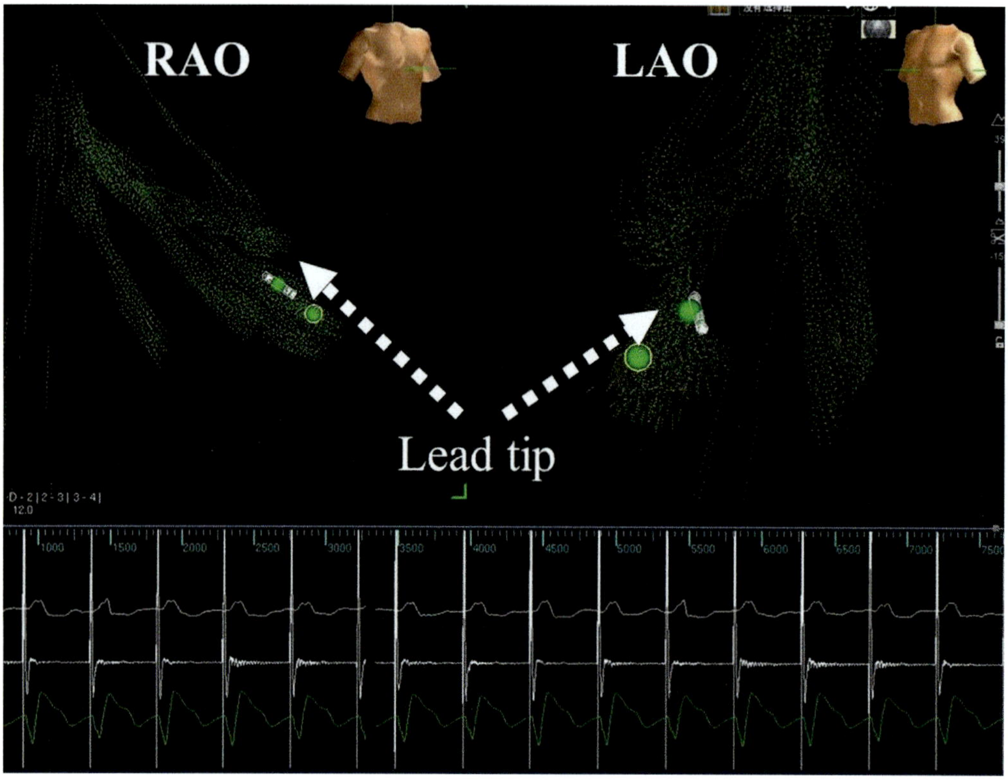

Fig. 18.7 Ventricular lead placed at a site with stable pacing capture. *Green* dot shows the position of the ventricular lead tip and the lower panel shows stable pacing capture at low voltage less than 1.0 V

Atrial Lead Implantation

(a) Replace the 6F sheath with an introducer sheath for the atrial lead; insert the atrial lead with an inner wire inside.
(b) Construct a geometry of the right atrium and the right atrial appendage with the atrial lead.
(c) Pacing 10–20 beats per minute faster than the patient's basic heart rate and set the pacing voltage at 1.0 V for seeking and screening an ideal site.
(d) Steer the tip of the atrial lead to an ideal site in the right atrial appendage in right anterior oblique plus left anterior oblique views.
(e) Observe and mark the length inserted when the lead just touch a target site and achieve stable pacing capture (Fig. 18.8).
(f) Withdraw the inner wire. Check the stability of the lead's tip and measure parameters as mentioned above.
(g) Fix the lead to the pectoral muscle with a suture once the parameters are acceptable. Collect the lead with a planned pulse generator.

Implantable Cardioverter Defibrillator (ICD)

The leads can be implanted according to the method mentioned above for the implantation of ventricular lead and atrial lead.

Cardiac Resynchronization Therapy/ Defibrillator (CRT/D)

Please refer to the dedicated chapter for further details. Similar to traditional method, left-sided vein is preferred for CRT implantation because left cannulation rout is more natural.

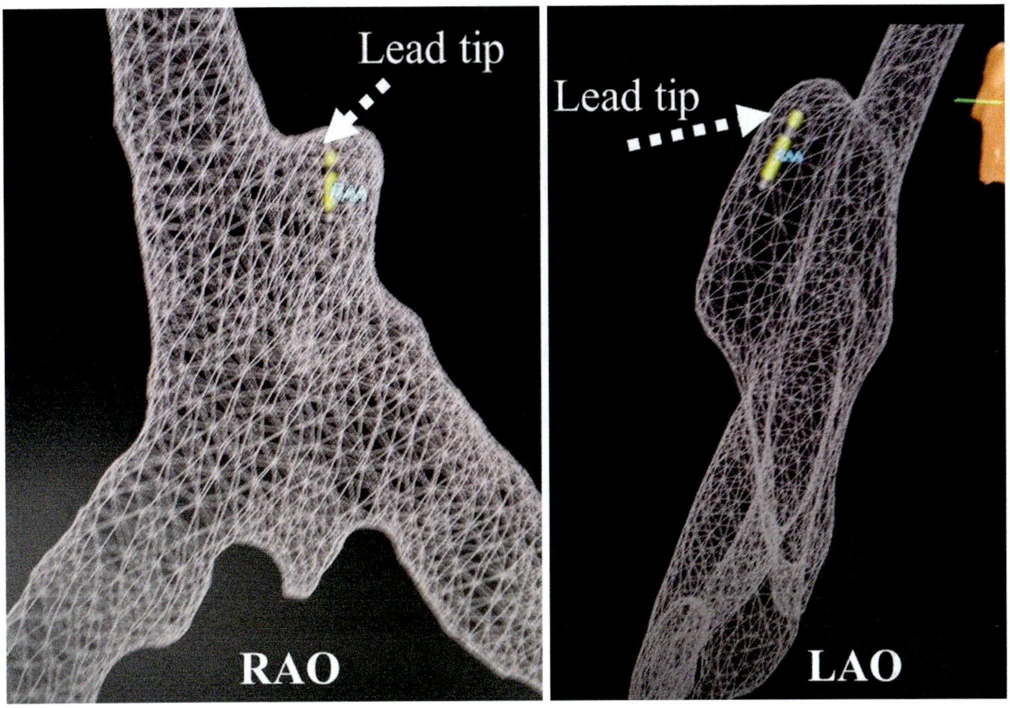

Fig. 18.8 Atrial lead placed at a site with stable pacing capture

(a) Puncture three different sites and insert three different guide wires.
(b) Under the guidance of Ensite NavX™ system, advance a 8F/10.5F introducer sheath along the medial guide wire according to the device type and insert a ventricular lead of active-fixation type; cannulate two 6F sheaths along other two guide wires, respectively; finally, withdraw all the guide wires.

Right Ventricular Lead

(a) Insert a right ventricular lead into the right ventricle via the 8F/10.5F sheath for CRT/CRTD; use the surface electrode patch as position reference; reconstruct a geometric model as the method mentioned above; steer and fix the right ventricular lead stably on the septum; label the position of the lead's tip with a point on the three-dimensional model.
(b) Set the fixed lead's tip as position reference during the following model reconstruction.
(c) Always keep the lead being connected to the three-dimensional navigation system so as to continuously monitor and confirm the spatial stability of the lead's tip.

Left Ventricular Lead

(a) Prepare the delivery system, which is designed for the insertion of left ventricular lead; check, flush, and assemble the delivery system in vitro.
(b) Replace the lateral 6F sheath with a 10.5F introducer sheath which can allow the delivery system to pass through.
(c) Choose a steerable ablation catheter to find the coronary sinus orifice; usually a catheter with big curve is recommended (e.g., Safire bidirectional ablation catheter, L-curve, St. Jude Medical or Celsius Ablation Catheters, B curve, Biosense Webster, Inc., Diamond Bar, CA, USA). Insert the steerable catheter via the delivery system, and connect the catheter with the three-dimensional navigation system; reconstruct a new geometric model mainly focused on anatomy nearby the CS orifice, and the CS.
(d) Leave the catheter in the distal part of the CS and leave a shadow of the CS location.
(e) Cautiously advance the delivery system; always keep the proximal electrode of the diagnostic or ablation catheter outside the tip

of delivery system so as to avoid the potential risk of cardiac perforation. The intracardiac electrogram recorded by the proximal electrodes will disappear and the image of ablation catheter will become deformed when the tip of delivery system begins to shield the proximal electrodes. Observe if there are manifestations mentioned above to guarantee a safe advancement of the delivery system.

(f) Tightly fix the delivery sheath with one or two suture knots once the delivery system reaches a proper position in the CS, usually at least 1–2 cm inside the orifice; withdraw the ablation or diagnostic catheter.

(g) Prepare a 0.014 in. wire, which is used for percutaneous transluminal coronary angioplasty; a wire with soft tip is preferred. Check the guide wire and the lead in vitro; make a mark on the wire with a knot or with sterile sticky paper at three fingers longer than the lead. A special-designed wire (VisionWire, Biotronik, Berlin, Deutschland) can be more convenient for reconstructing a detailed model of different branches of coronary sinus [13].

(h) Insert the wire into the lead and keep the wire extend outside the lead's tip at least 3–5 cm. Collect the tail of guide wire with Ensite NavX™ system.

(i) Insert the left ventricular lead with the marked inner guide wire into the distal part of CS via the delivery system.

(j) Reconstruct the geometric model of venous branches by gently moving the lead wire to-and-fro.

(k) Use another clip-pin cable to connect the cathode at the lead tail with the three-dimensional mapping system and to display the position of the lead's tip.

(l) Use the ventricular potential recorded by the right ventricular lead as reference; record the local ventricular activation time and the voltage amplitude at different sites in the cardiac vein; seek a position with the maximum conduction delay in the vein compared with the activation reference.

(m) Guarantee a safe advancement by applying the following tips: advance the lead gently; keep the lead cathode within two fingers away from the thread mark on the inner guide wire so as to keep the inner wire tip outside the lead's tip; observe whether the lead's tip move correspondingly with the operator's manipulation at any time.

(n) Perform an angiogram to reveal the venous branches if the three-dimensional model is incomplete or unsatisfactory. Utilize necessary fluoroscopic guidance just when the lead placement finds obstacles nearby the target site inside the vein.

(o) Advance the lead toward the target site after preliminary evaluation with the method mentioned above.

(p) Withdraw the guide wire to the coronary sinus to restore the natural shape of the lead's tip if the lead reaches the site.

(q) Evaluate the parameters, including pacing threshold, lead impedance, and sensitivity, and exclude the presence of diaphragmatic stimulation. Once acceptable parameters are obtained, tightly fix the lead to the pectoral muscle with a suture.

Atrial Lead

Replace the 6F sheath with a matched introducer sheath; insert the atrial lead and peel away the introducer sheath. Steer the lead's tip to an ideal site as mentioned above for the implantation of dual-chamber pacemaker. Fix the atrial lead to the pectoral muscle. Label the position of the lead's tip with a point on the three-dimensional model for continuous checking of the spatial stability of the lead's tip.

Device Placement

(a) Replace the 0.014 in. wire with a stiff inner wire routinely packed for steering the pacing leads. Keep the tip of inner wire just inside the coronary sinus.

(b) One staff stably hold the tail of left ventricular lead; another staff carefully cut off or peel away the delivery sheath; withdraw the inner wire; fix the left ventricular lead to the pectoral muscle. There are also peel-away left lead introducers that obviates the need to cut the delivery sheath.

(c) Check the position and parameters of all the three leads; collect them with the CRT device if all the parameters are satisfactory.

References

1. Fernandez-Gomez JM, Morina-Vazquez P, Morales Edel R, Venegas-Gamero J, Barba-Pichardo R, Carranza MH. Exclusion of fluoroscopy use in catheter ablation procedures: six years of experience at a single center. J Cardiovasc Electrophysiol. 2014;25:638–44.
2. Chen G, Sun G, Xu R, Chen X, Yang L, Bai Y, Yang S, Guo P, Zhang Y, Zhao C, Wang DW, Wang Y. Zero-fluoroscopy catheter ablation of severe drug-resistant arrhythmia guided by ensite navx system during pregnancy: two case reports and literature review. Medicine (Baltimore). 2016;95:e4487.
3. Yang L, Sun G, Chen X, Chen G, Yang S, Guo P, Wang Y, Wang DW. Meta-analysis of zero or near-zero fluoroscopy use during ablation of cardiac arrhythmias. Am J Cardiol. 2016;118:1511–8.
4. Lemery R. Interventional electrophysiology at the crossroads: cardiac mapping, ablation and pacing without fluoroscopy. J Cardiovasc Electrophysiol. 2012;23:1087–91.
5. Ventura R, Rostock T, Klemm HU, Lutomsky B, Demir C, Weiss C, Meinertz T, Willems S. Catheter ablation of common-type atrial flutter guided by three-dimensional right atrial geometry reconstruction and catheter tracking using cutaneous patches: a randomized prospective study. J Cardiovasc Electrophysiol. 2004;15:1157–61.
6. Wang Y, Chen GZ, Yao Y, Bai Y, Chu HM, Ma KZ, Liew R, Liu H, Zhong GQ, Xue YM, Wu SL, Li YF, Zhao CX, Liu QG, Lin L, Wang L, Wang DW. Ablation of idiopathic ventricular arrhythmia using zero-fluoroscopy approach with equivalent efficacy and less fatigue: a multicenter comparative study. Medicine (Baltimore). 2017;96:e6080.
7. Wittkampf FH, Wever EF, Derksen R, Wilde AA, Ramanna H, Hauer RN, Robles de Medina EO. Localisa: New technique for real-time 3-dimensional localization of regular intracardiac electrodes. Circulation. 1999;99:1312–7.
8. Merino JL, Peinado R, Silvestre J. Dual-chamber implantable cardioverter defibrillator implantation guided by non-fluoroscopic electro-anatomical navigation. Europace. 2008;10:1124–5.
9. Ruiz-Granell R, Ferrero A, Morell-Cabedo S, Martinez-Brotons A, Bertomeu V, Llacer A, Garcia-Civera R. Implantation of single-lead atrioventricular permanent pacemakers guided by electroanatomic navigation without the use of fluoroscopy. Europace. 2008;10:1048–51.
10. Ruiz-Granell R, Morell-Cabedo S, Ferrero-De-Loma A, Garcia-Civera R. Atrioventricular node ablation and permanent ventricular pacemaker implantation without fluoroscopy: use of an electroanatomic navigation system. J Cardiovasc Electrophysiol. 2005;16:793–5.
11. Tuzcu V, Kilinc OU. Implantable cardioverter defibrillator implantation without using fluoroscopy in a pregnant patient. Pacing Clin Electrophysiol. 2012;35:e265–6.
12. Guo P, Qiu J, Wang Y, Chen G, Proietti R, Fadhle AS, Zhao C, Wen Wang D. Zero-fluoroscopy permanent pacemaker implantation using ensite navx system: clinical viability or fanciful technique? Pacing Clin Electrophysiol. 2018;41:122–7.
13. Colella A, Giaccardi M, Colella T, Modesti PA. Zero x-ray cardiac resynchronization therapy device implantation guided by a nonfluoroscopic mapping system: a pilot study. Heart Rhythm. 2016;13(7):1481–8.

Cardiac Resynchronization Therapy (CRT) Guided by 3D Mapping System

19

Maurizio Del Greco, Massimiliano Marini, Fabrizio Guarracini, and Francesco Peruzza

Introduction

The transvenous devices implantation, such as pacemakers and defibrillators, is usually performed with the aid of fluoroscopy as the standard tool for lead visualization in the cardiac chambers. This implies radiation exposure for patients and operators. Furthermore, fluoroscopy allows only a two-dimensional view of catheter movements, making the placement of catheters challenging because of the complex anatomy of cardiac structures. Recently, systems for non-fluoroscopic 3D catheter navigation through the cardiac chambers and vascular structures have been developed [1–3]. In literature there are some reports demonstrating the possibility of implanting pacemakers by means of these tools and without the use of fluoroscopy. In the last 5 years the feasibility and the reliability of implanting a three-leads system (CRT device) guided by an electroanatomic navigation system were also explored [4, 5]. The use of the mapping system not only allows a significant reduction in fluoroscopy exposure, but also helps to identify segments of latest left ventricular electrical activation and to optimize CRT implantation in patients with and without left bundle branch block [6].

M. Del Greco (✉) · F. Peruzza
Department of Cardiology, Santa Maria del Carmine Hospital, Rovereto, TN, Italy
e-mail: maurizio.delgreco@apss.tn.it; francesco.peruzza@apss.tn.it

M. Marini · F. Guarracini
Department of Cardiology, S. Chiara Hospital, Trento, Italy
e-mail: massimiliano.marini@apss.tn.it; fabrizio.guarracini@apss.tn.it

Implantation Technique

The implantation is performed using the EnSite system (St. Jude Medical, Endocardial Solutions, Inc., St. Paul, MN, USA). Three pairs of adhesive electrodes are placed on the chest of the patient configuring an orthogonal axes and a low-power electrical potential (5.7 kHz) is generated across each pair of electrodes. The voltage gradient from each axis generates a three-dimensional navigation field. After the electrodes size and the inter-electrode spacing have been chosen for each catheter, the EnSite system can be used to create geometric models of the patient's cardiac chambers, showing in real time a 3D image of the catheters location. The EnSite system can also be used to measure the distance between points on the geometric model of the endocardial surface, using the Field Scaling algorithm. Field Scaling is based on geometrical points collected in continuous mode by catheters with defined inter-electrode spacing. Adjustments to the dimensions of the navigation field are made considering the known inter-electrode spacing of the catheters used to create the geometry of the 3-D model.

R. Proietti et al. (eds.), *Cardiac Electrophysiology Without Fluoroscopy*,
https://doi.org/10.1007/978-3-030-16992-3_19

Under local anesthesia with lidocaine, the left subclavian/axillary and cephalic veins are cannulated in order to introduce three different guidewires. The implantation method is performed as follows:

First, a standard electrophysiological catheter (usually a 5F deflectable 10 polar catheter), connected to the EnSite system, is introduced through a 10F valved sheath via delivery system and used to map reference points for the superior vena cava and then to create a rough 3D model of the right atrium (RA) and the right ventricle (RV). The catheter is used to cannulate the coronary sinus (CS) and to record local bipolar electrograms (filtered at 50–500 Hz) (Fig. 19.1).

The safe advancement of the delivery system is accomplished considering the deformation of catheters when not completely out of the delivery sheath with the proximal electrodes (Fig. 19.2). The electrophysiological catheter is withdrawn, leaving the delivery system in the CS.

Second, after creation of the 3D model, a bipolar RV lead for sensing/pacing and defibrillation connected to the EnSite system is introduced through a 9F sheath and the lead tip is positioned in the apex or in the mid-septum of the RV. A catheter "shadow" is recorded to check the position during the entire procedure, and it is also confirmed by a 12-lead electrocardiogram (paced QRS complex morphology) and a single shot of fluoroscopy. Sensed R-waves, impedances, and capture thresholds are evaluated. Once acceptable parameters have been obtained, the lead is sutured to the pectoral muscle (Fig. 19.3).

Third, through the delivery sheath, a quadripolar left ventricular (LV) lead is introduced into CS over the insulated guidewire (Vision Wire, Biotronik SE & Co. KG, Berlin, Germany), both connected to the EnSite System. The guidewire is completely insulated unless for the 15 mm distal tip and the 30 mm proximal end. This insulation enables to visualize the position of the distal end of the wire in the system once emerged from the delivery system. With small movements of the guidewire and a mixture of rotation and gentle pulling/pushing of the wire, it is possible to build the anatomy of the CS branches, to record the local unipolar electrograms (high-pass filtered at 30 Hz) and to perform unipolar pacing. At this moment of the procedure, the decision to perform CS angiography is left to the implanting physician. An activation map of the CS branches is performed during sinus rhythm and during the right ventricular pacing in order to locate the "electrophysiological target vessel" with the latest activation (LVED% > 75 in patients with left

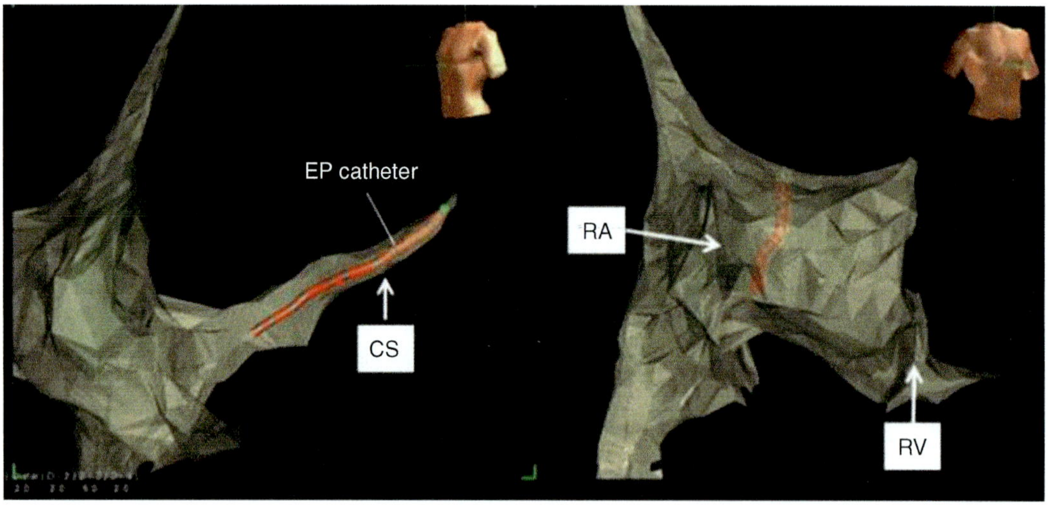

Fig. 19.1 After reconstruction of the right atrium (RA) and right ventricle (RV) anatomy by means of a 5F steerable electrophysiological catheter connected to the electroanatomic mapping system (EAMS), the catheter was inserted in the coronary sinus (CS)

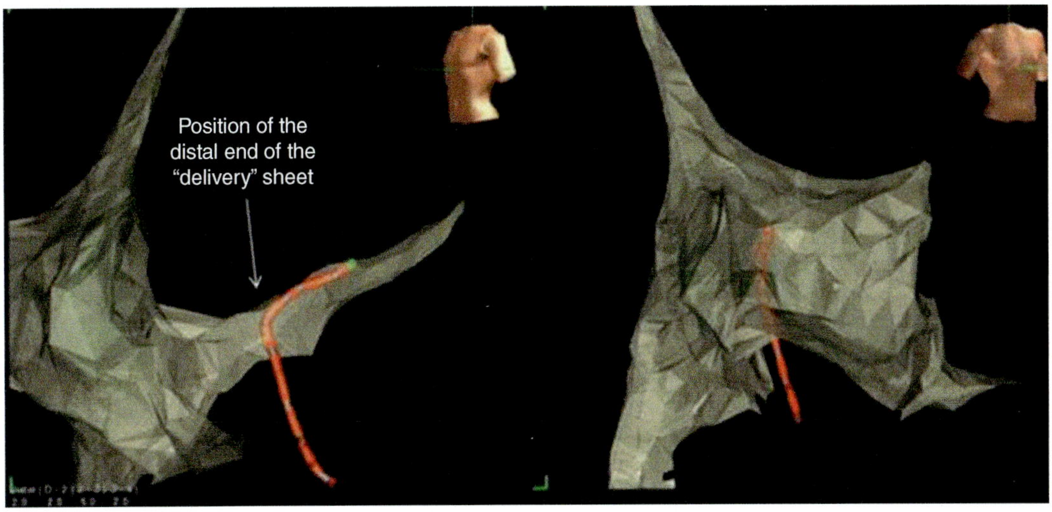

Fig. 19.2 The delivery sheath was then advanced inside the CS. The electrophysiologic catheter appears deformed when the distal end of the sheath reaches the proximal electrodes of the catheter

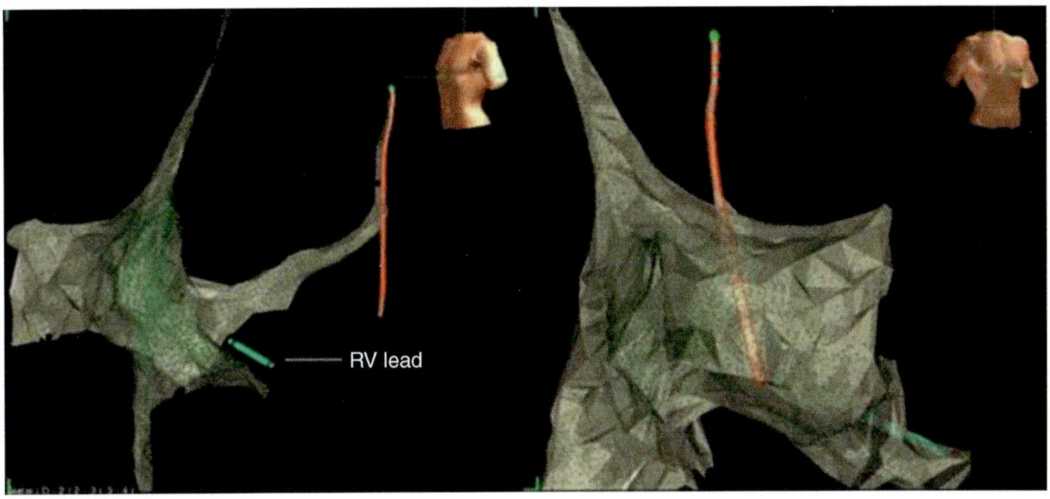

Fig. 19.3 A bipolar RV lead for sensing/pacing and defibrillation was inserted and placed in the RV apex under guidance by the EAMS

bundle branch block, LBBB). The right ventricular electrogram is used as reference during the activation map (Fig. 19.4a–d).

Fourth, once the CS anatomy has been reconstructed, the left ventricular lead (LV) is connected to the system and it is advanced over the insulated wire. The final position of the LV lead in the target vessel is chosen first in relation to the maximum activation LV delay but also considering the following factors: stable lead position in the vessel, absence of phrenic nerve stimulation, and an acceptable pacing threshold (Fig. 19.5). As is very often the case, the last three factors led to some compromise in the choice of the final LV lead position.

Finally, the right atrial lead, connected to the Ensite system, is placed in the right appendage by the guide of the navigation system, while a continued check of the catheter positions is carried out (Fig. 19.6a, b).

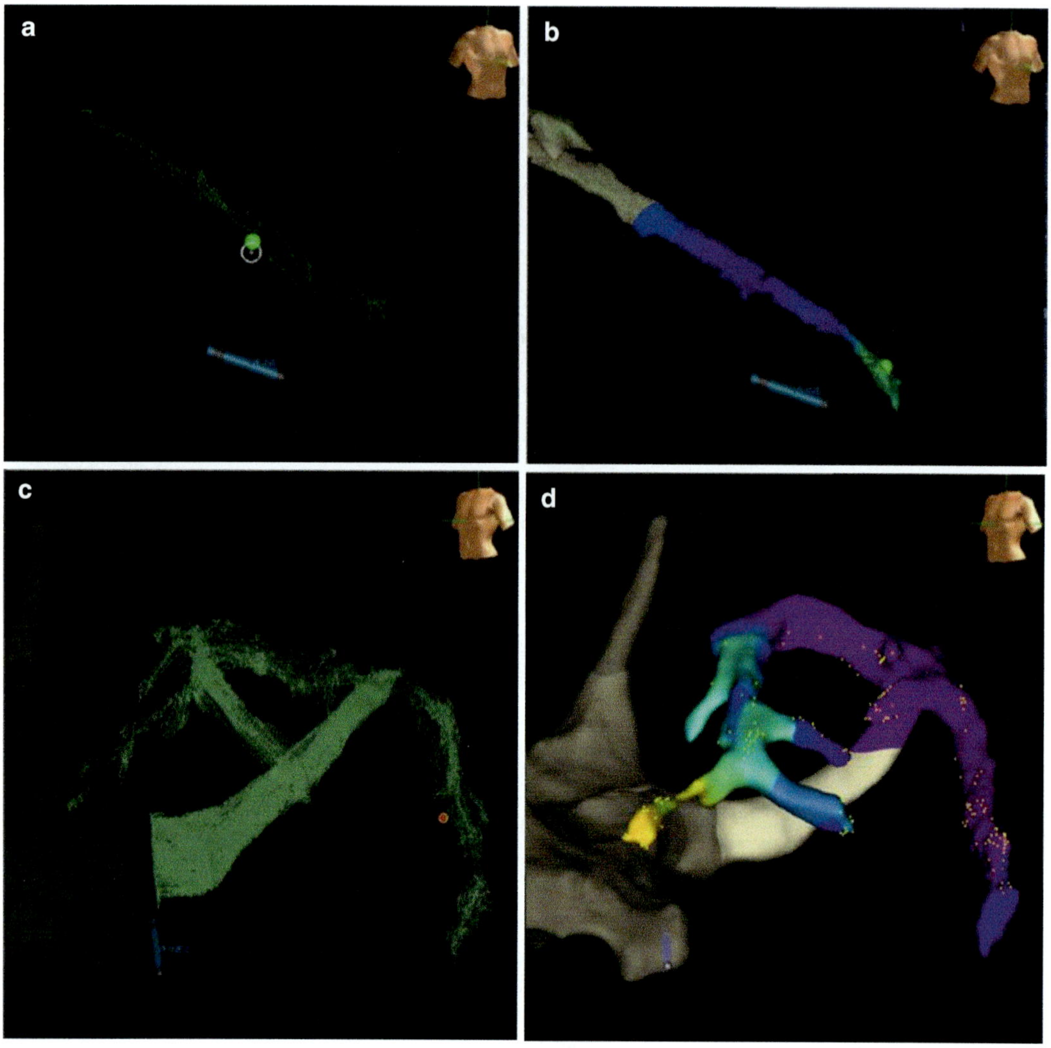

Fig. 19.4 (**a**) LV lead is introduced into CS over the insulated guidewire via delivery sheath. The tip of the guidewire is gently pushed, pulled, and rotated inside a CS branch. The electroanatomic mapping systems record lines of dots in the tridimensional space corresponding to the route of the guidewire tip. The dots will constitute the scaffold for anatomy reconstruction. (**b**) After multiple guidewire passages, the anatomy is finalized. At the same moment, activation times are recorded and displayed with a color-coded scale (in blue/violet the regions with late ventricular activation). (**c**) Tridimensional anatomy of the CS reconstructed using the dots recorded with multiple electrophysiological catheter and/or guidewire passages inside the vessels as a scaffold. (**d**) Finished model

General Considerations

The use of an electroanatomic navigation system in CRT implantation is feasible and safe. Del Greco et al. (2017) demonstrated in a multicenter registry that the CRT implantation by the use of a mapping system and with the technique described above was achievable both by centers with high (>10 procedures) and low experience (<10 procedure) [5]. The main findings of this study were the following: (1) the "electroanatomic-guided" CRT implantation allowed a reduction in fluoroscopy (about 75%) and angiography (about 70%) use as compared to "fluoroscopy-guided" CRT implantation; (2) the rates of implantation success and complications were similar between high- and low-experience centers; (3) the fluoroscopy and angiography use were lower in high-experience

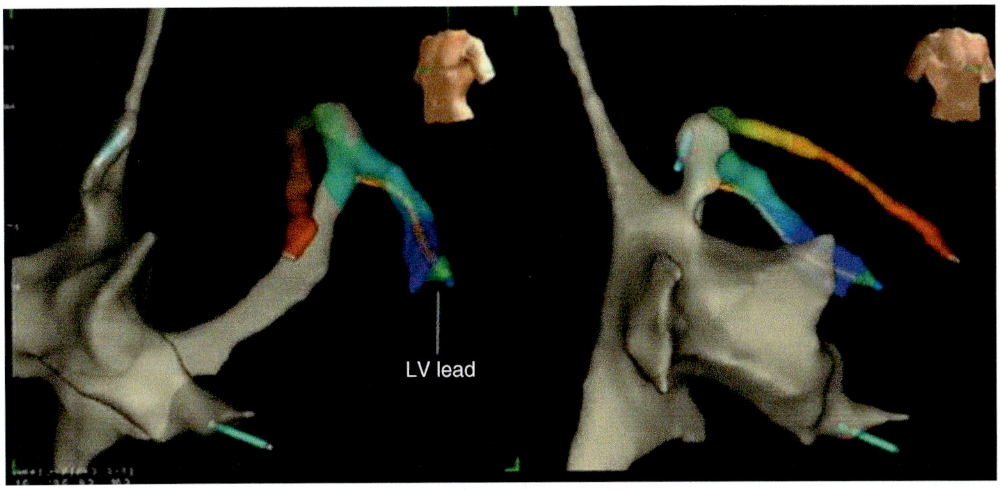

Fig. 19.5 After the identification of a branch with acceptable late activation, LV lead was advanced "over the wire"

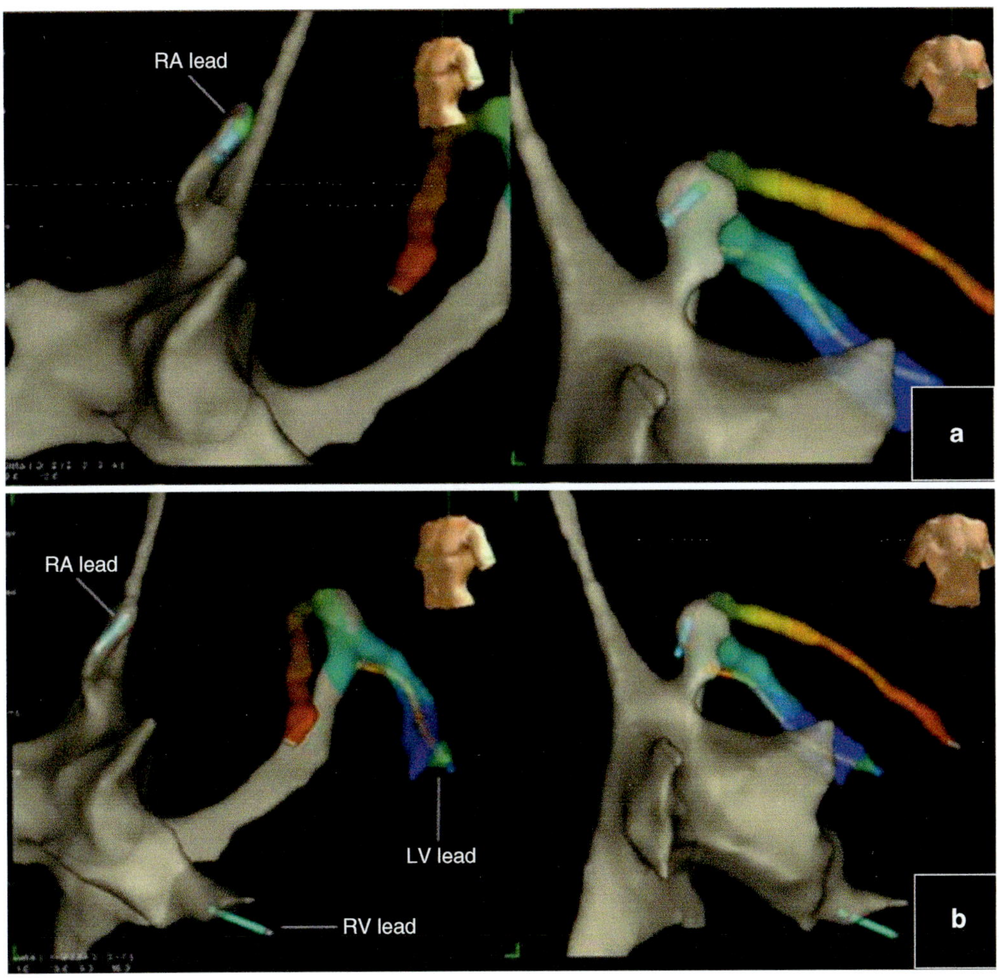

Fig. 19.6 (**a**) The right atrial lead was positioned in the right appendage under EAMS guidance. (**b**) Final position of the three electrodes

centers. However, in low-experience centers as well, the "electroanatomic-guided" CRT implantation resulted in a significant fluoroscopy and angiography reduction when compared with the "fluoroscopy-guided" CRT implantation; (4) the "electroanatomic-guided" CRT implantation enabled to map the LV activation, and to optimize LV lead implantation towards segments of delayed LV activation.

Fluoroscopy Time Reduction

The CRT device implantation is one of the interventional cardiology procedures with the highest radiation exposure, as average fluoroscopy time is several-fold higher than in standard pacemaker and ICD implantation [7]. The X-ray beam is often directed towards the operator, since the majority of CRT devices are implanted via a left subclavian access and CS navigation is usually performed in the left oblique view projection. The radiation risk is particularly high for CRT implanting physicians, and a conservative recommendation to perform a maximum of 4 CRT implantations per month per implanter has been suggested [8]. The increased awareness of the radiation risks for both patients and physicians have led many electrophysiologists to reduce the use of X-ray by implementing "near-zero fluoroscopy" procedures guided by an electroanatomic mapping system [9]. Recently, in the setting of device implantation, the first experiences of CRT devices implantation guided by electroanatomic mapping system have been published [6, 10–16]. The preliminary findings of these studies indicated that this approach significantly reduces radiation exposure and, even in centers performing their first electroanatomic-guided CRT implantation procedures, the radiation exposure dose is at least 50% lower than traditional fluoroscopic-guided CRT implantations [7].

LV Lead Positioning

A suboptimal LV pacing site is one of the reasons for non-response to CRT [17]. Several studies have suggested that pacing the LV in a site with late activation (either mechanical or electrical) may improve the hemodynamic response, reverse remodeling, and clinical outcome of CRT patients [18–21]. Although in the most cases the region of latest ventricular activation is the basal lateral LV wall, a significant variability among patients exists, especially in the presence of myocardial scars or intraventricular conduction delays other than left bundle branch block. Recently, it has been demonstrated that activation mapping of the CS by electroanatomic mapping system can be used to guide LV lead placement to regions of delayed activation (LV electrical delay percentage >75% of QRS duration in LBBB), and that the site with the latest electrical activation often does not correspond to the site of conventional "anatomical" LV lead placement, which targets a lateral CS branch regardless of the presence of myocardial scars or the type of conduction disturbance [22, 23]. Activation mapping appears important in patients with LBBB and even more in patients with no-LBBB, which showed a highly heterogeneous activation pattern. Del Greco et al. [6] demonstrated that in these patients, traditionally considered poor candidates to CRT implantation, an acceptable late activation (>50% of LV electrical delay %) can be found in the majority of cases with no-LBBB [6]. This finding may contribute to increase the rate of response to CRT of no-LBBB patients.

Limitations

The use of an electroanatomic mapping system during a CRT implantation can be useful and optimize the procedure; however some limitations are still present.

Indeed this technology was created and developed in order to provide a 3D image of the heart to interpret complex arrhythmias. The mapping system can significantly reduce the radiation exposure, but it does not allow us to visualize different wires, long sheaths, catheters curves, etc.

Further technological commitment from the industry is needed to overcome the limits still present in mapping systems.

References

1. Gepstein L, Hayam G, Ben-Haim SA. A novel method for nonfluoroscopic catheter-based electroanatomical mapping of the heart. In vitro and in vivo accurancy results. Circulation. 1997;95:1611–22.
2. Ventura R, Rostck T, Klemm HU, Lutomsky B, Demir C, Weiss C, et al. Catheter ablation of common type atrial flutter guided by three-dimensional right atrial geometry reconstruction and catheter tracking using cutaneous patches: a randomized prospective study. J Cardiovasc Electrophysiol. 2004;15:1157–61.
3. Novak PG, Macle L, Thibault B, Guerra PG. Enhanced left atrial mapping using digitally synchronized NavX three-dimensional nonfluoroscopic mapping and high-resolution computed tomographic imaging for catheter ablation of atrial fibrillation. Heart Rhythm. 2004;1(4):521–2.
4. Del Greco M, Marini M, Bonmassari R. Implantation of a biventricular implantable cardioverter-defibrillator guided by an electroanatomic mapping system. Europace. 2012;14:107–11.
5. Del Greco M, Maines M, Marini M, Colella A, Zecchin M, Vitali-Serdoz L, Blandino A, Barbonaglia L, Allocca G, Mureddu R, Marenna B, Rossi P, Vaccari D, Chianca R, Indiani S, Matteo ID, Angheben C, Zorzi A. Three-dimensional electroanatomic mapping system-enhanced cardiac resynchronization therapy device implantation: results from a multicenter registry. J Cardiovasc Electrophysiol. 2017;28(1):85–93.
6. Del Greco M, Zorzi A, Di Matteo I, Cima A, Maines M, Angheben C, Catanzariti D. Coronary sinus activation patterns in patients with and without left bundle branch block undergoing electroanatomic mapping system-guided cardiac resynchronization therapy device implantation. Heart Rhythm. 2017;14:225–33.
7. Picano E, Vano E, Rehani MM, Cuocolo A, Mont L, Bodi V, Bar O, Maccia C, Pierard L, Sicari R, Plein S, Mahrholdt H, Lancellotti P, Knuuti J, Heidelbuchel H, Di Mario C, Badano LP. A position document of the ESC associations of cardiovascular imaging, percutaneous cardiovascular interventions and electrophysiology. Eur Heart J. 2014;35:665–72.
8. Butter C, Schau T, Meyhoefer J, Neumann K, Minden HH, Engelhardt J. Radiation exposure of patient and physician during implantation and upgrade of cardiac resynchronization devices. Pacing Clin Electrophysiol. 2010;33:1003–12.
9. Giaccardi M, Del Rosso A, Guarnaccia V, Ballo P, Mascia G, Chiodi L, Colella A. Near-zero X-ray in arrhythmia ablation using a 3-dimensional electroanatomic mapping system: a multicenter experience. Heart Rhythm. 2016;13:150–6.
10. Ryu K, D'Avila A, Heist EK, Rosenberg SP, Chou J, Yang M, Singh JP. Simultaneous electrical and mechanical mapping using 3d cardiac mapping system: novel approach for optimal cardiac resynchronization therapy. J Cardiovasc Electrophysiol. 2010;21:219–22.
11. Mina A, Warnecke N. Near zero fluoroscopic implantation of BIV ICD using electro-anatomical mapping. Pacing Clin Electrophysiol. 2013;36:1409–16.
12. Valderrabano M, Greenberg S, Razavi H, More R, Ryu K, Heist EK. 3d cardiovascular navigation system: accuracy and reduction in radiation exposure in left ventricular lead implant. J Cardiovasc Electrophysiol. 2014;25:87–93.
13. Rad MM, Blaauw Y, Dinh T, Pison L, Crijns HJ, Prinzen FW, Vernooy K. Left ventricular lead placement in the latest activated region guided by coronary venous electroanatomic mapping. Europace. 2015;17:84–93.
14. Doring M, Sommer P, Rolf S, Lucas J, Breithardt OA, Hindricks G, Richter S. Sensor-based electromagnetic navigation to facilitate implantation of left ventricular leads in cardiac resynchronization therapy. J Cardiovasc Electrophysiol. 2015;26:167–75.
15. Thibault B, Mondesert B, Macle L, Dubuc M, Dyrda K, Talajic M, Roy D, Rivard L, Guerra PG, Andrade JG, Khairy P. Reducing radiation exposure during CRT implant procedures: single-center experience with low-dose fluoroscopy settings and a sensor-based navigation system (mediguide). J Cardiovasc Electrophysiol. 2016;27(11):1337–43.
16. Colella A, Giaccardi M, Colella T, Amedeo Modesti P. Zero X-ray cardiac resynchronization therapy device implantation guided by a nonfluoroscopic mapping system: a pilot study. Heart Rhythm. 2016;13(7):1481–8.
17. Gold MR, Birgersdotter-Green U, Singh JP, Ellenbogen KA, Yu Y, Meyer TE, Seth M, Tchou PJ. The relationship between ventricular electrical delay and left ventricular remodelling with cardiac resynchronization therapy. Eur Heart J. 2011;32:2516–24.
18. Singh JP, Fan D, Heist EK, Alabiad CR, Taub C, Reddy V, Mansour M, Picard MH, Ruskin JN, Mela T. Left ventricular lead electrical delay predicts response to cardiac resynchronization therapy. Heart Rhythm. 2006;3:1285–92.
19. Ypenburg C, van Bommel RJ, Delgado V, Mollema SA, Bleeker GB, Boersma E, Schalij MJ, Bax JJ. Optimal left ventricular lead position predicts reverse remodeling and survival after cardiac resynchronization therapy. J Am Coll Cardiol. 2008;52:1402–9.
20. Saba S, Marek J, Schwartzman D, Jain S, Adelstein E, White P, Oyenuga OA, Onishi T, Soman P, Gorcsan J 3rd. Echocardiography-guided left ventricular lead placement for cardiac resynchronization therapy: results of the speckle tracking assisted resynchronization therapy for electrode region trial. Circ Heart Fail. 2013;6:427–34.
21. Roubicek T, Wichterle D, Kucera P, Nedbal P, Kupec J, Sedlakova J, Cerny J, Stros J, Kautzner J, Polasek

R. Left ventricular lead electrical delay is a predictor of mortality in patients with cardiac resynchronization therapy. Circ Arrhythm Electrophysiol. 2015;8:1113–21.
22. Mafi Rad M, Blaauw Y, Dinh T, Pison L, Crijns HJ, Prinzen FW, Vernooy K. Different regions of latest electrical activation during left bundle-branch block and right ventricular pacing in cardiac resynchronization therapy patients determined by coronary venous electro-anatomic mapping. Eur J Heart Fail. 2014;16:1214–22.
23. Niazi I, Ryu K, Hood R, Choudhuri I, Akhtar M. Three-dimensional electroanatomic mapping of the coronary veins during cardiac resynchronization therapy implant: feasibility and possible applications. J Interv Card Electrophysiol. 2014;41:147–53.

20 Transesophageal Electrophysiological Study Without Fluoroscopy

Xiao Yun Yang, Jing Chen, and Mei Hu

Introduction

In the mediastinum, the esophagus is close to the posterior wall of left atrium. Due to the close proximity, the atrial waves can be clearly recorded by the catheter electrode placed in the esophagus. Therefore, the catheter electrode in esophagus can be used for electrophysiological study including the evaluation of sinoatrial node function, atrioventricular node function, and induction, termination, and differentiation of supraventricular tachycardia. This chapter will introduce the facilities required and the manipulation for transesophageal cardiac electrophysiological study and its' clinical application.

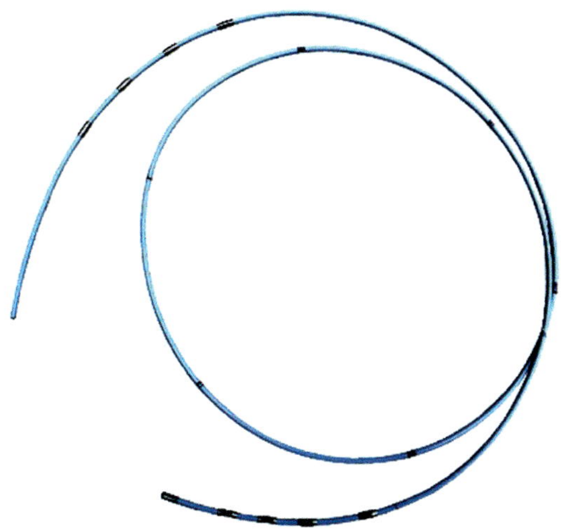

Fig. 20.1 Esophageal diagnostic catheter has four pairs of electrodes and its size is six or seven French

Facilities

1. Esophageal diagnostic catheter: it is used for recording the electrogram in esophagus and usually has four electrodes in pairs in both ends and its diameter is usually 6 French or 7 French; Its output can be adjusted from 0 to 50 V and pulse width 0–10 ms (Suzhou Dongfang Electronic Instrument Factory, Suzhou, China) (Fig. 20.1).
2. Cardiac electric stimulator: it can generate programmed stimulation or burst pacing; Cardiac Electric Stimulator (DF-5A, Suzhou Dongfang Electronic Instrument Factory, Suzhou, China) (Fig. 20.2).
3. Electrocardiograph machine or cardiac electrophysiological polygraph: it is collected to the esophageal diagnostic catheter with an alligator-style cable.
4. Clip-to-clip cable: it has alligator-style clips in both ends, which is generally used for pacing analysis during pacemaker implantation;

X. Y. Yang (✉) · J. Chen · M. Hu
Tongji Hospital, Tongji Medical College, Huazhong University of Science and Technology, Wuhan, China

R. Proietti et al. (eds.), *Cardiac Electrophysiology Without Fluoroscopy*,
https://doi.org/10.1007/978-3-030-16992-3_20

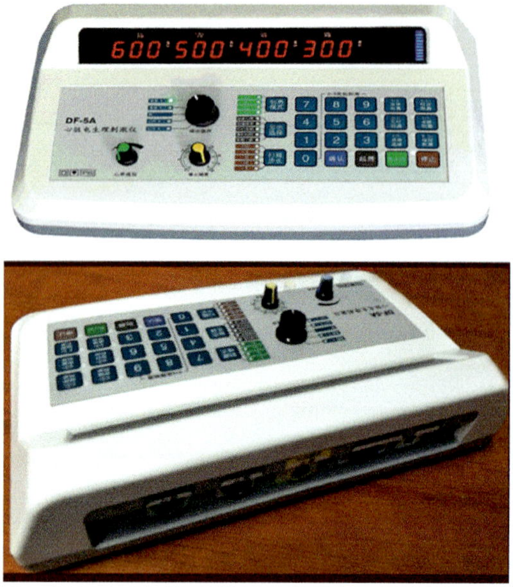

Fig. 20.2 Cardiac electric stimulator can generate programmed stimulation or burst pacing; Its output can be adjusted from 0 to 50 V and pulse width 0–10 ms

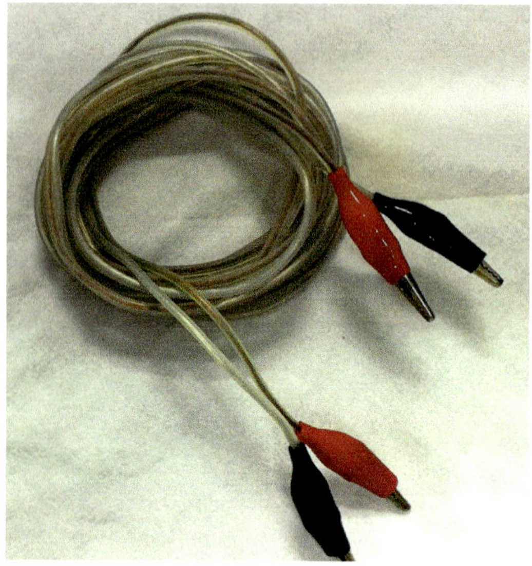

Fig. 20.3 Alligator style cable is used for collecting the esophageal diagnostic catheter and the electrocardiograph machine

it is used for collecting the esophageal diagnostic catheter with an electrocardiograph machine or a recording system (Fig. 20.3).

Patients Preparation

1. Discontinue antiarrhythmic drugs for at least five half-lives.
2. Fasting food for at least 4 h.

Indications

Transesophageal cardiac electrophysiological study can be applied in the following aspects:

1. Evaluate the function of sinoatrial node including the sinoatrial node recovery time and sinoatrial conduction time to confirm the presence of sick sinus syndrome.
2. Measure the refractory periods including sinoatrial node, atrial muscle, atrioventricular node, and ventricular muscle.
3. Use for the diagnosis, induction, and termination of supraventricular tachycardia.
4. Pace the heart temporally in patients with severe bradycardia in the ward in urgent situations.
5. Perform heart pacing loading test in patients who are not suitable for exercise test.

Contraindications

Transesophageal cardiac electrophysiological study is contraindicated in the following situations:

1. Acute upper respiratory tract inflammation.
2. Large aortic aneurysm.
3. Severe hypertension or uncontrolled hypertension.
4. Severe esophageal disease.
5. Severe cardiac disease, cachexia, or other status, which lead to the patient intolerant to catheter insertion.

Catheter Insertion

- Pre-shape the distal part of the diagnostic catheter, which is about 1.5 cm in length, makes it a blunt curve about in 120°.
- Daub the distal part with liquid paraffin.
- Insert the catheter into the patient's nose and advance the catheter till it reaches the epiglottis; then ask the patient swallow synchronously during advancement.
- Collect the proximal electrode to lead V1 of electrocardiograph machine with a clip-clip cable, which is routinely used for pacing analysis.
- Continue to advance the catheter until a clear atrial wave is visible in the recording system, and usually the depth varies from 37 to 40 cm.

Clinical Applications

Transesophageal cardiac electrophysiological study is a noninvasive approach for clinical electrophysiological diagnosis and treatment, which has been widely used since 1978 [1–3]. The atrial wave can be clearly recorded by a catheter inserted into the esophagus (Fig. 20.4). Transesophageal cardiac electrophysiological study can be easily applied and be helpful for the differentiation of atrioventricular reentrant tachycardia (Fig. 20.5) from atrioventricular nodal reentrant tachycardia (Fig. 20.6). In addition, it is also valuable in differentiating supraventricular tachycardia with fascicular block and ventricular tachycardia. As a catheter placed in esophagus can pace the left atrium and left ventricle indirectly, the transesophageal study can be applied for the termination of

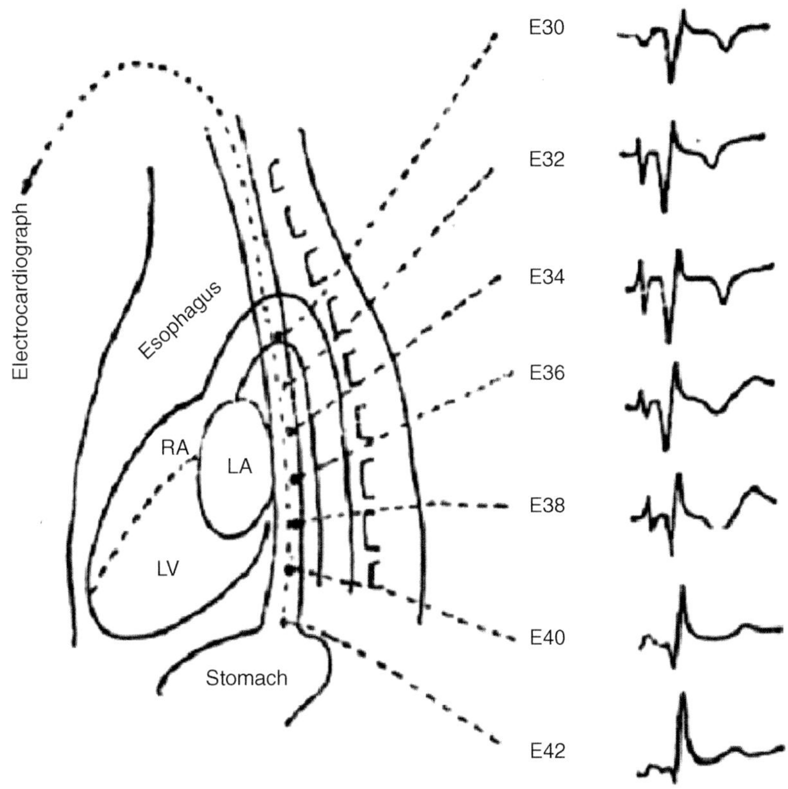

Fig. 20.4 Transesophageal electrogram was shown when the esophageal diagnostic catheter was placed in different position; *LA* left atrium, *LV* left ventricle, *RA* right atrium

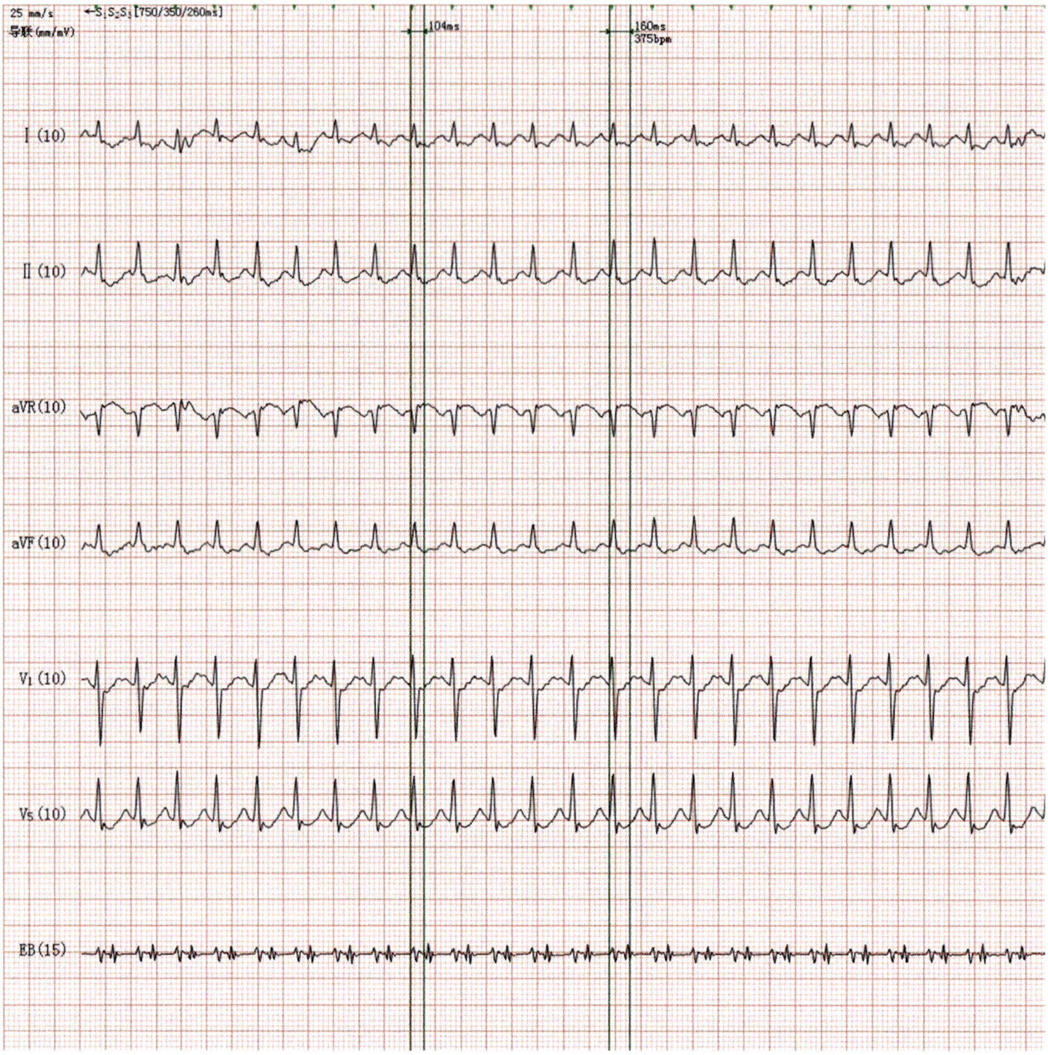

Fig. 20.5 Atrioventricular reentrant tachycardia was diagnosed with transesophageal cardiac electrophysiological study. The RP interval was greater than 70 ms in lead esophageal, which was shorter than it in lead V1, indicating that impulse travel antegrade through atrioventricular nodal and retrograde up the left concealed accessory atrioventricular bypass. The diagnosis of this tachycardia was atrioventricular reentrant tachycardia with left concealed accessory pathway

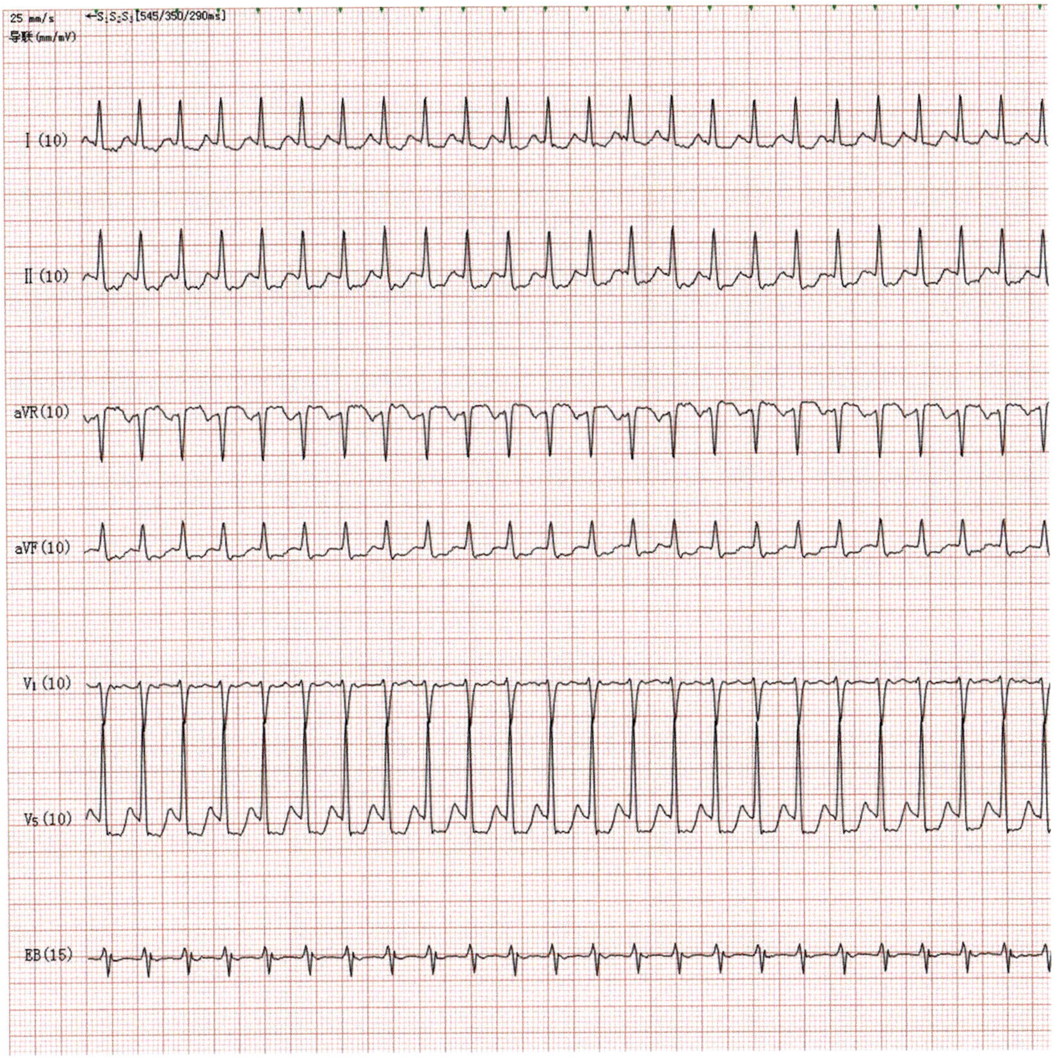

Fig. 20.6 Atrioventricular nodal reentrant tachycardia was diagnosed with transesophageal cardiac electrophysiological study. Synchronous recording of lead esophageal and V1 showed that retrograde P′ waves were merging with the QRS complex, which suggested an almost simultaneous depolarization of ventricle and atrium. As the RP′ interval was less than 70 ms in lead esophageal, it indicated that the tachycardia was atrioventricular nodal reentrant tachycardia

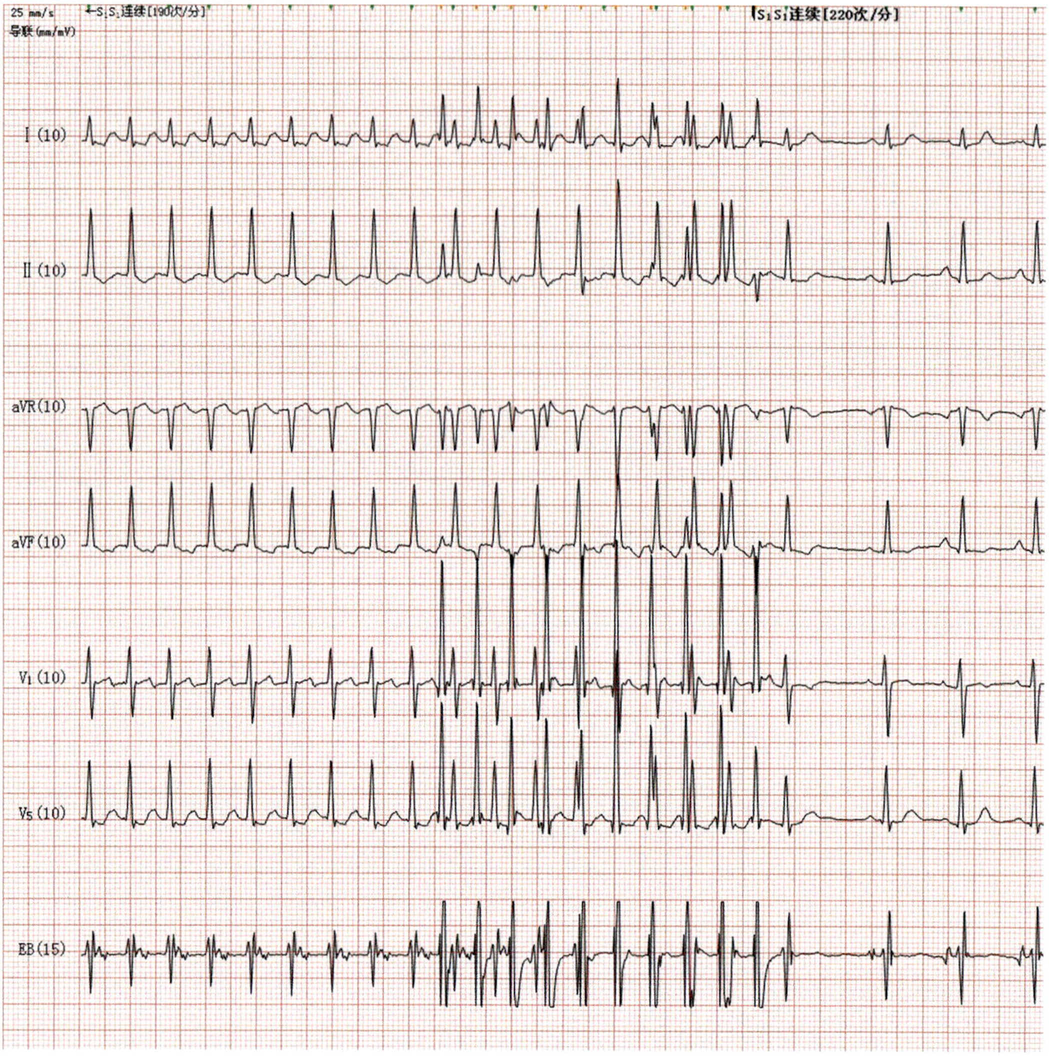

Fig. 20.7 The overdrive pacing effectively terminated the atrioventricular reentrant tachycardia in a 13-year-old female patient

supraventricular tachycardia in urgent situations or in special population (such as pregnant women and infants) (Fig. 20.7) [4]. Moreover, the electrophysiological features of the sinoatrial node can also be recorded (Fig. 20.8); it is helpful for evaluating the sinoatrial node function and determining the necessity of pacemaker implantation.

This study is noninvasive and only needs a catheter, a portable stimulator, a clip cable, and an electrograph machine. Thus, it is convenient for applying in outpatient department or in general hospitals for screening and treating cardiac arrhythmias in some special situations.

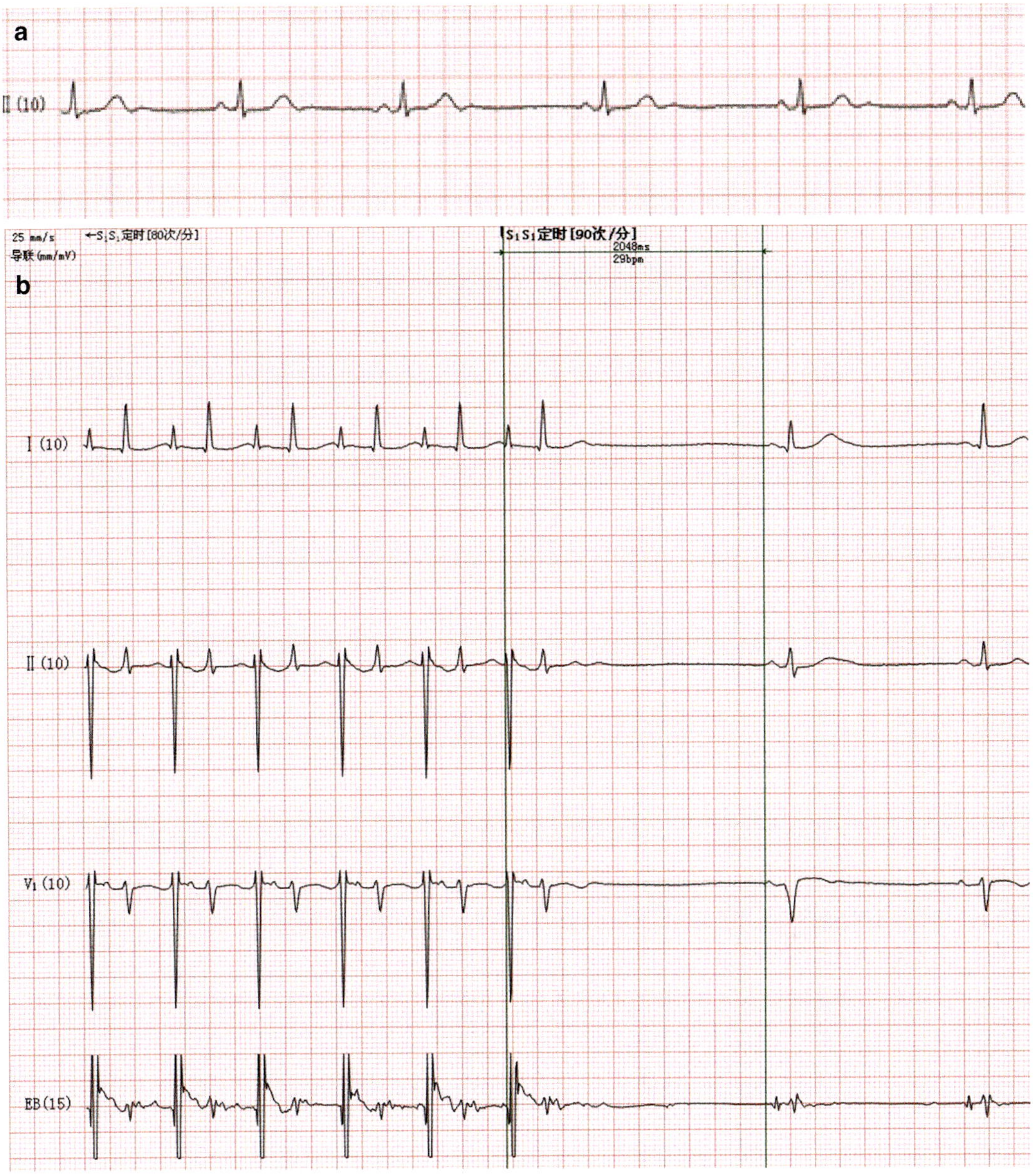

Fig. 20.8 (**a**) The sinus rhythm of the patient was approximately 40 beats per minute; (**b**) the sinus node recovery time (SNRT) was as long as 2048 ms after stimulation of atrium at 90 beats per minute and lasted for 30 s

References

1. Jiang WP. Electrophysiological studies of the accessory pathways by transesophageal atrial pacing. Zhonghua Xin Xue Guan Bing Za Zhi. 1983;11:11–4.
2. Volkmann H, Kuhnert H, Dannberg G. Electrophysiological evaluation of tachycardias using transesophageal pacing and recording. Pacing Clin Electrophysiol. 1990;13:2044–7.
3. He F, Zhao X, Cheng X. Evaluation of the clinical acute electrophysiological effects of propafenone using transesophageal atrial pacing. Zhongguo Yi Xue Ke Xue Yuan Xue Bao. 1994;16:239–41.
4. Blaufox AD, Warsy I, D'Souza M, Kanter R. Transesophageal electrophysiological evaluation of children with a history of supraventricular tachycardia in infancy. Pediatr Cardiol. 2011;32:1110–4.

Index

R. Proietti et al. (eds.), *Cardiac Electrophysiology Without Fluoroscopy*,
https://doi.org/10.1007/978-3-030-16992-3